Lasers in Head and Neck Surgery

Lasers in Head and Neck Surgery

Edited by

Edward C. Weisberger, M.D., F.A.C.S.
Associate Professor
Department of Otolaryngology—
Head and Neck Surgery
Co-Chairman, Laser Committee
Indiana University School of Medicine
Indianapolis, Indiana

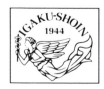

IGAKU-SHOIN   New York • Tokyo

Published and distributed by

IGAKU-SHOIN Medical Publishers, Inc.
One Madison Avenue, New York, N.Y. 10010

IGAKU-SHOIN Ltd.,
5-24-3 Hongo, Bunkyo-ku, Tokyo

Library of Congress Cataloging-in-Publication Data

Lasers in head and neck surgery / edited by Edward C. Weisberger.
    p.   cm.
   1. Head—Surgery. 2. Neck—Surgery. 3. Lasers in surgery.
I. Weisberger, Edward C.
   [DNLM: 1. Head—surgery. 2. Laser Surgery. 3. Neck—surgery.
WE 705 L343]
RD521.L27 1990
617.5'1059—dc20
DNLM/DLC
for Library of Congress   90-4132
                                              CIP

ISBN: 0-89640-181-2 (New York)
ISBN: 4-260-14181-3 (Tokyo)

Printed and bound in the U.S.A.

10 9 8 7 6 5 4 3 2 1

To Elizabeth and Alex,
and to Donna, Paul, Jason, Jennifer, and Ryan
for their guidance, understanding, and love.

Preface

Some of the first applications of laser technology to the treatment of human disease involved the head and neck area. We have witnessed a tremendous expansion in this field in the last 15 to 20 years. Whereas initially laser technology was found at only a few medical centers, now most hospitals and many outpatient treatment facilities have lasers available.

This book is a comprehensive review of laser applications in the head and neck area, providing information useful to otolaryngologists, head and neck surgeons, general surgeons, plastic surgeons, oral surgeons, dermatologists, gastroenterologists, pulmonologists, anesthesiologists, laser safety officers, and nurse laser coordinators. All of these specialties have some common interests in treating diseases of the head and neck with laser technology. I hope that this presentation of the state of the art in laser surgery of the head and neck will provide a firm foundation for further growth.

Acknowledgment

I deeply appreciate the invaluable assistance of Yona Urness in the preparation of this book. Without her dedication, hard work, and advice, the project could not have come to fruition.

My thanks to Craig Gosling, Chief of the Medical Illustration Department at Indiana University Medical Center, for his insightful illustrations used in the chapter on the larynx.

Finally, my deepest appreciation to my family for their support and understanding while I took the time away from them necessary to complete this work.

Contributors

Daniel P. Akin, M.D., Ph.D., F.A.C.S., A.A.F.P.R.S.
Director
Akin Medical Center
and
Chairman, Laser Committee
Memorial Hospital of Floyd County
New Albany, Indiana
and
Clinical Assistant Professor of
Otolaryngology
University of Louisville
Louisville, Kentucky

Sharon Collins, M.S., M.D., F.A.C.S.
Associate Professor of
Otolaryngology—Head and Neck
Surgery
Loyola University of Chicago
Medical Center
Maywood, Illinois
and
Chief, Section of Head and Neck
Surgical Oncology
Edward Hines Veterans
Administration Hospital
Hines, Illinois

Michael C. Dalsing, M.D., F.A.C.S.
Associate Professor
Director, General Vascular Surgery
Co-Chairman, Laser Committee
Indiana University Medical Center
Indianapolis, Indiana

Larry E. Dollens, C.E.
Laser Safety Officer
Indiana University Hospitals
Indiana University School of
Medicine
Indianapolis, Indiana

John D. Emhardt, M.D.
Assistant Professor of Anesthesia
Indiana University School of
Medicine
Indianapolis, Indiana

Ellen M. Friedman, M.D.
Assistant Professor of
Otolaryngology
Harvard Medical School
Children's Hospital Medical Center
Boston, Massachusetts

Jack L. Gluckman, M.D.
Professor of Otolaryngology and
Maxillofacial Surgery
Director, Division of Head and
Neck Surgery
University of Cincinnati Medical
Center
Cincinnati, Ohio

C. William Hanke, M.D.
Professor of Dermatology,
Pathology, and Otolaryngology—
Head and Neck Surgery
Indiana University School of
Medicine
Indianapolis, Indiana

Sherry Heller, B.S., R.N.
Clinical Service Facilitator, Lasers
Department of Surgery
Indiana University School of
Medicine
Indianapolis, Indiana

Arthur Klass, M.D.
Clinical Associate Professor of
    Medicine
Wayne State University School of
    Medicine
and
Chief, Endoscopy Unit
Sinai Hospital
Detroit, Michigan

Melissa W. Lee, B.S.
Research Associate
Department of Dermatology
Indiana University School of
    Medicine
Indianapolis, Indiana

S. George Lesinski, M.D., F.A.C.S.
Director, Department of
    Otolaryngology
The Bethesda Hospitals
and
Clinical Associate Professor of
    Otolaryngology and Maxillofacial
    Surgery
University of Cincinnati College of
    Medicine
Cincinnati, Ohio

Thomas A. Majcher, D.O.
Clinical Assistant Professor of
    Anesthesia
Indiana University School of
    Medicine
Indianapolis, Indiana

Praveen Mathur, M.B., B.S.
Clinical Assistant Professor of
    Medicine
Division of Pulmonary and Critical
    Care Medicine
Indiana University School of
    Medicine
Indianapolis, Indiana

Richard Milner, B.S.
Manager, Reichle Surgical Research
    Laboratory
Department of Surgery
Temple University School of
    Medicine
Philadelphia, Pennsylvania

Eugene Rontal, M.D.
Clinical Assistant Professor of
    Otolaryngology—Head and Neck
    Surgery
University of Michigan Medical
    School
Ann Arbor, Michigan

Michael Rontal, M.D.
Clinical Assistant Professor of
    Otolaryngology—Head and Neck
    Surgery
University of Michigan Medical
    School
Ann Arbor, Michigan

Steven D. Rowley, M.D., F.A.C.S.
Staff
Utah Valley Regional Medical
    Center
and
Otology-Neurotology, Private
    Practice
Provo, Utah

Scott Shapiro, M.D.
Assistant Professor of Neurosurgery
Indiana University School of
    Medicine
Indianapolis, Indiana

Mitchel B. Sosis, M.D.
Assistant Professor of
    Anesthesiology
Rush-Presbyterian—St. Luke's
    Medical Center
Chicago, Illinois

James A. Stankiewicz, M.D.
Vice Chairman and Professor of
    Otolaryngology—Head and Neck
    Surgery
Loyola University Medical School
Maywood, Illinois

Joseph L. Unthank, Ph.D.
Assistant Professor of Physiology
Departments of Surgery, Physiology
    and Biophysics
Indiana University School of
    Medicine
Indianapolis, Indiana

Edward C. Weisberger, M.D.,
    F.A.C.S.
Associate Professor
Department of Otolaryngology—
    Head and Neck Surgery
Co-Chairman, Laser Committee
Indiana University School of
    Medicine
Indianapolis, Indiana

John V. White, M.D., F.A.C.S.
Associate Professor
Director, Surgical Research
Department of Surgery
Temple University School of
    Medicine
Philadelphia, Pennsylvania

Jay Paul Willging, M.D.
Resident in Otolaryngology and
    Maxillofacial Surgery
University of Cincinnati College of
    Medicine
Cincinnati, Ohio

Robert P. Zitsch, III, M.D.
Assistant Professor of
    Otolaryngology and Maxillofacial
    Surgery
Division of Head and Neck Surgery
University of Missouri-Columbia
Columbia, Missouri

Contents

1
Fundamental Principles of Surgical Lasers

Joseph L. Unthank

A laser is a device that amplifies light to produce an extremely intense beam. Unlike other sources, lasers produce a beam of light that is coherent, monochromatic, and highly collimated. Each of these characteristics endows lasers with unique applications; the characteristics are discussed in detail later in this chapter. The word *laser* is actually an acronym for *l*ight *a*mplification by *s*timulated *e*mission of *r*adiation. To understand the principles of laser operation, it is necessary to understand all the terms in the laser acronym as they relate to the fundamental principles of light.

COMPONENTS OF THE *LASER* ACRONYM

Radiation

By the most strict interpretation of the acronym, the radiation emitted from a laser must be from within the light or optical portion of the electromagnetic spectrum (Fig. 1.1). This spectrum consists of near-ultraviolet, visible, and near-infrared radiation with wavelengths from approximately 200 to 400, 400 to 700, and 700 to 1000 nanometers (nm), respectively.[1] The principles of laser operation, however, are not limited to this portion of the electromagnetic spectrum. In fact, the first demonstration of the amplification of electromagnetic radiation by stimulated emission employed microwaves in a device called a *maser*.[2]

The three most common surgical lasers in current use emit wavelengths of 458 to 515 nm (argon laser), which is within the visible portion of the electromagnetic spectrum, and two wavelengths in the infrared spectrum—the neodymium:yttrium-aluminum-garnet laser (nd:YAG) at 1060 nm and the carbon dioxide (CO_2) laser at 10,600 nm. Excimer lasers, which are being tested for clinical application, extend the range of available wavelengths into the ultraviolet region (100 to 400 nm). Tunable-dye and free-electron lasers can produce wavelengths ranging from the

1

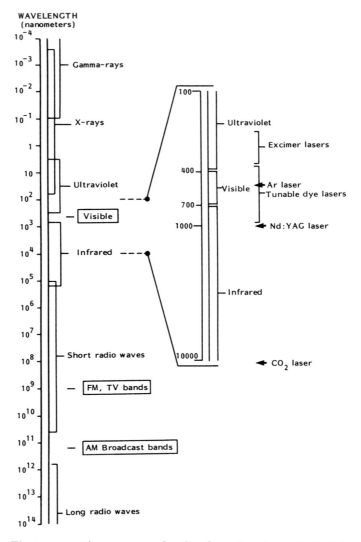

Figure 1.1. Electromagnetic spectrum. Section from the ultraviolet to infrared regions, which contains the wavelengths of current and potential surgical lasers, expanded.

ultraviolet to the infrared within the same laser and will provide distinct advantages in surgical techniques as they become more refined.

Stimulated Emission

The stimulated emission of radiation is the fundamental principle upon which all lasers are based. The phenomenon of stimulated emission was proposed by Einstein in his quantum theory of radiation in 1917,[3] but a number of major events preceded the development of this concept.

Until the seventeenth century, light was believed to consist of particles and was described by the corpuscular theory.[1] By the end of the nineteenth century, scientists had demonstrated that light is an electromagnetic wave and therefore part of the electromagnetic spectrum. At this time it was generally thought that knowledge regarding the nature of light was complete. Many of the phenomena of light, such as propagation, reflection, refraction, interference, diffraction, and polarization, were very adequately explained by the classical electromagnetic wave theory. By the beginning of the twentieth century, however, it was realized that the electromagnetic wave theory did not satisfactorily explain the absorption and emission of light by matter.

The process of photoelectric emission, which was discovered by Hertz in 1887, could not be accounted for by the wave theory.[1] In photoelectric emission, incident light induces the ejection of electrons from conductors. Investigators pursuing Hertz's discovery found photoelectric emission to be independent of the intensity of light but critically dependent upon the wavelength of the incident light.

The photoelectric effect was explained by Einstein in 1905 as the absorption of light energy by matter. Einstein extended the earlier proposal by Planck that light energy absorbed by matter must be transferred in discrete units, or quanta. Einstein postulated that the energy in the light beam was in discrete units called photons, and that the energy of a light photon was proportional to the frequency of the light. When a photon interacted with matter, either all or none of the photon's energy could be absorbed by an atom. The absorption of a photon of light energy could provide the atom enough energy to cause the emission of an electron.

The electromagnetic wave theory was also incapable of explaining the atomic emission spectrum.[1] Emission spectra refer to the wavelengths of radiant energy that are emitted from excited atoms. The emission spectra of elements are characterized by a limited number of distinct wavelengths rather than a continuous spectrum, and each element has its own characteristic spectrum. In 1913, Niels Bohr applied Planck's concept of light quanta to atomic theory in order to explain atomic emission spectra. Prior to the changes in atomic theory proposed by Bohr, the Rutherford model of the atom had generally been accepted. In Rutherford's model, electrons revolved around a positively charged nucleus. According to the electromagnetic wave theory, the revolving electrons would continually emit energy as they revolved. It was thought that as the electrons emitted energy, they spiraled inward toward the center of the atom and eventually collapsed into the nucleus. The electromagnetic wave theory predicted that all atoms would emit a continuous spectrum because the frequency of the electromagnetic radiation emitted by the revolving electrons would be equal to the frequency of revolution. This was obviously in contradiction to the line spectra that had been observed.

The first postulate of the atomic theory proposed by Bohr was that electrons can revolve around the nucleus of an atom in certain stable orbits without emitting radiant energy (Fig. 1.2).[1] Bohr's second postulate, which explained the emission of radiant energy, was that an electron can make a transition from one stable orbit to another of lower energy by emitting a photon having energy equal to the difference between the initial and final orbits.

The Bohr model was a major advance in our understanding of how atoms emit radiant energy. But Bohr's model explained only the emission spectra of hydrogen and a few other elements; it did not predict what energy levels elements should have nor explain the emission spectra of most elements and molecules. This required the development of quantum mechanics, which is able to predict energy levels and explain the frequencies of light observed in the atomic emission spectrum.

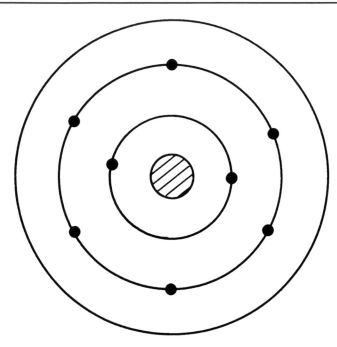

Figure 1.2. Bohr model of the atom. Electrons are located in discrete energy levels surrounding the nucleus. Energy is gained or lost by an electron only when the electron makes a transition from one energy level to another. The energy of the levels increases proportionally with the distance from the nucleus.

Although a description of quantum mechanics requires mathematics beyond the scope of this text, the following are major concepts of the quantum or wave mechanics theory of the atom. The electrons in an atom are visualized as a diffuse cloud that surrounds the nucleus. The position of the electrons within this cloud are within discrete energy levels and sublevels, or orbitals. These orbitals and energy levels are described by a set of quantum numbers.

According to our current understanding of how electrons within an atom or molecule interact with electromagnetic radiation, there are three types of radiative transitions—absorption, spontaneous emission, and stimulated emission (Fig. 1.3).[1] The absorption of a photon of energy by an atom occurs when an electron makes a transition to a higher energy level. In the normal or ground state of an atom, electrons occupy the lowest possible energy levels. Thermal, electrical, or optical energy can induce an excited state in which an electron makes a transition to a higher energy level farther from the nucleus. Such an excited state is not stable. Eventually, spontaneous emission occurs as the excited atom emits a photon of energy when the electron returns to its ground state.

Einstein proposed in 1917 that one photon of an appropriate wavelength or energy could interact with an excited atom to induce the emission of a second photon. This process of stimulated emission of radiation is the basic principle upon which lasers operate. In stimulated emission, the photon that is emitted from the excited atom has exactly the same frequency, direction, and phase as the incident photon.

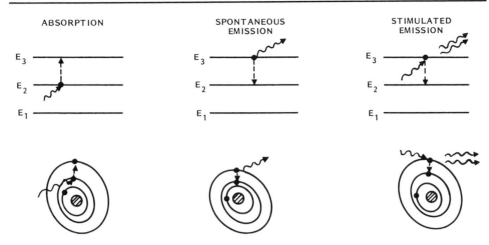

Figure 1.3. Radiative transitions. The three ways in which photons of light and matter can interact are illustrated by energy level diagrams and Bohr atomic models. An electron can absorb a photon and make a transition to a higher energy level. For this to occur in the illustration, the energy of the photon must be equal to $E_3 - E_2$. When absorption occurs, the atom goes from its normal or ground state to an excited state. The excited state is less stable than the normal state, and eventually the electron will return to ground state by the spontaneous emission of a photon with energy equal to $E_3 - E_2$. In stimulated emission, one photon of appropriate energy interacts with an excited atom to effect the release of a second photon. The incident and emitted photon have the same energy ($E_3 - E_2$) and are in phase.

Amplification

Although stimulated emission is the fundamental principle behind laser operation, the electromagnetic energy released by stimulated emission must be amplified for a laser to produce its characteristically intense beam of light. For the amplification of light to occur within a laser, the active laser medium must become a source of energy. Before the active medium of a laser is activated by an external power source, it contains more atoms in the normal state than in the excited state. As a laser operates, an external pump source reverses this situation so that more atoms exist in the excited state than in the ground state. When such a population inversion is induced, the number of photons is amplified as the photon released from one atom induces the emission of photons from other atoms through a chain reaction.

Light

The first term of the laser acronym (and the last to be considered) is light. As stated in the introduction, the light beam emitted from a laser has four distinguishing characteristics: It is intense, coherent, monochromatic, and highly collimated. Laser light is extremely intense, with immense energy in a very narrow beam. Unlike light emitted from other sources, light from a laser is very highly collimated. That is, all of the light waves are parallel and only minimal divergence occurs as the light beam is propagated from the laser. This characteristic permits the intense beam leaving the laser to be propagated over a considerable distance with minimal dissipation of energy.

The light originating from a laser is also coherent; the light is in phase both spatially and temporally.

Another distinct characteristic of laser light is that it is monochromatic. Although, technically, laser light is seldom composed entirely of a single wavelength—for example, argon laser light actually consists of several wavelengths—the output of a laser includes only a relatively narrow band of electromagnetic radiation and is therefore said to be monochromatic. The importance of monochromaticity from a surgeon's perspective lies in the fact that tissue components absorb electromagnetic wavelengths selectively.

COMPONENTS OF A SURGICAL LASER SYSTEM

Some components of surgical lasers are essential for the operation of any laser. Other components provide additional features that are important or necessary in the application of the laser to surgical technique.

Essential Components of All Lasers

Three components are absolutely essential for laser operation: an active medium, a laser pump or power source, and an optical or resonating chamber (Fig. 1.4).

The Active Medium

The first major component of all lasers is the active medium, which may be in a liquid, a solid, or a gaseous phase. The name of the laser is generally derived from the active medium.

Examples of solid-state lasers include the ruby laser and the neodymium:yttrium-aluminum-garnet laser (Nd:YAG). The ruby laser, which was the first to be developed, uses a ruby crystal as the active medium. The neodymium:yttrium-aluminum-garnet laser is one of the common surgical lasers and is also named by its active medium. Another type of solid-state laser is the semiconductor or diode laser.

Common gas lasers include the argon laser, the carbon dioxide (CO_2) laser, and the helium-neon laser. Together with the Nd:YAG laser, the carbon dioxide and argon lasers are the lasers most commonly used in surgery. The helium-neon laser is generally used as an aiming beam in lasers that have an output not visible to the human eye. Excimer lasers, which are undergoing clinical evaluation, have an active medium consisting of a mixture of rare and halide gases.

There are also liquid lasers that employ a complex organic dye in the active medium. Regardless of its state, the function of the active medium in a laser is to provide the source of excited atoms, molecules, or ions from which the emission of photons can be stimulated and amplified.

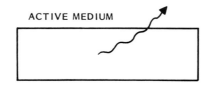

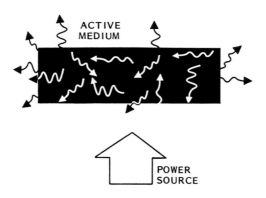

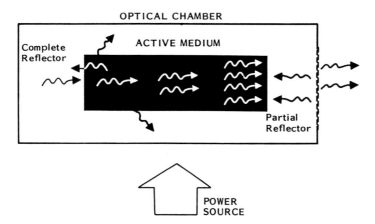

Figure 1.4. Essential components of lasers. The top panel represents the active medium of the laser in its nonactivated state, which is characterized by few if any excited atoms. In the middle panel, a power source has been applied to the active medium to produce a population inversion with many excited atoms. Spontaneous emission may occur, but there is no directionality to the emitted photons and little amplification. The addition of an optical chamber with two reflective surfaces in the bottom panel provides for directed output and feedback and amplification between the back reflector and the front partial reflector.

The Power Source

All lasers require an external power source to activate the laser medium by generating a population inversion. The most common types of laser pumps or power sources are optical pumps or flash lamps and electric discharge pumps.

The Optical Cavity (Resonating Chamber)

All lasers also must have an optical cavity, or resonating chamber to provide directed output and feedback for amplification and collimation. The active medium is contained within the optical cavity. Photons within the active medium are reflected by a complete and a partial reflector for both collimation and amplification. The partial reflector at the front of the laser directs the output.

Additional Components for Surgical Lasers

The active medium, laser pump, and optical chamber are essential in the operation of any laser. Lasers that are used for surgical procedures have several additional requirements.[4]

Surgical lasers require high power to produce the appropriate tissue effect because of their inefficiency. The CO_2 lasers are approximately 20% efficient, the argon laser has an energy efficiency of much less than 1%. The relatively high power input and low efficiency produce considerable heat, so surgical lasers require either an internal or external cooling system.

An aiming beam is required for surgical lasers that do not have visible outputs. Helium-neon lasers are commonly used for this purpose. The aiming beam is coaxial with the surgical laser beam, and, in general, when the aiming beam is in focus, one can assume that the surgical laser beam is focused.

The output of all surgical lasers must be transmitted from the laser to the desired site on the patient. Available delivery systems include hand-held probes attached to the end of fiberoptics or an articulated arm and direct coupling to a surgical microscope. Not all delivery systems are available for all lasers; fiberoptics are not yet available for the CO_2 laser.

A control panel is necessary so that the power output and the frequency and duration of the laser beam exposure can be regulated. A remote switch, either on the microscope or foot operated, is also needed to control the laser and free the hands for the surgical procedures.

SELECTION OF LASERS FOR SURGERY

The ability of a laser to incise, vaporize, and coagulate tissue is determined by the wavelength of the laser beam, the mode of operation of the laser (continuous, pulsed, or Q-switched), and the energy fluence upon the tissue.

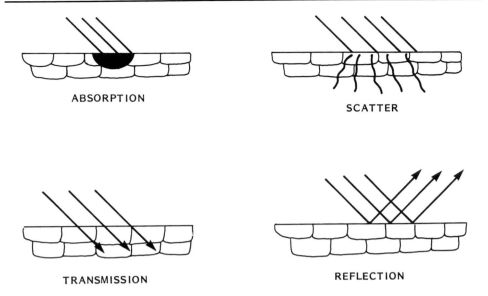

Figure 1.5. Laser beam interaction with tissue: absorption scatter, transmission, and reflection of the laser beam by tissue. The relative degree to which these phenomena of light occur is dependent upon the wavelength of the laser and the tissue characteristics.

Wavelength

A major consideration in selecting a laser for a specific function is the wavelength of the laser beam. As illustrated in Figure 1.5, the laser beam can be absorbed by the tissue, scattered or dispersed throughout the tissue, transmitted through tissue, or reflected from the tissue surface. The degree to which each of these phenomena occur is determined largely by the wavelength of the laser and the absorptive characteristics of the tissue being treated. The almost total absorption of the laser beam of the CO_2 laser within 0.2 mm of the tissue surface makes this laser well suited for cutting and tissue ablation.[2] The argon laser is used to treat port wine hemangiomas because its 514-nm wavelength is selectively absorbed by hemoglobin.[2] The deeper and more diffuse effects of the Nd:YAG laser beam are related to its greater degree of transmission and dispersion in tissue.[2] The potential of new lasers for surgical applications will depend primarily upon their wavelength.

Mode of Operation

Lasers operate either in a continuous or a pulsed mode. In a continuous type, a steady flow of photons is emitted with little fluctuation in intensity, providing a constant and stable delivery of energy. Continuous output requires a constant power source to keep the active medium in an excited state so that stimulated emission, amplification, feedback, and direct output occur continuously.

Pulsed lasers use an intermittent power source such as a flash lamp to provide sudden bursts of energy to the active medium. The population inversion of the active medium only lasts for a very short time after each impulse of energy from the intermittent power source. Consequently the laser beam occurs as a pulse rather than a continuous wave.

The average power output of a continuous wave laser is generally greater than that of a pulsed laser, but pulsed lasers develop a much higher maximum instantaneous energy. For example, a 25-W continuous wave CO_2 laser may be electronically gated to produce a power output of 125 to 500 W at 50 to 250 Hz, while a pulsed CO_2 laser has a peak maximum power output of up to 4000 W. A pulsed CO_2 laser has the advantage of achieving a much deeper cutting effect with less thermal effect than the continuous type, because tissue can cool between pulses.

Both pulsed and continuous wave lasers can also be operated in a Q-switched mode.[5] A fast shutter is positioned between the active medium and the partial reflector that allows output from the optical chamber. The external pump is activated while the shutter is closed. Energy builds up within the active medium to levels far above the threshold required for lasing and produces greater than normal excitation of the active medium. When the shutter is opened this excess excitation is discharged as a very short pulse with extreme intensity that is orders of magnitudes greater than the energy ordinarily produced by either a continuous or a pulsed beam. The pulse duration of a Q-switched laser is between 10^{-6} and 10^{-9} second, and the power during this short duration may be as high as 10 million watts.

Energy Fluence

In addition to the wavelength of the laser beam and the mode of laser operation, the effect of the laser beam on tissue is determined by the power density of the laser and the length of time the tissue is exposed to the laser beam.[6] The power density, or irradiance, of the laser beam is simply the amount of energy that is incident upon a specific unit of tissue area; it is expressed as W/cm^2. The power of the laser beam is regulated by the control box. The area of the laser beam incident upon the tissue is determined largely by the focal length of the laser optics and the distance of the laser probe from the tissue.

Laser beams can be focused to spot sizes much less than a millimeter in diameter (in special applications, less than a micrometer) or defocused to increase the area of tissue exposed. An important concept to remember in any application of lasers is that power density is inversely proportional to the square of the laser beam radius:

$$\text{Power density} = \frac{\text{laser power output in watts}}{\text{cross-sectional area of incident beam}}$$

$$\text{Power density} = \frac{\text{laser power output in watts}}{\pi r^2}$$

Consequently, for a laser beam with a specific power output, changes in spot size can have a tremendous effect on power density, as illustrated in Figure 1.6. In practice, a focused beam of high intensity is used for cutting and a defocused beam for ablation or coagulation.

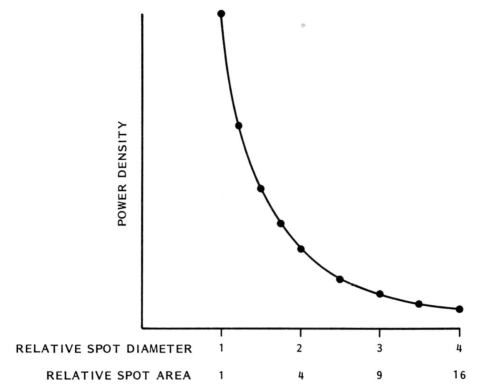

Figure 1.6. The relationship between the power density of the laser beam and the spot diameter and area of the incident beam. Power density is inversely proportional to the spot area, which is directly proportional to the square of the spot radius.

The product of the power density of the laser beam and the time to which tissue is exposed to the beam is the energy fluence, usually expressed as joules/cm^2. For a continuous wave laser, the energy fluence is simply the power density multiplied by the duration of the exposure. For pulsed and Q-switched lasers, the actual exposure time must be calculated from the pulse duration and the number of pulses (pulse frequency multiplied by the total duration of exposure).

For the purpose of standardization and reproducibility, the report of any studies of tissue responses to laser exposure should include the specific laser and wavelength, the power setting of the laser, spot size, power density, energy fluence, the exposure time, and, if the laser is pulsed or Q-switched, the pulse rate and duration.[6]

Major events in the development of laser theory and technology are summarized in Table 1.1. Specific lasers with surgical applications are discussed below. The major characteristics of the lasers most commonly used in surgery are summarized in Table 1.2.

The Carbon Dioxide Laser

The CO_2 laser is the most commonly used for general surgery. It was developed by C. K. N. Patel in 1964 at Bell Laboratories.[5] The wavelength of the CO_2 laser

TABLE 1.1. *Major Events in the Development of Laser Theory and Technology*

1905	Einsteins's explanation of photoelectric emission by absorption[1]
1913	Bohr model of the atom and explanation of atomic emission[1]
1917	Einstein's proposal of the process of stimulated emission of radiation[1]
1955	Microwave amplification by stimulated emission of radiation (Gordan and-coworkers)[2]
1958	Schawlow and Townes' proposal that stimulated emission could be used to amplify light[4]
1960	First laser demonstrated by Maimin—pulsed ruby laser[4]
1961	Helium-neon laser by Javan. First gas laser, first continuously operating laser[4] Development of Nd:YAG laser by Johnson[2]
1962	Development of argon laser by Bennett and coworkers[2]
1964	CO_2 laser developed by Patel and coworkers at Bell Laboratories[4]
1966	First dye laser, developed by IBM Laboratories[5]
1967	First laser commercially available for medical applications—CO_2 laser byAmerican Optical[4]
1975	Excimer lasers developed by AVCO, Inc.[5]

is in the midinfrared region at 10,600 nm. The power of CO_2 lasers available for surgical use ranges from approximately 100 mW to 100 W. The operation of the CO_2 laser combines the use of carbon dioxide, nitrogen, and helium. In the activation process a nitrogen atom is first excited and its energy transferred to CO_2. After stimulated emission has occurred, collisions with He return the CO_2 to ground state. The carbon dioxide laser has a high efficiency compared to other gas lasers, but it requires cooling because of the high powers used. Its high efficiency permits the use of an internal heat exchanger for cooling. An aiming beam is necessary because the beam of light from the CO_2 laser is not visible to the human eye. A helium-neon laser is usually used for this purpose.

One of the disadvantages of the CO_2 laser is the delivery system. Fiberoptics for transmitting the infrared radiation of the CO_2 laser are not yet commercially available. Consequently, the CO_2 laser must either be used as a hand-held probe at the

TABLE 1.2. *Major Characteristics of Surgical Lasers*

Characteristics	CO_2	Nd:YAG	Argon
Wavelengths (nanometers)	10,600	1060	458–515
Chromophore	Water	—	Hemoglobin, melanin
Power (watts)	0.1–100	5–120	0.001–25
Mode	CW, P, Q	CW, Q	CW, P
Delivery	Articulated arm, microscope	Fiberoptics	Fiberoptics
Penetration depth	<0.2 mm	3–5 mm	1 mm

CW = continuous wave; P = pulsed; Q = Q-switched.

end of an articulated arm with multiple reflective mirrors or coupled to an operating microscope.

The CO_2 laser employs a 110-V electric discharge pump as a power source. Scattering of the laser light is negligible because most of the beam is absorbed at the tissue surface. Because the absorption coefficient of water at 10,600 nm is high, essentially all the incident energy is absorbed within 0.2 mm of tissue surface.

At low power densities and large spot sizes the CO_2 laser can be used to vaporize tissue, and the heat conducted to adjacent tissue coagulates blood and lymph vessels up to approximately 500 μm. For incision, a small spot size with a high power density is used. Milliwatt CO_2 lasers are used for vascular anastomosis at power settings of 250 mW or less and laser beam diameters up to 250 μm. Both continuous and pulsed CO_2 lasers are available.

The Argon Laser

An aiming beam is not necessary for the argon laser, which has a light output within the visible region from 458 to 515 nm, primarily 488 and 515 nm.[4] Up to 25 W of blue-green light can be emitted, although medical lasers are usually limited to 15 W.

Argon gas is the active medium for this laser. The argon atoms are converted to argon ions by a high electric current. A 220-V input is required and about 5 gallons of water per minute must be supplied for cooling because of the laser's inefficiency. The beam is delivered by fiberoptics.

The primary wavelength of the argon laser is near the maximal absorption for hemoglobin, melanin, and myoglobin. The penetration depth is variable, depending upon the amounts of these tissue chromophores, but is typically about 1 mm. The deeper penetration of the argon laser makes it less effective than the CO_2 laser as a cutting device. The argon laser is used principally in plastic surgery, ophthalmology, and dermatology. Specific applications include treatment of diabetic retinopathy and port wine hemangiomas.

Neodymium:Yttrium-Aluminum-Garnet (Nd:YAG) Laser

The active medium of the neodymium:yttrium-aluminum-garnet laser is 1 to 3% neodymium (Nd) ions in an yttrium-aluminum-garnet (YAG) matrix.[4] The light emitted from this laser is in the near-infrared region at 1060 nm. The power range of medical Nd:YAG lasers is up to 100 W. The pump source for the active medium is a xenon or krypton arc lamp, which requires 220 V.

The Nd:YAG laser is a very inefficient system, and therefore a great deal of heat is generated in energizing the laser crystal medium. The available plumbing must supply adequate water flow to achieve the necessary cooling. The laser beam is delivered by fiberoptics with a He-Ne or xenon laser aiming beam.

The near-infrared light from the Nd:YAG laser is not strongly absorbed by water or body pigments. Consequently its penetrating depth (3 to 5 mm) is much greater than that of other surgical lasers. Because of the relatively low absorption coefficient of tissue components for the Nd:YAG laser beam, there is considerable tissue scatter and reflection from the tissue surface. Focusing is of little value with the Nd:YAG laser because of the large amount of scattering, and the zone of damage is more diffuse than with the other surgical lasers. Also because of the scattering, a higher power is generally needed for a specific tissue effect such as coagulation. With the Nd:YAG laser, thermal coagulation is possible in blood vessels up to approximately 3 mm in diameter.[4]

This laser is ineffective as a cutting tool because of its relative lack of precision. A cone-shaped area of coagulation extends into the tissue, producing deep thermal necrosis, even though surface effects may not be apparent. The Nd:YAG laser can be used either in a continuous wave or pulsed manner.

Excimer Lasers

The first excimer lasers were developed by AVCO, Inc., in 1975.[5] The term excimer was derived from "excited dimer," which describes the active medium of this type of laser. The active medium of excimer lasers consists of molecules of two atoms: one atom from the noble gas family and one from the family of halogen gases. The gas medium is activated by an electric discharge pump and produces intense ultraviolet radiation. The most popular excimer lasers and their wavelengths in nanometers are argon-fluoride (193), krypton-fluoride (248), xenon-chloride (308), and xenon-fluoride (351).[5] The average power output of these lasers ranges from about 7 to 20 W. Excimer lasers are operated only in the pulsed mode.

A major difference between the excimer lasers and other surgical lasers is the manner in which the ultraviolet light interacts with tissue. Unlike light of longer wavelengths, which produces a thermal effect upon the irradiated tissue, ultraviolet light is thought to disrupt molecular bonds in a photochemical process that expels disrupted molecular fragments from the laser field with minimal thermal effect upon the underlying tissue. Because of this difference in the tissue effect of ultraviolet laser light, it is thought that excimer lasers may be capable of removing atherosclerotic plaque without any associated thermal damage of the artery. Clinical trials are currently in progress to evaluate this potential of excimer lasers. Unique concerns of the excimer lasers are the possible leakage of toxic gas and the potential mutagenic effects of ultraviolet radiation.[5]

Dye Lasers

The first dye laser was a pulsed type developed by Sorkin and coworkers of IBM Laboratories in 1966 and was powered by a ruby laser.[5] The first continuous wave dye laser was developed in 1970 by Kodak Research Laboratories.[5] The active medium of dye lasers is a complex organic dye, which is dissolved in water or alcohol. A distinct advantage of dye lasers is that the wavelength of the output can be selected or "tuned" according to the dye that is used.

An example of a dye laser available for medical applications is the Candela SPTL-1 laser. The wavelength of this laser, 585 nm, is determined by a proprietary mixture of dyes. The dye is excited by a flash lamp. This wavelength has proven much more suitable for treating vascular lesions of the skin in children than the

488-nm output of the argon laser.[7] The ability to determine specific wavelengths of laser energy output should improve treatment of several medical disorders.

Free-Electron Lasers

A type of laser that appears to hold great potential for future surgical applications is the free-electron laser.[8,9] It has a high efficiency, and its beam can be tuned from the far ultraviolet to the far infrared. The gain medium of the free-electron laser is an electron beam in a vacuum. The electrons are forced to vibrate as they pass through alternating magnetic fields. The wavelength of the resulting laser beam is varied by altering the magnetic field characteristics or the velocity of the electrons. Free-electron lasers are very expensive but provide a combination of wavelengths and pulselengths that are not otherwise available.

REFERENCES

1. Sears FW, Zemansky MW, Young HD: *University Physics.* Reading, MA, Addison-Wesley, 1980.
2. Fuller TA: Fundamentals of lasers in surgery and medicine. In Dixon JA (ed): *Surgical Application of Lasers.* Chicago, Year Book Publishers, 1987.
3. Apfelberg DB: Biophysics, advantages, and installation of laser systems. In Apfelberg DB (ed): *Evaluation and Installation of Surgical Lasers,* New York, Springer-Verlag, 1987.
4. Enderby CE: Laser instrumentation. In Dixon JA (ed): *Surgical Application of Lasers.* Chicago, Year Book Publishers, 1987.
5. Fuller TA: Fundamentals of Laser Surgery. In Fuller TA (ed): *Surgical Lasers: A Clinical Guide.* New York, Macmillan, 1987.
6. Arndt KA, Noe JM, Northam DBC, et al: Laser therapy: basic concepts and nomenclature. *J Am Acad Dermatol* 5:649–654, 1981.
7. Tan OT, Carney JM, Margolis R, et al: Histologic responses of portwine stains treated by argon, carbon dioxide and tunable dye lasers. *Arch Dermatol* 122:1016–1022, 1986.
8. Brau CA: Free-electron lasers. *Science* 239:1115–1121, 1988.
9. Winburn DC: *What Every Engineer Should Know About Lasers.* New York, Marcel Dekker, 1987.

2
Laser–Tissue Interaction

John V. White
Richard Milner

The scalpel is a simple, elegant surgical instrument. It cleanly divides tissue more precisely than any other device. It produces only a single reaction in soft tissues, that of tissue separation. The laser is somewhat more complex. As a precisely controlled energy delivery device, the laser is capable not only of dividing tissue but of altering its biology. There is a significant laser-tissue interaction that, when appropriately applied, can produce tissue reactions ranging from division to fusion repair.

Understanding the basis of the laser–tissue interaction is essential to appropriate laser use. The interaction of laser and viable tissue is regulated by the individual characteristics of each. Laser wavelength, power, power density, and energy fluence all serve to regulate and modify the input of laser energy into tissues. Tissue composition and chromophore content modify the biologic response to laser energy. This chapter examines how some of the concepts of laser physics introduced in Chapter 1 relate to the biologic effect of lasers on tissue.

LASER CHARACTERISTICS

The electromagnetic spectrum represents the array of wavelengths that can be emitted from electrical or magnetic fields. The spectrum itself can be divided into five major areas based upon the wavelengths. Moving from the shortest to the longest wavelengths, these spectral regions are the x-ray, ultraviolet, visible, infrared, and radiowave. The shorter the wavelength, the greater the tissue disruption.

Electromagnetic radiation within the x-ray portion of the spectrum causes materials to ionize rapidly. The impact of energy within this spectral band can induce instant atomic and molecular disruption. The immense theoretical power of x-ray lasers has made them an area of intense investigation by the U.S. military as part of the "Star Wars" defense initiative. These lasers are not available for experimental or clinical medical use.

Lasers within the ultraviolet region (100 to 380 nm) also have an ionizing effect

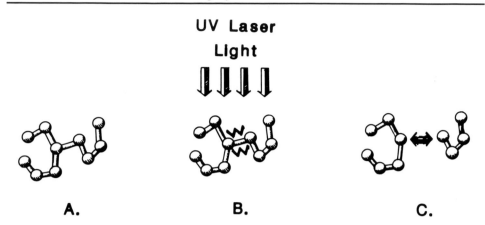

Figure 2.1. Photochemical effect. (*A*) Weaker molecular bonds are subject to disruption. (*B*) Ultraviolet laser light (190 to 380 nm) is absorbed by weaker bonds. *(C)* The excited molecular bonds rupture and the molecular fragments are ejected from the field.

on tissue.[1,2] The major target of tissue interaction is the chemical bond, which reacts through a photochemical process (Fig. 2.1). The incident short-wavelength light energy is directly absorbed by molecular bonds. The excited electronic bonds rupture, fragmenting the molecule. The molecule fragments are ejected from the field, carrying with them the absorbed energy and thereby terminating the laser–tissue interaction. This energy dissipation is known as *photochemical desorption.*

Lasers with shorter wavelengths may disrupt bonds of a number of different strengths, whereas those with wavelengths closer to 380 nm have a more pronounced impact on weaker bonds. Because the process of ultraviolet laser energy absorption and desorption occurs rapidly, little heat is generated. Low heat generation is clearly seen as the hallmark of laser–tissue interaction mediated by a photochemical process. Examination of tissue divided by an ultraviolet laser reveals cleanly divided tissue edges with minimal coagulation necrosis due to heat (Fig. 2.2).

Minimal ionization but significant tissue heating occurs with lasers of longer wavelengths, such as those within the visible (380 to 700 nm) and infrared (700 to 1 mm) portions of the electromagnetic spectrum. Most currently available medical lasers fall into this group and comprise the family of *thermal lasers* (Table 2.1). Interaction of these lasers with biologic materials is mediated by a photothermal process (Fig. 2.3). On contact with tissue, the laser light energy is converted to thermal energy, causing a rapid rise in tissue temperature. As tissue temperature reaches the range of 43 to 60°C, protein and collagen begin to denature and uncoil. As the temperature continues rising to 60 to 99°C, these tissue components begin to decompose. Tissue temperatures of 100°C or greater cause rapid vaporization of intracellular water with cellular explosion, which explosion expels the heated material from the field, dissipating the absorbed energy. Depending on laser wavelength and tissue composition, this process may occur rapidly or slowly. Slower heating of tissue affects a larger volume of tissue.

The photothermal effect just described produces a characteristic lesion in viable tissue (Fig. 2.4).[3] At the epicenter of laser impact, a crater is formed. This *zone of*

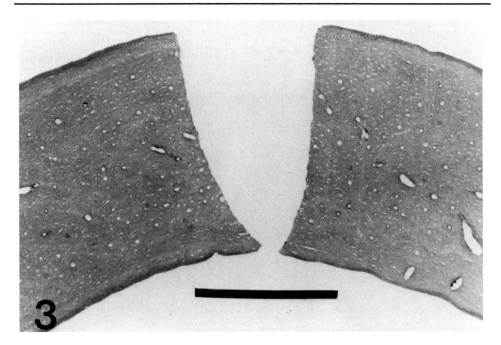

Figure 2.2.   Excimer laser osteotomy. The division of rabbit long bone with a XeCl (380 nm) laser produces a clean cut with minimal thermal injury of divided edges. (With permission: Yow L, et al: Ablation of bone and polymethylmethacrylate by a XeCl (308 nm) excimer laser. *Lasers Surg Med* 9:141–147, 1989.)

vaporization is easily recognized on histologic sections by the absence of previously existing tissue. The region is created by the immediate vaporization of intracellular water and decomposition of cellular components resulting in cellular explosion and expulsion. The walls of the cavity are lined by a fine carbonaceous debris consisting of the charred remnants of cellular and noncellular structural components.

Immediately surrounding this cavity is the *zone of coagulation,* which can be recognized histologically by the coarsened appearance of the interstitial collagen and the absence of cells. This zone is created by the diffusion of heat from the area of laser impact. Temperatures in this zone generally range between 45 and 99°C. Beyond

TABLE 2.1   *Currently Available Thermal Lasers*

Lasers	Wavelength (nm)
Argon	488, 514
KTP	532
Copper vapor	578
Gold vapor	630
Krypton	647–676
Nd:YAG	1,060
CO_2	10,600

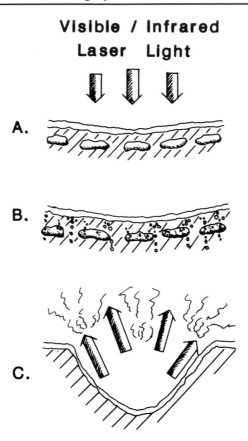

Figure 2.3. Photothermal process. (*A*) Thermal laser light (380 nm to 1 mm) is converted to heat upon absorption in tissue. (*B*) The heat causes a rapid rise in tissue temperature with vaporization of intracellular water. (*C*) Cellular explosion ejects tissue components from the field.

this zone is an area of mild thermal injury recognized histologically be edema of the cells without cell loss or alteration in collagen stroma. This *zone of edema* generally resolves within 24 to 48 hours.

The magnitude of the laser–tissue interaction is regulated by the laser's power output, the power density at point of impact, and the energy fluence (Table 2.2). The *power output* of a laser is defined as the time rate at which energy is emitted; it is expressed in watts. Laser power is directly regulated by setting the power meter of the laser prior to its use. This power is delivered into a spot created by the focusing lens. The *power density,* a measure of the intensity of the beam, is determined by the quotient of the power and the area of the spot size and is reported as watts per square centimeter (W/cm^2).

$$\text{Power density (PD)} = \frac{\text{power (watts)}}{\pi r^2 (\text{cm}^2)},$$

where r = spot radius in centimeters.

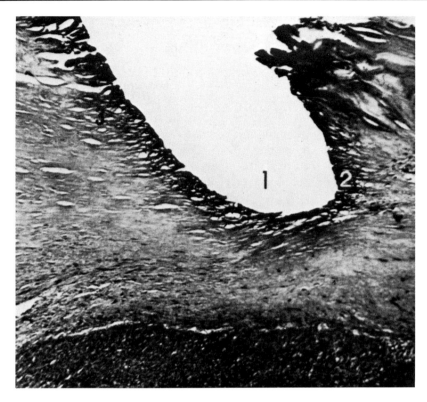

Figure 2.4.   Thermal laser injury. The central crater (1, zone of vaporization) is formed by the heat-induced explosion of tissue. The surrounding tissue demonstrates cell death and thermal coagulation of the protein and collagen stroma (2, zone of coagulation). Beyond this are mildly edematous cells. (With permission: Abela GS, et al: Effects of carbon dioxide, Nd:YAG, and argon laser radiation on coronary atheromatous plaques. *Am J Cardiol* 50:1199–1205, 1982.)

For any given power, a smaller spot area produces a greater power density. A greater power density causes more intense laser–tissue interaction. Very low power densities have little immediate ablative effect on tissue. The depth of the zone of vaporization is most directly dependent upon the power and power density of the incident laser beam. The extent of tissue effect is determined by the total amount of laser energy imparted to the tissues. This is defined as the *energy fluence* and is

TABLE 2.2.   *Determinants of the Magnitude of Laser–Tissue Interaction*

Parameter	Calculation	Units
Power		Watts (W)
Power density	$\dfrac{\text{Power}}{\text{Spot area}}$	W/cm^2
Energy fluence	Power density $\times$ time	j^*/cm^2

*1 joule = 1 watt × second (i.e., one watt of power applied for 1 second).

calculated by multiplying the power density by the time of laser energy application. It is expressed as joules per square centimeter (j/cm²).

$$\text{Energy fluence} = \text{PD} \times \text{time} = \frac{\text{power (watts)} \times \text{time (sec)}}{\text{spot area (cm}^2)}.$$

As energy fluence increases, the volume of tissue affected also increases. The volume of the zones of coagulation and edema is proportional to the total time of energy transfer from the laser to the tissue. Longer radiance causes more extensive thermal energy diffusion through the tissue. Thus, the parameters of energy delivery can be set to provide precise and reliable control of laser affects upon tissues.

TISSUE CHARACTERISTICS

Tissue composition and chromophore content can alter the pattern of laser energy uptake and thermal responsiveness. Each tissue type has a specific pattern of light absorption. Absorption peaks occur at those wavelengths most absorbed by the several tissue components. Tissue has a high responsiveness when it is irradiated by laser energy at a wavelength that corresponds its light absorption peak. Tissues are relatively more resistant to laser energy when irradiated at a wavelength that demonstrates low absorption in the tissue. One application of these principles is the use of argon laser energy for the treatment of port-wine stains (Fig. 2.5). The dermis overlying these cutaneous lesions is translucent and has little absorption of light at 514 nm, whereas the pigmented lesion itself has a strong absorption peak at this wavelength. Thus, argon laser energy can pass through the overlying dermis without inducing significant thermal damage. The energy is readily absorbed in

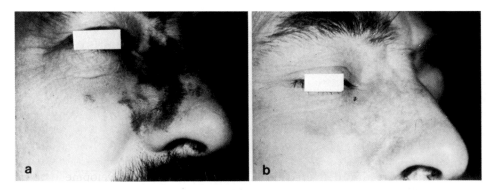

Figure 2.5. Argon laser treatment of port-wine stain: (*A*) before and (*B*) after. Because the overlying epidermis is relatively translucent to the argon wavelength, coagulation of the vascular lesion can be accomplished with minimal overlying skin destruction. (With permission: Mordon SR, et al: Comparative study of the ''point-by-point technique'' and the ''scanning technique'' for laser treatment of port-wine stain. *Lasers Surg Med* 9:398–404, 1989.)

the pigmented lesion which undergoes photothermal coagulation. During healing, the coagulum is replaced by more cosmetically appealing nonpigmented fibrous tissue.[4,5]

Photothermal effect and tissue responsiveness to laser energy can also be modified by the presence of chromophores within the tissue.[6] *Chromophores* are endogenous compounds that have limited distribution and demonstrate a high affinity for light at specific wavelengths. This affinity enhances the photothermal impact upon the tissue in the immediate vicinity of the chromophore even if the tissue itself has limited absorption of that specific laser wavelength. The treatment of port-wine stain with argon laser energy also demonstrates the application of this principle. The endothelial cells of the capillary tufts within the lesion have only moderate affinity for light at the 514-nm wavelength. However, hemoglobin acts as a chromophore for this light, rapidly absorbing it and enhancing the photothermal effect on the surrounding capillary tufts.

Knowing the pattern of absorption of light and the presence of chromophores within a specific type of tissue permits the clinician to perform more selective photoablation. In addition, an understanding of the laser parameters governing energy delivery enables the clinician to select and use lasers according to a reasonable prediction of the laser–tissue interaction. This approach to laser use may broaden the applications of the laser in treating patients. It may also lead to new, more selective, and less disruptive techniques in patient care.

SPECIFIC LASER–TISSUE INTERACTIONS

Argon Laser

The argon laser can be used at a number of different wavelengths between 488 and 514 nm. It operates within the visible portion of the electromagnetic spectrum, and the emission appears as blue-green light. Because of energy conversion inefficiencies, the peak power output is in the range of 20 W. Argon laser radiation is strongly absorbed by the tissue chromophores melanin and hemoglobin. Its moderate tissue penetration and optical scatter make the argon laser suitable for photocoagulation without vaporization. Therefore, it has been widely used in ophthalmology and dermatology. Treatment of retinal lesions,[7] port-wine stains,[8] and other pigmented lesions[8-10] are applications of the argon laser, appropriate to the characteristics of its laser-tissue interaction.

Perhaps the most widely publicized use of the argon laser is for the treatment of arterial occlusive disease. This application demonstrates an attempt to modify the laser–tissue interaction to extend the usefulness of the laser. The argon was the first laser to be readily delivered through fiberoptics. The development of this fiberoptic delivery system in the early 1970s sparked the imagination of physicians around the world because it permitted the delivery of laser energy to sites within the body that had previously been inaccessible without major surgical exposure.

Almost immediately, the treatment of occlusive disease of the coronary arteries was attempted.[11,12] Acute or chronic arterial occlusion was created in experimental animals by ligating a vessel and allowing it to thrombose.[13-15] An argon laser catheter

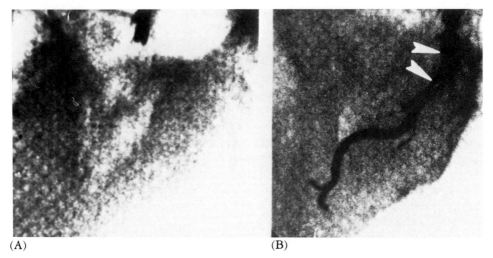

(A)   (B)

Figure 2.6. Effect of argon laser energy on thrombus. (*A*) The chronically occluded vessel was treated with argon laser energy delivered through a bare fiber. (*B*) The majority of the plaque and thrombus was vaporized with little injury to the artery wall. (With permission: Choy DSJ, et al: Laser coronary angioplasty: experience with 9 cadaver hearts. *Am J Cardiol* 50:1209–1211, 1982.)

was passed from a distant site to the area of occlusion, and the laser was triggered to emit argon energy from the bare argon fiber. The early results from these investigations demonstrated remarkable clearing of the occlusion with minimal injury to the vessel wall (Fig. 2.6).

Clinical application of argon laser vaporization of atherosclerotic plaque, however, was not successful.[16] Although the laser energy was capable of clearing soft atherosclerotic plaque, calcified areas were relatively resistant, and the use of greater energy fluences caused a high incidence of vessel perforation.[17,18] Experimenters then attempted to control the photothermal effect and optical scatter within the vessel by placing a metal tip over the end of the argon fiber (Fig. 2.7),[19] thereby converting the photothermal process from a tissue-level interaction to a laser-biomaterial interaction. The metal tip is heated by the argon laser. The heat is conducted to the tissues in a limited, predictable area. With this alteration, the argon laser has been successfully used to recanalize stenotic and occluded arteries and has improved the physician's ability to treat atherosclerosis.[20,21]

Carbon Dioxide (CO₂) Laser

The CO_2 laser emits energy at 10,600 nm (10 μm), which is in the mid-infrared portion of the electromagnetic spectrum. The emission is invisible to the eye and therefore requires a separate red beam of the helium-neon laser for targeting. The CO_2 laser is capable of high power outputs, with currently available medical lasers delivering up to 100 W. The 10.6-μm wavelength is readily absorbed by water, which results in a chromophore-independent, uniform pattern of energy uptake with little optical scatter within tissues. Because soft tissue is 60 to 70% water by weight, the CO_2 laser–tissue interaction is superficial, with limited penetration and

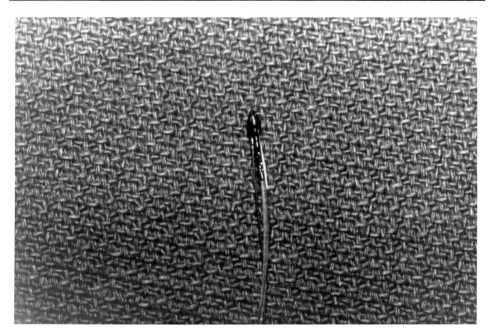

Figure 2.7. The Laser Probe (Trimedyne), used clinically for peripheral laser angioplasty, has an olive-shaped metal tip placed over the end of the argon fiber.

optical scatter. It has relatively little effect on anhydrous tissue, such as bone. Its controlled, superficial tissue effect makes the CO_2 laser suitable for a wide variety of applications in the surgical specialties of otorhinolaryngology. As the beam cannot, at the present, be delivered through fiberoptics, it must be delivered through an articulating arm. Through this delivery system it can be used to make precise incisions or to ablate tumors a layer at a time.

The effect of superficial vaporization makes the CO_2 laser an ideal instrument for the treatment of infected wounds and ulcers.[22-24] The laser is capable of vaporizing the surface of ulcers in a layer-by-layer fashion. The high temperature of the incident CO_2 beam, 1500°C, sterilizes all tissue in its path. The zone of coagulation underlying this superficial vaporization seals small vessels and lymphatics. By sealing lymphatics, lymphborne bacteria are prevented from leaking onto the wound. This method of debridement of infected ulcers and wounds minimizes tissue loss and provides immediate sterilization. If the sterile surface represents the only area of infection, primary closure, immediate skin grafting, and healing by secondary intent are all acceptable therapeutic choices. This method of treating persistent and often debilitating infections using the inherent characteristics of the CO_2 laser permits significantly improved patient care (Fig. 2.8).

The superficial action of the CO_2 laser also makes it quite suitable for tissue repair, one of the truly unique applications of a thermal laser. At power densities of 1000 W/cm^2, the laser produces the three zones of tissue injury. A power density in the range of 150 W/cm^2 reduces the photothermal effect below the vaporization threshold and produces a zone of coagulation at the epicenter of laser impact.[25] As previously stated, collagen can denature and reanneal within this zone. When divided collagen elements are in close apposition, they may intertwine and reanneal in a fashion that produces tissue repair or tissue "welding" (Fig. 2.9).[26]

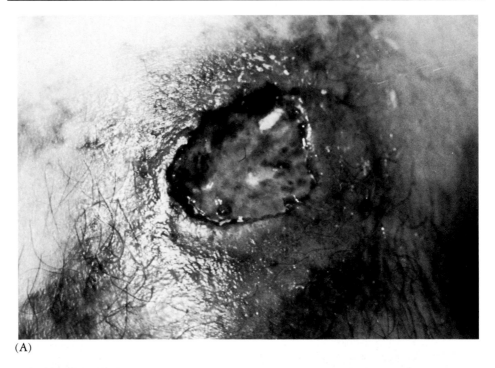

(A)

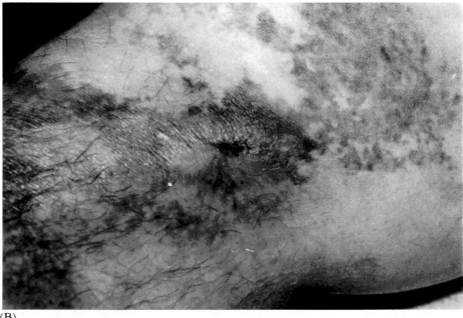

(B)

Figure 2.8. CO_2 laser sterilization of an infected ulcer. (*A*) The CO_2 laser was set at 40 W in continuous mode; the beam was defocused to a diameter of 5 mm (PD = 204 W/cm^2) to vaporize the purulent surface of the ulcer. (*B*) Eight weeks after laser therapy, the ulcer was healed.

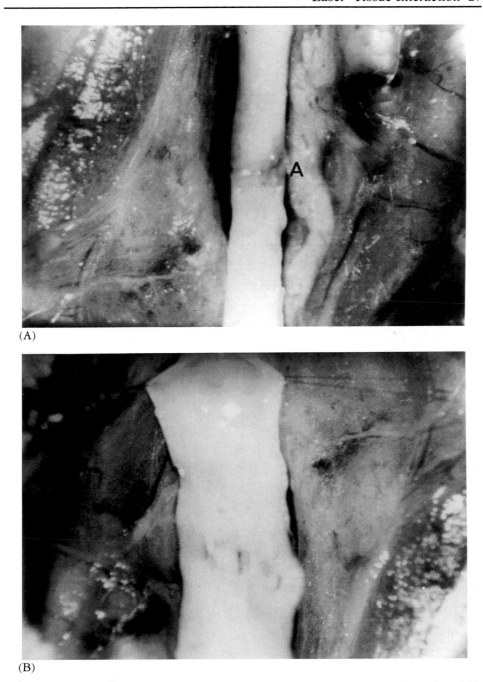

(A)

(B)

Figure 2.9. CO_2 laser tissue fusion. (*A*) Gross appearance of external surface of a rabbit carotid artery end-to-end anastomosis 4 weeks after fusion. (*B*) Flow surface of vessel is smooth with excellent healing between stay sutures. (With permission: White JV, et al: Laser fusion tissue repair with the CO_2 laser. *Proc Photo-Opt Instrum Eng* 1066:35–40, 1989.)

TABLE 2.3. *Applications of Laser Tissue Repair*

Tissue Fused	Laser
Blood vessels	CO_2,* Argon, Nd:YAG
Skin	CO_2, Argon, Nd:YAG
GI tract	CO_2, Nd:YAG
Pleura	CO_2, Nd:YAG
Biliary tree	CO_2
Fallopian tube	CO_2
Nerve	CO_2*
Tendon	CO_2
Ureter	CO_2
Vas deferens	CO_2*

*Clinical trials have begun.

This application of the inherent characteristics of the CO_2 laser–tissue interaction has been exploited to repair a wide variety of tissues experimentally and clinically (Table 2.3).

These same characteristics are responsible for a major limitation of the CO_2 laser. Because the 10.6-μm wavelength is so well absorbed by water, the CO_2 laser is relatively ineffective for photocoagulation of blood vessels greater than 1 mm in diameter.[27] Although this laser is excellent for the division of soft tissue, its applications are limited in highly vascularized tissues, such as liver and spleen.[28] Once CO_2 laser energy penetrates the anterior surface of a blood vessel, its energy is immediately dissipated by the water contained in the flowing blood. Understanding this characteristic of the CO_2 laser–tissue interaction permits the laser surgeon to extend the benefits of the laser by eliminating blood from the lumen before applying laser energy. Selective clamping of vessels before division extends the CO_2 laser photocoagulation to vessels up to 2 mm in diameter. Its characteristic laser–tissue interaction, when knowledgeably applied, make this laser the most versatile of the medical lasers currently available.

Neodymium:Yttrium-Aluminum-Garnet (Nd:YAG) Laser

The Nd:YAG laser emits energy at 1060 nm, which is in the near-infrared portion of the electromagnetic spectrum. Most available YAG lasers are capable of delivering up to 100 W of power in a continuous mode. The near-infrared wavelength is less absorbed by blood than either argon or CO_2 and is deeply penetrating into tissues. The deep penetration and scatter of Nd:YAG radiation in soft tissues causes the zone of necrosis to expand for up to 24 hours after the delivery of laser energy has stopped. These properties make the Nd:YAG laser suitable for deep photocoagulation in soft tissue. The laser has been widely used in the treatment of vascular lesions and tumors of the mucosa of the gastrointestinal tract to cause them to slough without bleeding.

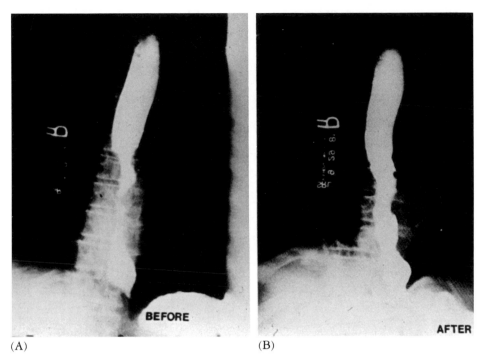

(A)   (B)

Figure 2.10.   Treatment of occluding esophageal cancer with Nd:YAG laser therapy. (*A*)
The occluding lesion is exposed to fiberoptically delivered Nd:YAG laser energy. (*B*)
After 48 hours, tissue slough is complete and patient is able to tolerate oral intake. (With
permission: Fleischer D, et al: Endoscopic Nd:YAG laser therapy for carcinoma of the
esophagus: a new palliative approach. *Am J Surg* 143:280–283, 1982.)

The palliative treatment of patients with unresectable carcinoma of the esophagus and stomach has been significantly improved by use of the Nd:YAG. Previously, these patients required esophageal bypass surgery to permit swallowing of
saliva and small amounts of food. These palliative operations carried a high morbidity and mortality. The Nd:YAG laser has been used to recanalize the occluded
portion of the gastrointestinal tract because it can penetrate deeply into soft tissues
and induce a relatively large zone of tissue slough without bleeding.[29,30] Most frequently, the endoscope can be gently pushed past the occlusive lesion. The portion
of the tumor projecting into the lumen of the esophagus is irradiated as the scope
is withdrawn. A slowly progressive circumferential slough of the tumor to a depth
of several millimeters occurs over the subsequent 48 hours, after which the patient
is generally able to swallow saliva and small amounts of food (Fig. 2.10). This
endoscopic procedure can be accomplished with low morbidity and mortality on an
outpatient basis and provides true palliation without disability.

The use of Nd:YAG energy to resect liver is an example of the adverse effects
of the inherent laser–tissue interaction. The deep penetration of Nd:YAG energy,
which allows photocoagulation of blood vessels well below the surface of the tissue,
was thought to be of particular benefit to the surgeon in major hepatic resections.
However, the sinusoidal structure of the liver without discrete vessel walls and the
delayed slough of tissue has led to significant immediate blood loss[31] and postopera-

tive bleeding and bile leakage. Therefore, the photothermal effect of the Nd:YAG laser was modified to prevent deep tissue penetration. This was accomplished by placing a sapphire tip on the end of the laser fiberoptic.[32,33] The sapphire tip, like the metal cap on the argon fiber, changes the laser energy transformation from a tissue-level process to a materials interaction. The sapphire tip converts some of the YAG energy to heat and highly focuses the beam so that it is emitted only to those tissues in contact with the tip. With this modification of the Nd:YAG laser–tissue interaction, this near-infrared wavelength can be used successfully to resect not only liver but also a wide variety of soft tissues such as spleen and pancreas.

Excimer Laser

The term *excimer* is derived from "excited dimer," which refers to the molecular composition of the medium contained in lasers that emit in the ultraviolet waveband (100 to 380 nm). Lower wavelengths within the ultraviolet portion of the electromagnetic spectrum can profoundly affect cellular contents, cleaving and injuring protein and DNA structure without lysing the cell. This property has led to the suggestion that lasers emitting wavelengths <190 nm have carcinogenic potential. However, the "cold"-cutting capability of the excimer laser may be of significant benefit in a variety of clinical settings situations that require division or surgical modification of bone.

The benefit of "cold" cutting is well demonstrated in dental applications. The photothermal effects exerted by the CO_2 laser energy on tooth enamel lead to cracks and fissures (Fig. 2.11). The enamel cracks as the dentin expands during heating; fissures occur during rapid cooling.[34] Ultraviolet laser energy (XeCl, 308 nm) does not induce such changes (Fig. 2.12). During dental procedures such as root canal therapy, the XeCl laser can induce photochemical decomposition of dentin without heat.[35] The end result is controlled, smooth ablation of dental tissues without irregularities. This method of laser–tissue interaction holds promise for improvement in patient care.

Lasers that interact with tissue through a photothermal process are effective for ablation of cellular material. However, they have relatively little effect upon anhydrous material such as bone. Midinfrared-wavelength thermal lasers are capable of producing pyrolysis of bone, but they delay healing because they cause thermal injury of cellular elements. The erbium:YAG laser creates a zone of necrosis of 5 to 11 μm, whereas the CO_2 laser produces a zone of thermal necrosis greater than 600 μm.[36] The 308-nm XeCl excimer laser can cleanly divide the molecular bonds without significant thermal injury (Fig. 2.2). These applications of the excimer laser demonstrate an improvement in surgical technique using the native laser–tissue interactive properties of the ultraviolet wavelength.

The pace of laser development continues to increase, and physicians are constantly introduced to more sophisticated technology. It remains the obligation of the laser surgeon to understand the specific characteristics of the laser–tissue interaction of each device. Only in this way can the promise of the laser to extend and improve our ability to care for patients be fulfilled.

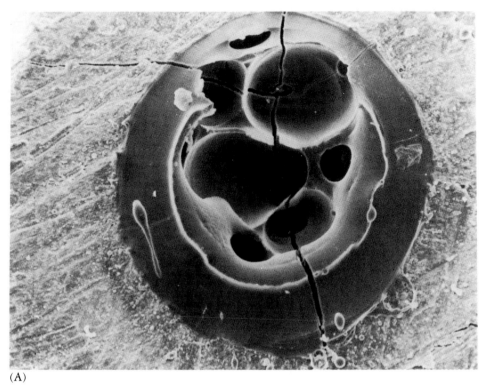

(A)

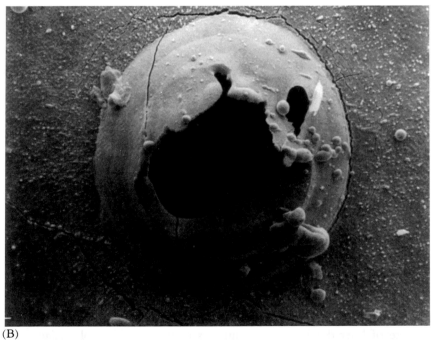

(B)

Figure 2.11. Effects of CO_2 laser on tooth structure. (*A*) On scanning electron microscopy (SEM) the enamel surface of a tooth after a single 0.5-sec 2-W pulse demonstrates cracks. (*B*) The dentin reveals conical and radial fissures. (With permission: Keller U, Hibst R: Experimental studies of the application of the Er:YAG laser on dental hard substances: II. Light microscopic and SEM investigations. *Lasers Surg Med* 9:345–351, 1989.)

31

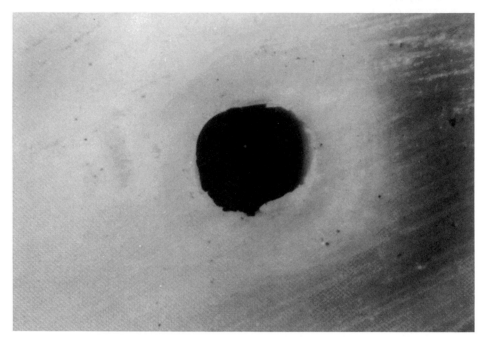

Figure 2.12.   Effect of UV laser on tooth structure. The XeCl (308 nm) laser produces a clean ablative lesion in dentin with minimal thermal injury. (With permission: Pini R, et al: Laser dentistry: a new application of excimer laser in root canal therapy. *Lasers Surg Med* 9:352–357, 1989.)

REFERENCES

1. Laudenslager JB: Ion-molecule processes in lasers. In Ausloos P (ed) *Kinetics of Ion-Molecule Reactions*. New York, Plenum, 1978.

2. Brau CA: Rare gas halogen excimers. In Rhodes CK (ed) *Excimer Lasers*. New York, Springer-Verlag, New York, 1979.

3. Beck OJ, Wilske J, Schoenberger JL, et al: Tissue changes following applications of lasers to the rabbit brain: results with CO_2 and neodymium:YAG laser. *Neurosurg Rev* 1:31–36, 1979.

4. Noe JM, Barsley S, Gerr D, et al: Port-wine stains and the response to argon laser therapy: successful treatment and the predictive role of color, age, and biopsy. *Plast Reconstr Surg* 65:130–136, 1980.

5. Finley J, Barsley S, Greer, et al: Healing of port-wine stains after argon laser therapy. *Arch Dermatol* 117:486–489, 1981.

6. Parrish JA: Laser photomedicine: selective laser-tissue interaction. In Dixon JA (ed): *Surgical Applications of Lasers*. Chicago, Year Book Medical Publishers, 1987, pp 34–51.

7. Bloom LH, Brucker AJ: Lasers in ophthalmology. *Surg Clin North Am* 64(5): 1013–1024, 1984.

8. Cosman B: Experience in the argon laser therapy of port-wine stains. *Plast Reconstr Surg* 65:119–129, 1980.

9. Dolsky RL: Argon laser skin surgery. *Surg Clin North Am* 64(5):861–870, 1984.

10. Keller GS, Doiron D, Weingarten C: Advances in laser skin surgery for vascular lesions. *Arch Otolaryngol* 111(7):437–440, 1985.

11. Lee G, Ikeda RM, Kozina J, et al: Laser-dissolution of coronary atherosclerotic obstruction. *Am Heart J* 102:1074–1075, 1981.

12. Choy DSJ, Stertzer SH, Rotterdam HZ, et al: Laser coronary angioplasty: experience with 9 cadaver hearts. *Am J Cardiol* 50:1209–1211, 1982.

13. Choy DSJ, Stertzer S, Rotterdam HZ, et al: Transluminal laser catheter angioplasty. *Am J Cardiol* 50:1206–1208, 1982.

14. Crea F, Fenech A, Smith W, et al: Laser recanalization of acutely thrombosed coronary arteries in live dogs: early results. *J Am Coll Cardiol* 6(5):1052–1056, 1985.

15. Abela GS, Conti CR, Normann S, et al: A new model for investigation of transluminal recanalization: human atherosclerotic coronary artery xenografts. *Am J Cardiol* 54: 200–205, 1984.

16. Choy DSJ, Stertzer SH, Myler RK, et al: Human coronary laser recanalization. *Clin Cardiol* 7:377–381, 1984.

17. Lawrence PF, Dries DJ, Moatamed F, et al: Acute effects of argon laser on human atherosclerotic plaque. *J Vasc Surg* 1(6):852–859, 1984.

18. Dries DJ, Lawrence PF, Syverud J, et al: Responses of atherosclerotic aorta to argon laser. *Lasers Surg Med* 5(3):321–326, 1985.

19. Sanborn TA, Faxon DP, Haudenschild CC, et al: Experimental angioplasty: circumferential distribution of laser thermal energy with a laser probe. *J Am Coll Cardiol* 5:934–938, 1984.

20. Yang Y, Hashizume M, Arbutina D, et al: Argon laser angioplasty with a laser probe. *J Vasc Surg* 6:60–65, 1987.

21. Wright JG, Belkin M, Greenfield AJ, et al: Laser angioplasty for limb salvage: observations on early results. *J Vasc Surg* 10:29–38, 1989.

22. Stellar S, Meijer R, Walia S, et al: Carbon dioxide laser debridement of decubitus ulcers: followed by immediate rotation flap or skin graft closure. *Ann Surg* 2:230–235, 1974.

23. Glantz G, Korn A: The use of CO_2 laser in general surgery. In Kaplan I (ed): *Laser Surgery III*. Tel Aviv, Ot-Paz, 1979, p 179.

24. Eltorai I, Glantz G, Montroy R: The use of the carbon dioxide laser beam in the surgery of pressure sores. *Int Surg* 73:54–56, 1988.

25. White JV, Leefmans E, Stewart GJ, et al: Laser fusion tissue repair with the CO_2 laser. *Proc Photo-Opt Instrum Eng* 1066:35–40, 1989.

26. White JV, Dalsing MC, Yao JST, et al: The tissue fusion effect of the CO_2 laser: analysis of application to the vascular anastomosis. *Surg Forum* 36:455–457, 1985.

27. Dixon JA: General surgical applications of lasers. In Dixon JA (ed): *Surgical Applications of Lasers*. Chicago, Year Book Medical Publishers, 1987, pp 119–143.

28. Goldenberg A, Goldenberg S, Neto JG, et al: CO_2 laser and suture in splenic parenchyma: an experimental study. *Lasers Surg Med* 5:405–413, 1985.

29. Pietrafitta JJ, Dwyer RM: Endoscopic laser therapy of malignant esophageal obstruction. *Arch Surg* 121:395–400, 1986.

30. Karlin DA, Fisher RS, Krevsky B: Prolonged survival and effective palliation in patients with squamous cell carcinoma of the esophagus following endoscopic therapy. *Cancer* 59:1969–1972, 1986.

31. Tranberg KG, Rigotti P, Brackett KA, et al: Liver resection—a comparison using the Nd:YAG laser and ultrasonic surgical aspirator in blunt dissection. *Am J Surg* 151: 368–374, 1986.

32. Daikuzono N, Joffe SN: An artificial sapphire probe for control of photocoagulation and tissue vaporization using the Nd:YAG laser. *Med Instrum* 19:173–178, 1985.

33. Joffe SN, Brackett KA, Sankar MY, et al: Resection of the liver with the Nd:YAG laser. *Surg Gynecol Obstet* 163:437–442, 1986.

34. Keller U, Hibst R: Experimental studies of the application of the Er:YAG laser on dental hard substances: II. Light microscopic and SEM investigations. *Lasers Surg Med* 9:345–351, 1989.

35. Pini R, Salimbeni R, Vannini M, et al: Laser dentistry: a new application of excimer laser in root canal therapy. *Lasers Surg Med* 9:352–357, 1989.

36. Yow L, Nelson JS, Berns MW: Ablation of bone and polymethylmethacrylate by XeCl (308 nm) excimer laser. *Lasers Surg Med* 9:141–147, 1989.

3A

Principles of Laser Safety: Organization, Administrative Controls, and Standard Operating Procedures

Sherry Heller

The safe use of medical lasers requires that certain administrative controls and standard operating procedures be created to organize an appropriate hospital laser program. Also, all personnel dealing with this technology must be made aware of the hazards specific to it. This chapter provides guidelines for establishing an organizational structure for a laser program and discusses specific policies and procedures that should guarantee an appropriate level of laser safety.

Twenty years ago only a few hospitals were using lasers. In the last few years, laser technology has spread rapidly, and even the smallest hospitals are now ordering lasers. This rapid growth has created problems for hospitals regarding standards of care: Lasers in industry have long been regulated by government standards, but no such standards have existed for lasers used in medicine.

The future of laser surgery and medicine depends on the user.[1] Therefore it is imperative that all personnel involved have adequate training and education. The American National Standards Institute (ANSI) has published mandatory safety requirements for lasers in industry. *American National Standard for the Safe Use of Lasers* (ANSI Z136.1) is the precursor to the recently published *Laser Safety in the Health Care Environment* (ANSI Z136.3). Both publications contain guidelines for setting up a laser program and can be used in conjunction with each other. These guidelines are not currently mandatory for the medical community but future standard of practice will be based on it.

ANSI Z136.3 is intended for use by anyone involved with the installation, operation, maintenance and service of lasers in the medical setting. Control mechanisms, safety, and training guidelines are described in detail.

THE LASER COMMITTEE

Administrative controls outlined in ANSI Z136.3 are based on the formation of a laser controlling committee. The membership, the functions and the authority of this committee should be established in its charter. Having these in writing avoids conflicts about the functions of the committee. This committee should be in place and fulfilling its functions before lasers are put into use in the institution.

Membership

A chairperson for the committee should be named by the chief of staff. Membership should include representatives from each specialty service interested in laser use—anesthesiology, administration, nursing (usually operating room), clinical engineering—and the laser safety officer (see second part of this chapter). All members of the committee should be interested in promoting the use of lasers within the facility and should have some knowledge about lasers.

Functions

A principal function of the laser committee is to establish credentialing criteria for physicians who will use lasers. The guidelines set up by the American Society of Laser Medicine and Surgery are those proposed in ANSI Z136.3 (Table 3.1). The steps to follow in applying for laser privileges should be listed in detail (Table 3.2).

A process by which technical support personnel can obtain certification to work with lasers must also be established. This would include resident physicians, nurses, or technicians who are expected to operate the lasers and clinical engineering personnel who will service the equipment. All other staff who are present during laser

TABLE 3.1. *ANSI Z136.3 Guidelines for Physician Credentialing*[2]

Physician Training Program
1. Review pertinent literature and audiovisual aids
2. Laser course attendance (8 to 10 hours)
   a. Basic laser physics
   b. Laser tissue interaction
   c. Discussion of clinical specialty field
   d. Hands-on experience
3. Consultation with experienced laser physician
   a. 6 to 8 hours observation/hands-on experience
      OR
   b. Accredited residency including laser use
4. Laser safety training
   a. Potential hazards
   b. Requirements for laser safety
   c. Standard operating procedures

TABLE 3.2. *Suggested Flowchart for Physician Credentialing*

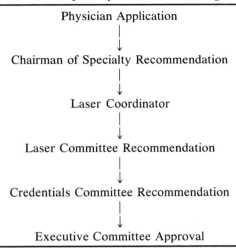

Physician Application

Chairman of Specialty Recommendation

Laser Coordinator

Laser Committee Recommendation

Credentials Committee Recommendation

Executive Committee Approval

operation need to have safety training, and the laser committee should specify what is included in that training (Table 3.3).

Development of Policies and Procedures

All safety measures, emergency procedures, and preventive maintenance policies need to be addressed by the laser committee. These will be covered in detail later in this chapter and in the chapter discussing anesthesia for laser surgery (Chapter 4).

Development of Documentation

Documents such as laser usage report forms, safety audits, credentialing application forms, and maintenance records need to be developed.

TABLE 3.3. *ANSI Z136.3 Guidelines for Support Staff Certification*[2]

Technical/Support Staff Training Program
1. Laser bioeffects
2. Potential hazards
   a. Eye and skin hazards
   b. Fire hazards
   c. Hazards of laser plume
   d. Other hazards
3. Requirements for laser safety
   a. Laser eye protection
   b. Elimination of explosion hazards
   c. Smoke evacuation
   d. Reduction of reflected beam
4. Standard operating procedures

Appointment of the Laser Safety Officer

The laser safety officer (LSO) is the person assigned the day-to-day responsibility of enforcing the policies and procedures developed by the laser committee. The person selected should have attended a training program covering laser principles, laser safety, and their practical application.[2]

Development of Training Programs

The laser committee may conduct programs to educate other physicians in laser surgery. A library of laser materials can be established to assist in the education of physicians, residents, nurses, and technicians.

Recommendations for Laser Purchases

The laser committee is an ideal group to evaluate and recommend laser purchases. Representatives of all interested specialties are now involved in laser activities and are promoting the use of lasers. Areas that need to be addressed are potential usage, purchase alternatives, physical plant modifications needed, and the specific manufacturers' equipment and service agreements.

The installation of a YAG laser provides a good example of the planning required for implementation of a specific laser modality. The operating room or treatment room where the YAG laser will be employed must be provided with the proper electrical outlets and an adequate plumbing system. The YAG laser is a very inefficient modality and requires a high current capability and large heat dissipation capabilities.[3] The electrical outlets must provide 208 V, three-phase power. The plumbing system should be capable of providing water flow at a rate of 8 liters per minute to provide adequate cooling of the YAG laser. Acquisition of a certain type of laser without providing the appropriate physical plant modifications can result in unnecessary delay in activation of the system for clinical use and in unnecessary expense to the hospital.

An effort should be made to acquire equipment that will have multiservice use so that there will be a faster return on the initial investment.

Feasibility studies should help determine what type of laser should be considered first.[4] If the initial investment will be more than is affordable, renting or leasing lasers might be considered. Other areas that need to be considered are:

What services will be offered by the vendor?

What accessories will be covered in the purchase?

What kind of service contract is offered and how much turnover time will be promised for repairs?

Will the vendor provide training for personnel as part of the purchase price?

After gathering all this information, the laser committee can make recommendations to the administration on the types of lasers to be acquired.

3B
Principles of Laser Safety: Hazards and Specific Safety Measures

Larry E. Dollens

The usefulness of health care laser systems (HCLS) lies in their ability to concentrate a relatively large amount of energy into a very small area. By varying the spot size, the pulse width, and the pulse repetition rate, to control the rate at which energy is delivered, the surgeon can achieve physiological reactions ranging from tissue warming through complete cellular destruction. Unfortunately, the very characteristic that makes the HCLS so useful also makes it easily the most dangerous piece of equipment in the operating room. It qualifies for this distinction for two reasons. First, it is capable of causing injury not only to the patient but also to the surgeon, to the operating team, and even to observers at some distance from the operating table. Second, the mechanisms of potential injury are not readily apparent to the uninformed. Medical lasers are even more hazardous than comparably powered industrial laser systems.[5] In the industrial setting the beam path is usually enclosed and inaccessible during laser operation. The opposite is necessarily true in the medical setting.

The following discussion reviews the most salient issues about laser safety for the clinical practitioner. Any institution using lasers in surgery should have in place a comprehensive laser safety program directed by a trained medical laser safety officer. Additionally, the physician credentialing process should require training in laser safety. The ANSI document Z136.3[6] is an excellent reference resource for a safety program, and medical laser safety officer courses are available from organizations such as Rockwell Associates, Inc., P.O. Box 43018, Cincinnati, Ohio, 45243.

Let us now examine several types of hazards and the relevant safety measures. HCLS hazards fall into two broad categories: (1) hazards directly associated with the beam, including retinal, corneal, and skin burns, and (2) secondary hazards including fire, electrocution, toxic waste, and plume radiation. There are some references in the industrial literature to ionizing radiation hazards, but that issue is not addressed except to state that no HCLS device in current production poses a threat of that nature. Likewise, the electrocution hazard is predominantly associated with service procedures[7] during which access panels are removed and interlock switches are defeated. This is not to imply that the hazard is of little consequence, since several fatal industrial accidents have been documented.

BEAM HAZARDS

The predominant HCLS hazard is eye injury resulting either from a direct beam or from a specular beam reflection striking the eye.[8] The actual site of injury may be either the cornea or the retina, and is a direct function of where the beam energy is dissipated. In the visible and near-infrared portions of the light spectrum (400 to 1400 nm), a photon will pass through the ocular media with little loss of energy through conversion to thermal or chemical energy. Lasers such as the Nd:YAG and argon, which operate within that portion of the spectrum, present a retinal hazard, since energy from them passes through the cornea and is dissipated at the retina. Energy from lasers operating outside the 400 to 1400 nm portion of the spectrum (i.e., the CO_2 laser) is converted to thermal energy at the cornea, which is effectively opaque to those wavelengths.

If a single thought regarding laser safety were to be remembered, it should be this: Nearly every visible to near-infrared spectrum HCLS is easily capable of producing a beam of sufficient power to cause irreversible damage to the retina in a time period so short that blink or aversion response will afford no protection. The only reliable method of eye protection is to require *all individuals* in the operating suite to wear *approved* laser safety glasses at all times when the laser is turned on and *in the operate mode*.[9] This should be an inflexible rule even if operating through an endoscope using a light fiber or through an operating microscope equipped with a mechanical shutter. Light fibers can break and mechanical shutters can malfunction! Reports documenting such incidents already exist.

Early safety glasses embodied the optical characteristics of welders' goggles. They did a poor job of blocking laser energy and were often cast aside because they severely obstructed the surgeon's vision. Modern optical technology has produced safety glasses that are highly efficient screens, effectively blocking light at a laser's specific frequency while passing nearly all photon energy at other visible wavelengths. This fact gives rise to a crucial safety point. Glasses designed for use with one type (wavelength) of laser may afford absolutely no protection if used with another type. The potential hazard presented by the multiwavelength lasers should be of concern. These hybrid lasers make it easy to switch from one wavelength to another—but will it be so easy to remember to switch glasses also?

ANSI-approved safety glasses have their effective wavelength and optical density (o.d.) stamped on the frame.[10] Make certain the wavelength stamped on the glasses matches the operating wavelength of the laser to be used. If the information doesn't appear on the glasses—*don't wear them!*

One final recommendation about glasses: Most laser safety glasses are available in either plastic or glass versions. Those with glass lenses are strongly recommended because they will withstand the impact of a much more powerful beam. Glass-lensed safety glasses are a bit on the expensive side (about $400 for a set of prescription YAG glasses). However, retinal replacements aren't available at any price.

The rule "always wear eye protection" must also include the patient.[11] For the conscious, alert patient, it is appropriate to provide the same eyewear used by the surgical team. For the unconscious patient (or for the conscious patient in whom the laser safety glasses would interfere with the procedure), the closed eyelids should be covered with moistened sterile cotton eyepads that are in turn covered with moistened towels or metallic eye protectors. A stainless steel eyeshield is available as an alternative for use during dermatologic and plastic surgery.

An unfocused laser beam loses very little energy in traversing distance. There exists, therefore, a high potential for injury in being struck by either a direct or a reflected beam even at some distance from the laser. We must therefore also provide for the safety of individuals who may be just outside the operating room and for those individuals who may be entering it. All windows to the operating room must be covered with a material that is opaque at the operating laser wavelength. For situations in which theater viewing during surgery is required, there are window coverings that allow relatively normal viewing by blocking only light energy that is at or near the laser wavelength. Unless there is a specific need for this type of window covering, however, a material that is opaque to light is recommended. Materials which are designed to occlude light at a specific wavelength can be quite expensive and are of no protective value if a laser of another wavelength is moved into the room.

It is also important to provide ANSI-approved warning signs, blocking screens, and safety glasses at *each* entrance to the operating suite.

The ANSI-approved *warning sign* as seen in Figure 3.1[12] conveys information required for individuals about to enter an operating room to protect themselves adequately (i.e., the fact that a laser is in use and its operating wavelength and power). The signs should be placed in lighted sign holders that are controlled by a switch located inside the operating suite. The signs should be lit only when the laser is in the operate mode.

The *blocking screens* reduce the probability of laser light exiting the surgical suite when a door is open. They can be made of the same material as the window blinds and should be placed as shown in Figure 3.2.

Safety glasses must be put on before one enters the room. It is a good practice to have one or two pairs hanging near each laser warning sign.

One final thought about beam hazards: The laser should be placed in the operate mode only when actually targeted on the operative site. If the surgeon releases the handpiece, even for a moment, the laser should be placed in standby. Many devices in the operating room, including most lasers, may be controlled by a footswitch— electrosurgery units, operating lights, table positioning units, microscopes, suction, etc. It is very easy to confuse the laser-activating footswitch with other footswitches and thereby to activate it unintentionally.

PLUME HAZARDS

Health care laser systems, in particular the CO_2 laser in continuous mode, are capable of producing a smoke plume containing particulate matter from the operating site. The plume presents two hazards, plume radiation and plume content biohazard.

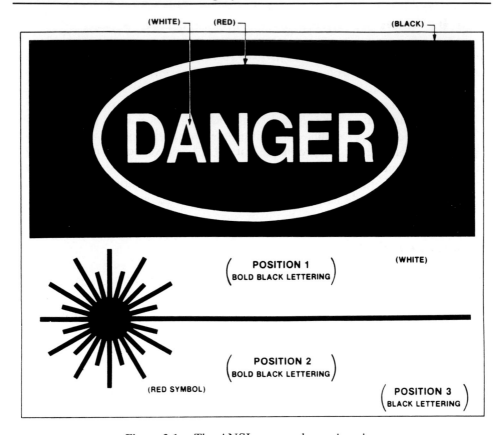

Figure 3.1. The ANSI approved *warning sign*.

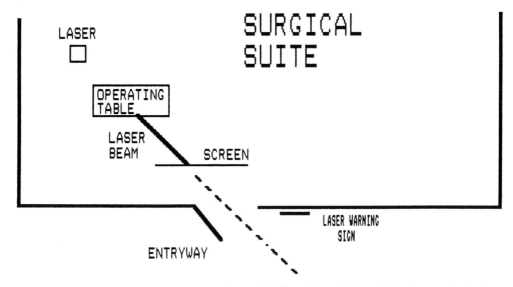

Figure 3.2. Blocking screens reduce the probability of laser light exiting the surgical suite when a door is open.

Plume Radiation

If the laser beam contacts the smoke plume, some of the energy may be shifted in wavelength through a phenomenon known as *Raman scattering.* This secondary emission is often in the visible white or blue-white portion of the light spectrum and of sufficient intensity to cause temporary blindness. Since this secondary emission is not at the same frequency as the laser beam, the laser safety glasses will not afford any protection. Adequate smoke evacuation, using a laser smoke evacuator, is the only effective solution to this problem. Normal surgical suction is inappropriate. First, due to the small bore diameter of most connecting tubing, the flow volume will be entirely inadequate; second, the fluid trap is ineffective for particulate matter suspended in air. The result can be clogged wall vacuum lines and hostile administrators.

Plume Content Biohazard

The plume biohazards to operating room personnel fall into three general categories:

1. A direct toxic effect of the particulate matter might affect the distal tracheobronchial tree and pulmonary parenchyma. The particle size of material in the laser plume has been measured to be as small as .1 mm and as large as .8 mm. The average size is approximately .3 mm.[13] Acute inflammatory changes have been demonstrated in rats after exposure to a laser plume.[14] Some authors have alluded to a possible toxic effect from laser smoke analogous to black lung disease that might take place after prolonged exposure.[14-15]

2. Viral particles may be inhaled, with possible transmission of viral diseases.[16,17] The transmission of human papilloma virus might induce benign papillomatous changes,[18,19] and has been implicated in some malignant change.[20] Other potential risks include transmission of the hepatitis virus and the AIDS virus.

3. Viable cells from malignant tumors may be inhaled by personnel in the operating room.[16,21,22]

Viral particles can be significantly smaller than .1 mm.[13] However, viral DNA and whole viruses usually attach to larger size particles and the filtration of these larger particles may effectively prevent disease transmission. There is data to suggest that whole cells are too large to be actually conveyed in the laser plume.[13,23]

Potential risks posed by the laser plume to the patient being treated are dissemination of malignant cells and a "vacuum" effect that might convey malignant cells and bacteria to the depths of a wound.[24] There is evidence to suggest that malignant cells might be scattered for a short distance during laser tissue interaction.[25] However, they do not exist in the smoke plume, itself.

Certain measures should be taken to minimize the hazards of laser plume inhalation. A standard operating room mask probably filters .3 mm particles with a 50% efficiency level. Masks are currently available that advertise the ability to filter .3 mm particles at a 95% efficiency level and products will soon be available that are said to filter .1 mm particles at a 95% efficiency level. However, one independent study conducted by a Department of Energy Filter Test Facility showed that some "laser masks" filtered at a significantly lower efficiency than 95% (i.e. 45%–60%). This is in the same efficiency range as a standard surgical mask.[26] To be maximally effective, the laser mask must be worn properly. The adhesive strip that is located along the superior edge of the mask must be tightly applied to the nose and cheeks. If there is not an adhesive strip, one can be fashioned using double-sided adhesive tape applied to the upper border of the inside of the mask. The remainder of the mask must be molded carefully around the facial contours. These measures prevent "blow-by" that diminishes particle filtration efficiency.

Laser smoke evacuators should be employed that have the flow capacity to effectively exhaust the laser plume and the filtration capacity to filter particles down to sub-micron size. The collecting tubing that is used to evacuate the laser plume should be approximately 2 cm in diameter and should be placed as close as possible to the operative site. When the CO_2 laser is used with the articulating arm and attached handpiece, a stream of nitrogen gas is often employed to blow the plume away from the operative area and therefore prevent smoke from obscuring the operator's view. However, this practice has the effect of disbursing the laser plume into the room and makes efficient and effective evacuation more difficult.

FIRE HAZARDS

Surgical lasers are associated mainly with two kinds of fire hazards: airway burns from endotracheal tube fires and sterile surgical drape fires.

A laser beam striking a conventional polyvinylchloride (PVC) endotracheal tube containing an oxygen-enriched atmosphere can instantly result in an endotracheal tube fire.[27,28] The magnitude of this particular hazard has been born out in recent years by a rapidly increasing number of incident reports. The precautionary steps are straightforward:

Don't use PVC endotracheal tubes, wrapped or otherwise, during laser surgery.

Do use either rigid metallic tubes or Rusch red rubber tubes wrapped with a reflective metallic tape such as 3M #425 aluminum tape.

Do test the wrapped tube for its ability to withstand being struck by a laser beam. Since these tapes are not FDA approved for medical applications, there may be differences between a manufacturer's production runs. One should not assume that because the same brand of tape worked the last time, it will work again.

Don't secure the tube to the patient with tape, which interferes with rapid extubation in case of fire.

Drapes that are employed during laser operations should be moistened or made of flame retardant material. It is also of significant value to have a halon-type fire extinguisher available. Halon will quickly extinguish most fires and does not pose the contaminant problem presented by chemical-type extinguishers.

In summary:

Wear appropriate approved safety glasses at all times the laser is in the operate mode.

Use ANSI recommended warning signs at all entrances to the operating suite.

Put the laser in the operate mode only when actually targeted on the operative site.

Use suction designed specifically for laser applications during any procedure in which a plume is generated.

REFERENCES

Organization, Administration, and Standard Operating Procedures

1. Absten GT, Joffe SN: *Lasers in Medicine, An Introductory Guide,* 2nd ed. London, Chapman and Hall, 1989.
2. American National Standards Institute. *Laser Safety in the Health Care Environment.* Laser Institute of America, Z136.3, 1988.
3. Lasers: facilitating their acquisition and wider use, *Med Laser Buyer's Guide.* ECRI, 1988, pp 118–123.
4. Mackety CJ: *Perioperative Laser Nursing: a Practical Guide,* 2nd ed. Cincinnati, Laser Centers of America, 1989.

Hazardous and Specific Safety Measures

5. Goldman L: *The Biomedical Laser,* New York, Springer-Verlag, 1981, p 11.
6. *American National Standard for the Safe Use of Lasers in Health Care Facilities* (ANSI Z136.3). Toledo, Laser Institute of America, 1988.
7. Breedlove B, Schwartz D: *Clinical lasers: expert strategies for practical and profitable management.* Atlanta, GA, American Health Consultants, 1984, chap 3.
8. Rockwell J: *Laser Safety in Surgery and Medicine.* Cincinnati, Rockwell Associates, 1985, pp 6–11.
9. *American National Standard for the Safe Use of Lasers in Health Care Facilities* (ANSI Z136.3, sect 4.5). Toledo, Laser Institute of America, 1988.
10. *American National Standard for the Safe Use of Lasers in Health Care Facilities* (ANSI Z136.3, sect 4.6.2.5). Toledo, Laser Institute of America, 1988.
11. Spaeth D: Selecting proper laser eyewear is worth the headache. *Clin Laser Monthly* 5:78, 1987.
12. *American National Standard for the Safe Use of Lasers* (ANSI Z136.1). Toledo, Laser Institute of America, 1986.
13. Nezhat C, Winer WK, Nezhat, et al: Smoke from laser surgery: is there a health hazard? *Lasers Surg Med* 7:376–382, 1987.
14. Baggish MS, Elbakry M: The effects of laser smoke on the lungs of rats. *Am J Obstet Gynecol* 156(5):1260–1265, 1987.
15. Jacques A: The laser plume: is it a health hazard? *Canadian Operating Room Nursing Journal* 7(3):5–9, 1989.
16. Oosterhuis JW, Vershueren RCJ, Eibergen R, et al: The viability of cells in the waste products of CO_2 laser evaporation of Cloudman mouse melanomas. *Cancer* 49:61–67, 1982.
17. Walker NPJ, Matthews J, Newsom SWB: Possible hazards from irradiation with the carbon dioxide lasers. *Lasers Surg Med* 6:84–86, 1986.

18. Garden JM, et al: Papilloma virus in the vapor of carbon dioxide laser-treated verrucae. *JAMA* 259(8):1199, 1988.

19. Garden J, Baggish M: Laser plume danger: questions remain, caution advised. *Clin Laser Monthly* (Clinical Laser Management Conference Coverage) 6(10):109–112, 1988.

20. Bradford CR: Squamous cell carcinoma of the head and neck in organ transplant recipients: one possible role of oncogenic viruses. *Laryngoscope* 100:190–194, 1990.

21. Bellina JH, Stejernholm RL, Kurpel JE: Analysis of plume emissions after papovavirus irradiation with the carbon dioxide laser. *J Reprod Med* 27(5):268–270, 1982.

22. Bellina JH, Stejernholm RL, Kurpel JE: Biochemical analysis of carbon dioxide plume emission from irradiated tumors. In Bellina JH: *Gynecologic Laser Surgery.* New York, Plenum Press, 1981.

23. Lapple CE: Particle Technology. *Stanford Res Inst J* Vol. 5 (3rd quarter) 1961, pp. 95–102.

24. Frenz M, Mathezloic F, Stoffel MHS, et al: Transport of biologically active material in laser cutting. *Lasers Surg Med* 8:562–566, 1988.

25. Hoye RC, Ketcham AS, Riggle GC: The air-borne dissemination of viable tumor by high-energy neodymium laser. *Life Sci* 6:119–125, 1967.

26. Kneedler JA, Purcell SK: Face masks as protection from laser plume. *AORN J* 50(3):520–521, 1989.

27. Sosis M: Danger: special endotracheal tubes burn, disintegrate under laser fire. *Clin Laser Monthly* 6(12):135–140, 1988.

28. Breedlove B, Schwartz D: *Clinical lasers: expert strategies for practical and profitable management.* Atlanta, GA, American Health Consultants, 1984, chap 16.

SUGGESTED READING

Organization, Administration, and Standard Operating Procedures

Dixon JA: *Surgical Application of Lasers,* ed 2. Chicago, Year Book, 1987.

Kauffman KC, Silveira LA: The successful key to a laser program: the laser coordinator, *Med Laser Buyer's Guide.* 1989, pp 82–83.

Mackety CJ: Administrative responsibilities for laser surgery. *Med Laser Buyer's Guide* 102–110, 1988.

Pfister J: Purchasing a laser, *Med Laser Buyer's Guide,* Tulsa, OK, Pen Well Publishing Company, pp 111–112, 1988.

Rockwell RJ: *Laser Safety in Surgery and Medicine,* ed 2. Cincinnati, Rockwell Associates, 1987.

4A
Anesthesia: Pediatric Applications

John D. Emhardt
Thomas A. Majcher

The ability to provide precise bloodless surgery has made the laser a valuable tool for the ablation of obstructive pediatric airway lesions. The anesthetic management of laser surgery entails a number of considerations. First, since the laser is commonly used in conjunction with the microscope, the surgical field must be virtually immobile to allow the precision required for this surgery. Second, the patients requiring laser airway surgery are usually anesthetic challenges, ranging from the near totally obstructed neonate to the anxious toddler presenting for his twentieth surgery.

The carbon dioxide (CO_2) laser, frequently used for the treatment of juvenile laryngeal papillomatosis, reduced the morbidity and mortality of the disease.[1] The most common age at diagnosis of juvenile laryngeal papillomatosis is between 2 and 5 years, and therapy usually requires several operations.[2] The anesthetic management of this disease can serve as a prototype for most laser operations, involving the pediatric airway.

The slightly different anatomy of the pediatric airway, the increased metabolic rate and anesthetic requirements of children, and the difficulty of atraumatically and safely anesthetizing a child many times all influence the anesthetic management of juvenile laryngeal papillomatosis.

ANATOMIC AND PHYSIOLOGICAL CONSIDERATIONS

The maturation process of several organ systems has direct bearing on the conduct of anesthesia for laser surgery. Some salient differences exist between the infant and the adult. Typically, the patient with juvenile laryngeal papillomatosis falls somewhere in between.

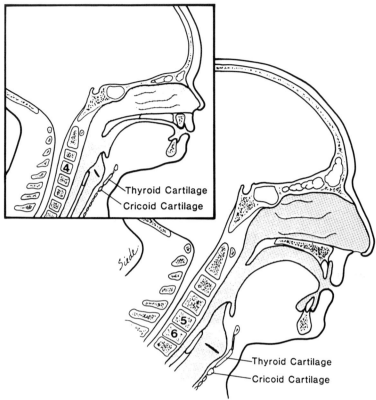

Thyroid Cartilage
Cricoid Cartilage

Thyroid Cartilage
Cricoid Cartilage

Figure 4.1. Comparative structural differences between the newborn (*inset*) and the adult upper airway. (From Diaz JH, et al: Newborn vs adult upper airway. In Goldsmith JP, et al: *Assisted Ventilation of the Neonate*. Toronto, W.B. Saunders, 1988, pg 359.)

The Airway

Five major anatomic differences exist between the infant and the adult airway (Fig. 4.1).[3]

1. The infant has a relatively large tongue, which more easily obstructs the airway and may be more difficult to maneuver with the laryngoscope.
2. The larynx is more cephalad in the infant than the adult, and this position may interfere with glottic visualization during laryngoscopy.
3. The infantile epiglottis is floppy and difficult to lift with a laryngoscope.
4. The infantile vocal cords are angled with respect to the trachea versus a perpendicular orientation in the adult; this angularity may impede the passing of an endotracheal tube beyond the anterior commissure.
5. Finally, the narrowest part of the infantile airway is the cricoid ring. Surgical trauma or a snugly fitting endotracheal tube may cause subglottic edema at the cricoid ring, which could lead to postoperative airway obstruction in a patient with a smaller trachea (Fig. 4.2).

The anterior, more cephalad position of the infantile glottis makes mask ventilation more difficult in that a finger placed under the chin or the body of the mandible

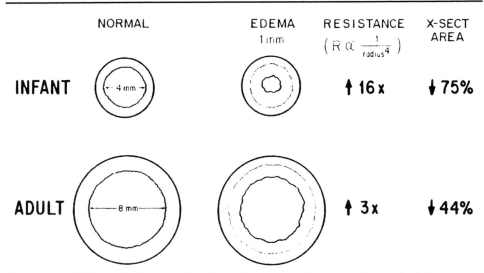

Figure 4.2. Effects of edema in the subglottis on the resistance to flow in the infant versus adult airway. Note that resistance to flow is inversely proportional to the radius of the lumen to the fourth power for laminar flow (to the fifth power for turbulent flow). The same principle holds for resistance to gas flow through tubes of decreasing diameter. (From Cote CJ, et al: The pediatric airway. In Ryan JF, et al (eds): *A Practice of Anesthesia for Infants and Children.* Orlando, FL, Grune and Stratton, 1986, pg 39.)

to provide jaw thrust may deform the soft tissues of the glottis enough to cause airway obstruction (Fig. 4.3). Also, infants less than 6 months of age are obligate nasal breathers and are prone to airway obstruction. By 10 to 12 years of age the pediatric airway becomes a small version of the adult.[3]

Respiratory Mechanics

The infant's a more compliant chest wall, less compliant lungs, and immature mechanics of diaphragmatic breathing mean that infants must work hard to breathe relative to their overall energy expenditure.[4] These features also make the infant prone to atelectasis during anesthesia. Controlled or assisted ventilation, usually with endotracheal intubation, is generally used during anesthesia to help offset the effects of infantile physiology. During airway laser surgery, however, an endotracheal tube could interfere with surgical exposure.

Laryngeal Sensitivity

The infantile larynx is richly innervated and sensitive to stimulation.[5] Infantile glottic reflexes are very active, making the infant prone to laryngospasm at light levels of anesthesia. Reflex laryngospasm can be triggered by an foreign material that comes into contact with the larynx, including secretions and laryngoscopes; thus care must be taken to avoid the combination of light anesthesia and foreign material in the airway. Older children are also prone to laryngospasm. Should partial airway obstruction occur, gentle continuous positive airway pressure should be instituted.

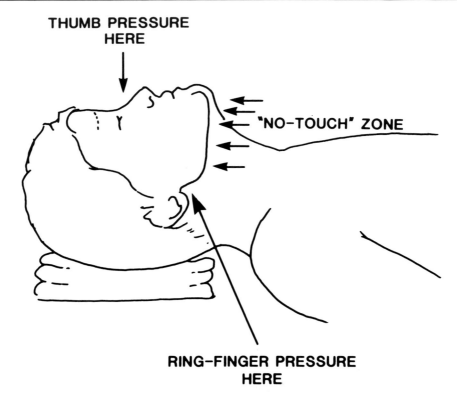

THUMB PRESSURE HERE

"NO-TOUCH" ZONE

RING-FINGER PRESSURE HERE

Figure 4.3. Correct pressure points to obtain a proper mask fit for an infant. Note that a finger placed over the chin in an attempt to provide jaw thrust might obstruct the anterior, cephalad infantile glottis. By using the angle of the mandible to lift the jaw anteriorly with the thumbs on the mask, a patent airway can be provided.

If obstruction is complete and positive airway pressure is ineffective, an intravenous injection of succinylcholine may be required to relieve laryngospasm. If intravenous access has not been secured, succinylcholine can be administered intramuscularly (4 mg/kg in children, 5 mg/kg in infants).[6]

Metabolic Rate

The metabolic rate in infants is twice that of the adult,[7] thus increasing oxygen consumption and carbon dioxide production. A more rapid rate of fluid turnover related to an increased surface: volume ratio renders the infant and toddler susceptible to dehydration with prolonged preoperative fasting. Guidelines for preoperative NPO periods vary between institutions but are usually similar to those in Table 4.1.

Since infants have a higher ratio of oxygen consumption to functional residual capacity, they have less reserve in the case of inadequate gas exchange. Short periods of airway obstruction may produce profound deoxygenation. Their higher metabolic rate may also play a role in the increased anesthetic requirements—that is, minimum alveolar concentration (MAC)—of older infants and children (Fig. 4.4).

TABLE 4.1. *Preoperative Fasting Guidelines for Pediatric Patients*

Age	Fasting Time	
	Clear Liquids	Milk/Solids
< 2 mon	2 h	4 h
2 mon–3 yr	4 h	6 h
> 3 yr	6 h	8 h

Cardiac Output

The infant myocardium is immature and contains a lower percentage of contractile tissue when compared with adults.[8] This feature makes the heart noncompliant and more dependent on the heart rate to maintain cardiac output. Atropine (10 μ/kg) or glycopyrrolate (5 μg/kg) can maintain heart rate if an anesthetic with negative chronotropic effects is used[9] or if vagal stimulation occurs. The antisialagogue effect of these drugs is also valuable for laser surgery. Although anesthesia may reduce the heart rate, bradycardia in a child should be considered due to hypoxemia until proven otherwise.

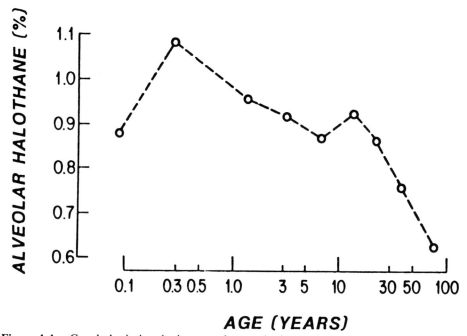

Figure 4.4. Graph depicting the increase in anesthetic requirement (MAC) with decreased age. Note that in the premature infant and neonate the anesthetic requirement is actually less than at 6 months of age. (From Cote CJ, et al: The pediatric airway. In Ryan JF, et al (eds): *A Practice of Anesthesia for Infants and Children.* Orlando, FL, Grune and Stratton, 1986, pg 82. As modified from Gregory GA, et al: *Anesthesiology* 30:488–491, 1969 and Lerman J, et al: *Anesthesiology* 59:421–424, 1983.)

Emotional Maturity

Although not a problem in neonates, emotional status plays a key role in the conduct of anesthesia for children. Separation anxiety, the fear of needles, and parental concerns frequently influence the preoperative treatment and anesthetic induction. Psychological considerations must be balanced with principles of safe airway management for the induction of anesthesia in children with juvenile laryngeal papillomatosis.

ANESTHETIC MANAGEMENT

The anesthetic goals for pediatric microlaryngeal laser surgery are listed in Table 4.2. An essential aspect of management is teamwork.The anesthesiologist and the surgeon share the airway, so communication and cooperation is critical. Information about the relative severity of the disease or the possible presence of tracheal involvement should be readily available to the anesthesiologist. Changes in oxygen saturation and depth of anesthesia should be communicated to the surgeon. This team approach is important at all phases of the surgery, from preoperative evaluation to postoperative care.

Preoperative Evaluation

The most important aspect of the preoperative evaluation of children with juvenile laryngeal papillomatosis deals with airway obstruction, which all these patients have to some degree. One indicator is a change in phonation or hoarseness. Other signs include the development of stridor and/or decreased exercise tolerance. Parents are usually attuned to the degree of obstruction that the patient is experiencing. The older child can also reliably describe the degree of airway obstruction.

Most patients with juvenile laryngeal papillomatosis are scheduled for numerous laser excisions during their lifetime. Many are on a routine operating room sched-

TABLE 4.2. *Anesthetic Goals for Pediatric Microlaryngeal Laser Surgery*

Maintain oxygenation.
Maintain adequate depth of anesthesia.
Prevent the progression of a partial airway obstruction to a complete airway obstruction.
Provide an immobile surgical field.
Prevent distal seeding of the papilloma virus.
Minimize psychological trauma.
Protect against aspiration of gastric contents.
Protect the patient and operating room personnel from the laser.
Minimize postoperative tracheal edema.
Decrease airway secretions.
Provide technique suitable for outpatient surgery.
Provide adequate lung ventilation.

ule. These children often request, or at least prefer, certain induction techniques. Some may benefit from preoperative medications such as a sedative-hypnotic, an H_2-blocker (cimetidine 7.5 mg/kg p.o. or ranitidine 1–2 mg/kg p.o.), and/or an antisialagogue (atropine 20 μg/kg p.o.).[10] Many of these operations are being done on an outpatient basis, which may have some bearing on the choice of premedicant.

Some patients with more aggressive forms of the disease require emergent treatment. On presentation, these patients are stridorous and dyspneic and may have the appearance of a patient with acute epiglottitis. In such cases, spontaneous ventilation must be preserved throughout the induction period to be sure of a patent airway. Narcotic and sedative premedication should be avoided in the severely obstructed patient because of the respiratory depressant effects of these drugs.

The age of the child and the degree of emotional maturity of both the patient and the parents are important to the conduct of anesthesia. The anesthesiologist should try to allay anxiety by personally reassuring the patient and family and briefly describing anticipated procedures in simple terms. The anesthesiologist must stress that no surprises will occur in the operating room. If an intravenous line is to be established with local anesthesia while the patient is awake, the patient should be warned. Honesty is crucial in establishing trust, and trust is especially important with patients who have juvenile laryngeal papillomatosis. They will be anesthetized many times over the course of the illness.

Monitoring

In addition to monitoring the delivery of anesthetic gases and oxygen to the patient, patients are routinely monitored by electrocardiography, blood pressure cuff, precordial stethoscope, and temperature probe. Monitors should be positioned and volumes set so that they can be seen and heard by the entire surgical team.

Over the last five years pulse oximetry has developed into the most important operating room monitor. Pulse oximetry provides a noninvasive, simple, continuous measure of a patient's oxygenation and is essential for anesthetizing the child for microlaryngeal laser surgery. Pulse oximetry is based on the difference in light absorption between reduced hemoglobin and oxyhemoglobin and requires light of two wavelengths to pass through a vascular bed to photodiode. Commonly the monitor is placed over a finger. Operating room lights can interfere with the probe sensitivity, requiring that the probe be shielded. Results can be altered by intravascular dyes, hyperbilirubinemia, and certain hemoglobin abnormalities such as the presence of carboxyhemoglobin, methemoglobin, or sulfhemoglobin.

Monitoring of end-tidal carbon dioxide tension (capnography) is also becoming more common.[11] This can be done by infrared analysis, mass spectrometry, or Ramen spectroscopy. Capnography is especially valuable in detecting inadequate ventilation or airway obstruction. The shape of the capnogram can provide much information about the ventilatory state of the patient (Fig. 4.5). The use of this monitor is limited for microlaryngeal laser surgery, since an accurate reading requires an undiluted alveolar gas sample. This requires either a snug mask fit or an endotracheal tube, both of which offer a significant impediment to surgery.

Transcutaneous oxygen (tcO_2) tensions are also used in some cases. This monitor has a slower response than the pulse oximeter,[12] and the transcutaneous measure-

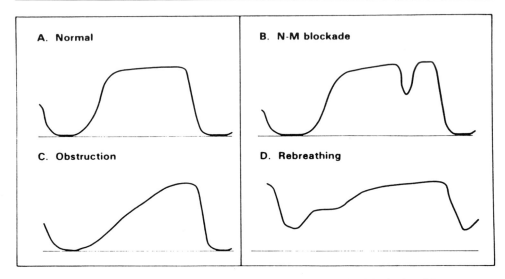

A. Normal

B. N-M blockade

C. Obstruction

D. Rebreathing

Figure 4.5. (*A*) A normal capnogram. (*B*) Partial neuromuscular blockade with spontaneous diaphragmatic movement results in a cleft due to the inrush of carbon dioxide free gas as the diaphragm contracts. (*C*) Prolonged exhalation due to endotracheal tube kink or small airway obstruction. (*D*) Rebreathing of carbon dioxide due to faulty ventilating valves or inadequate fresh gas flow. Note that the capnogram does not return to baseline. (Reprinted with permission: Swedlow DB: Mass spectrometers and respiratory gas monitoring. In Barash PG (ed): *American Society of Anesthesiologists Annual Refresher Courses*, Philadelphia, JB Lippincott, 1985.)

ment of oxygen depends on variables other than oxygen tension, such as skin perfusion.[13] tcO_2 is more accurate in infants than in adults, owing to differences between adult and infant skin.[14] High levels of oxygen tension that are recognized as 100% saturated by the pulse oximeter can be measured by tcO_2. For example, suppose a patient ventilated with 100% oxygen had an arterial oxygen tension of 500 torr. The transcutaneous monitor would detect a drop to 250 torr, whereas a pulse oximeter would not detect a problem because hemoglobin is 100% saturated at both 500 and 250 torr.

Normally, tcO_2 reads about 20% less than paO_2,[14] but several studies have suggested spuriously high readings of this monitor when halothane is used.[15-17] Others have demonstrated that halothane interference occurs in vitro and not in vivo.[18] Clinically, transcutaneous oximetry can be taken as a direct reflection of paO_2, even in the presence of halothane.

Monitors that measure both tcO_2 and transcutaneous carbon dioxide ($tcCO_2$) are available as well. Transcutaneous CO_2 is always somewhat greater than $pcCO_2$,[19] and the response time is slower than that of tcO_2[20] This method of monitoring carbon dioxide tension is especially valuable during ventilation techniques that do not employ an endotracheal tube and thereby preclude the use of end-tidal carbon dioxide assessment.

A transcutaneous nerve stimulator is also an important monitor, especially if the intraoperative ventilation technique relies heavily on muscle relaxants. The nerve stimulator can detect when neuromuscular blockade is adequate for surgery and when recovery of neuromuscular transmission is complete.

Induction of Anesthesia

In Moderate to Severe Airway Compromise

Children presenting for laser surgery of the airway with signs of marked upper airway obstruction are managed similarly to those with acute epiglottitis. It is critical to maintain spontaneous ventilation until the airway is secured so that a partial airway obstruction does not become complete. Administration of muscle relaxants to facilitate intubation, or overriding the child's own respiratory drive, may cause changes in upper airway ventilatory dynamics that could lead to obstruction. Visualization of air bubbles during laryngoscopy may be a valuable marker of the location of the glottic opening in the patient with very abnormal airway anatomy.

Spontaneous ventilation can be maintained by using a halothane inhalation technique, which is a preferred method of induction even if intravenous access is present. If a child strongly resists mask induction, small doses of intravenous barbiturates may be administered incrementally until the child accepts the inhalation induction. These must be titrated slowly to avoid apnea or airway obstruction. Ketamine may be an alternative, but it can increase secretions and may make the larynx more sensitive to stimulation.[21] Atropine or glycopyrrolate are used to offset the cardiac depressant effects of halothane[9] and to act as an antisialogogue.

For the partially obstructed patient with juvenile laryngeal papillomatosis, laryngospasm on induction could prove disastrous. Halothane is a volatile anesthetic that is least irritating to the airways when compared to isoflurane or enflurane and will cause less coughing or laryngospasm than the other drugs.[22] In our experience the incremental addition of halothane with 30% oxygen in nitrous oxide provides a rapid, smoother induction with a lower risk of laryngospasm than if high initial doses of halothane are used.

After the incremental achievement of a high level of inspired halothane ($\sim$3 to 4%) one must wait an appropriate time to have adequately anesthetized the patient for laryngoscopy. The delayed rise of anesthetic partial pressure in the central nervous system and the exquisite sensitivity of the larynx sometimes necessitate a wait of 10 minutes or longer before halothane is expired at the level necessary for good intubating conditions (1.8 to 2.25%).[23] Before insertion of the laryngoscope lidocaine is administered laryngotracheally (no more than 4.0 mg/kg)[24] or intravenously[25] (1.5 to 2.0 mg/kg) to prevent coughing. The glottis will be ready for manipulation (intubation or suspension laryngoscopy) about 60 seconds later. Only after the airway is established should a muscle relaxant be given.

In Minimal Airway Compromise

Different considerations exist in children presenting for airway laser surgery without significant airway obstruction. Most commonly, this population consists of patients with papillomatosis who regularly present for laryngoscopy, bronchoscopy, and laser surgery. Some of these patients require continued therapy throughout their childhood, forming close emotional ties with members of the surgical team and very strong preferences about the type of induction technique used. Preferably, the anesthesiologists most familiar to the patient participate in the anesthetic, using an induction method of the child's choosing. The presence of a familiar face, and the feeling of autonomy gained by having some choice about the induction technique, will go far in reducing the psychological stress of repeated surgeries. Many induction techniques are available, depending on the age and disposition of the child on the day of surgery.

Once induction has been accomplished, the anesthesiologist must determine the need for and the safety of succinylcholine if a muscle relaxant is to be used. Because succinylcholine is a potent triggering agent for malignant hyperthermia, some anesthesiologists have stopped using this drug except for very strong indications, that is, bowel obstruction or laryngospasm. Others have used this drug for years and will continue to do so because they consider it safe and valuable. In a child with papillomatosis, a muscle relaxant may be indicated to facilitate endotracheal intubation. Succinylcholine may be the muscle relaxant of choice since it is so short-acting. If airway obstruction occurred with relaxation, spontaneous ventilation would return much faster with this short-acting agent.

Management of Ventilation

The initial anesthetic management of a patient with juvenile laryngeal papillomatosis centers on the difficulties of safely anesthetizing the child with a compromised airway. After anesthesia has been induced and the airway secured, the focus is on the problems and dangers associated with microscopic laryngeal surgery and the laser. These latter considerations underlie the development of the many ventilation techniques that have been used for this surgery. Five types of ventilation have been described for the management of anesthesia, all but one of which have been used in children. Each technique has associated advantages and disadvantages, which are summarized in Table 4.3.

Positive Pressure Ventilation via an Endotracheal Tube

Delivery of anesthetic gases and oxygen via a wrapped or armored endotracheal tube is probably the most common method of ventilation for laryngeal laser surgery in adults. An extensive review of endotracheal tube protection is provided later in this chapter. This protection also applies to tracheostomy tubes that may be present in patients with juvenile laryngeal papillomatosis. Measures that decrease the risk

TABLE 4.3.   *Disadvantages of Ventilation Techniques Currently Used for Pediatric Microlaryngeal Laser Surgery*

Disadvantage	Positive Pressure Ventilation	Spontaneous Ventilation	Jet Injector Ventilation	High-Frequency Ventilation	Apneic Ventilation
Specialized equipment			X	X	
Precludes capnography		X	X	X	
Risk of fire	X				
Risk of pneumothorax			X		
Risk of aspiration		X	X	X	X
Anatomy obscured	X				
Vocal cord motion		X			
Operating room pollution		X			

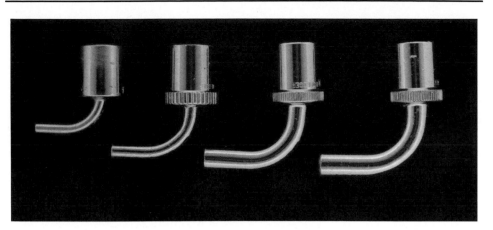

Figure 4.6. Metal elbow connectors that are available in a number of sizes can be used in place of a tracheostomy tube for airway laser surgery.

of endotracheal tube fire should also include minimizing gases that support combustion. For this reason one must reduce the concentration of oxygen as much as is safely possible by diluting the gas with air, usually to 30%. Nitrous oxide will support combustion and should not be used to reduce the oxygen concentration.[26] Anesthetic gases have been safely diluted with helium, even in unwrapped polyvinyl chloride endotracheal tubes.[27] Endotracheal tube ignition is impeded by the high thermal diffusivity of helium, which decreases heat of materials in contact with the laser.[28] Another advantage of helium dilution in pediatric patients may be that the lower density of helium allows more gas to flow through small tubes.

In the child with a tracheostomy, the plastic tracheostomy tube should be removed from the airway before airway laser surgery and replaced by a commercially available metal tracheostomy tube that has a standard-sized anesthesia connector. These metal tubes come in a variety of sizes to accommodate all but the smallest of pediatric airways. A less expensive alternative is to insert an appropriately sized metal curved endotracheal adapter (Fig. 4.6) into the stoma to which the breathing circuit is attached (personal communication, Marvin Jewell, M.D.).

Using an endotracheal tube for positive pressure ventilation facilitates conventional ventilation techniques and capnography as well as administration of anesthetics and muscle relaxants. In adults a small tube that the surgeon can manipulate may be placed. Ventilation through an endotracheal tube during microlaryngeal laser surgery is not ideal in children, however. Space in the pediatric airway is already restricted, and ventilation through very small (2.5- or 3.0-mm) tubes is difficult because of their resistance to high gas flows. Laryngeal pathology, especially of the posterior commissure, may be obscured by the endotracheal tube (Fig. 4.7). Furthermore, most of the specialized endotracheal tubes are not available in very small sizes.

One must be careful with the foil tape commonly used to shield endotracheal tubes because ridges in the tape can damage the glottis, and unseen holes may render the tube vulnerable to ignition. The tube should be wrapped spirally from the distal end proximally, since the laser is fired at a tangent to the tube. Tubes taped in this fashion will be better shielded than if taped from the proximal end

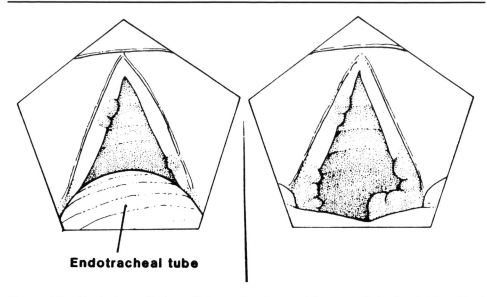

Endotracheal tube

Figure 4.7. Posterior pathology that can be obscured by an endotracheal tube. (From Weisberger EC, et al: Apneic anesthesia for improved endoscopic removal of laryngeal papillomata. *Laryngoscope* 98:693–697, 1988.)

distally. Pieces of metallic tape can break off and lodge in the airway as a foreign body. Finally, a test using the laser to check flammability should be done on all tapes to be used for this purpose, since manufacturing specifications may change without notice.

Spontaneous Ventilation

A number of techniques using spontaneous ventilation and local anesthesia have been described.[24,29-31] Anesthesia is induced either via intravenous thiopental or face mask and a combination of oxygen, nitrous oxide, and halothane, is used for maintenance. These techniques rely heavily on adequate topical anesthesia with lidocaine. To avoid toxic serum levels of lidocaine following topical application in the larynx, the dose should be limited to no more than 4 mg/kg.[24] Lidocaine is applied from the pharynx to the carina. Muscle relaxants are not used, and premedication is used sparingly to enusre spontaneous ventilation. Intravenous administration of procaine may be used to supplement anesthesia, suppress the cough reflex, and decrease laryngeal sensitivity.[32] Oxygen and anesthetic gases are insufflated during the procedure, either via a catheter in the pharnyx,[31] via a port of the operating laryngoscope, or by nasopharyngeal insufflation.[29] Another technique is via an Andrews anterior commissure retractor.[30]

Adding methoxyflurane to the gas mixture via a second vaporizer will create an even smoother technique owing to its long duration of action, high potency, and ability to sustain spontaneous ventilation. Methoxyflurane is a potent nonflammable agent that provides excellent analgesia with minimal ventilatory depression.[24] This agent is no longer in common use, owing to its potential for nephrotoxicity, but it does provide a smooth intraoperative anesthetic. The potency of methoxyflurane (MAC = 0.17%) allows less agent to be used. A major drawback of this technique is that the newer anesthetic machines are not able to accommodate the dual vaporizer setup required.

An advantage of spontaneous ventilation is that it requires neither endotracheal intubation nor positive pressure ventilation, which could cause distal seeding of the papilloma virus. The patient's ventilatory pattern can also provide a clue to the depth of anesthesia. The absence of an endotracheal tube obviates any problems associated with the flow of gases through a narrow tube or the flammability of the endotracheal tube. Furthermore, the surgeon is able to work in an uncluttered airway.

Disadvantages of spontaneous ventilation include the potential for hypoventilation or apnea under deep anesthesia. This risk is especially important in the small infant with altered ventilatory mechanics. Secondary cardiac dysrhythmias might occur with too deep or too light a level of halothane anesthesia especially when associated with hypercarbia. The pollution of the operating room with anesthetic gases can also be problematic, as scavenging is very difficult. Spontaneous ventilation might also produce motion in the surgical field. Finally, since muscle relaxants must be avoided, the depth of anesthesia is especially critical. Light anesthesia could lead to coughing and laryngospasm, although both of these should be minimized by tracheal topicalization.

Jet Injector Ventilation

Terms used to describe jet ventilation techniques are confusing. *Venturi jet injector* and *Sanders jet ventilation* both refer to the technique of manually jetting intermittent bursts of gases into the airway. This can be done via a special laryngoscope or bronchoscope. Metal tubes specially designed for jet injector ventilation below the level of the vocal cords[33,34] have been developed, but their use in children is limited by the small size of the pediatric airway. *High frequency jet ventilation,* in contrast, refers to mechanical ventilation of the lungs at rates exceeding 60 breaths per minute. High frequency ventilation may be administered through a bronchoscope or an endotracheal tube, or directly into the trachea by means of a catheter or laryngoscope port.

Supraglottic insufflation of a high pressure source of oxygen aimed at the trachea may be used to ventilate patients undergoing laser surgery of the airway. High pressure oxygen is controlled by an adjustable regulator connected to an air gun like those commercially used for spray painting (Fig. 4.8). The anesthesiologist triggers the air gun to provide intermittent bursts of oxygen.[35-37] Some anesthesia departments have assembled their own jet injector systems with equipment purchased from a local hardware store. Of critical importance to avoid barotrauma is the reducing valve between the high pressure wall oxygen source and the air gun. Furthermore, tubes leading from the air gun to the larynx might best be connected without Luer lock adapters to ensure a popoff response in the event of reducing-valve failure. A typical system can be assembled for $100 to $200 (personal communication, Geoffrey Lane, M.D.). Commercially available systems designed for jet injection are available at a slightly higher cost.

The laryngoscope, blade, larynx, and trachea must be aligned in a straight line and the anterior part of the larynx must be clear of obstructing lesions before using jet injector ventilation.[38] Adequacy of ventilation is gauged by observing chest

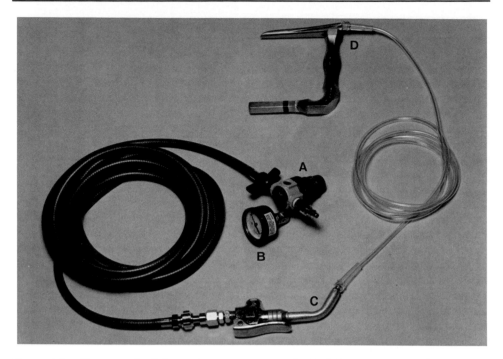

Figure 4.8. Photograph of the equipment necessary for jet injector ventilation. (*A*) Reducing valve that plugs to the wall source of oxygen. (*B*) Manometer dial. (*C*) Jet injector device. (*D*) Suspension laryngoscope with the injector tubing plugged into one of the side channels.

expansion and by noninvasive monitoring such as pulse oximetry and transcutaneous cooximetry. Indirect measurements of tidal volume and hyperinflation during jet injector ventilation have been made with "pneumobelts," straps that are placed around the thorax and abdomen whose excursion is calibrated to a known tidal volume.[39]

The jet injector has been evaluated in children during bronchoscopy.[40] The size of the jet, the length and angle of the jet, and the size of the bronchoscope are important. Tidal volume can be varied by adjusting the driving pressure of the injector (usually between 30 and 50 psi). Even the smallest bronchoscope delivers 6 to 9 ml/kg tidal volumes if the higher driving pressures are used. Foot pedal triggering devices are available to free the hands of the anesthesiologist.[41]

Advantages of jet injector ventilation include an uncluttered airway, the absence of combustible material in the airway, and a virtually motionless field. Disadvantages include the inability to deliver 100% oxygen, since air is entrained via the venturi principle. Barotrauma, specifically pneumomediastinum and pneumothorax, has been reported. This may pose a higher risk in children with noncompliant lungs, such as prematurely born infants with bronchopulmonary dysplasia. Jet injector ventilation may be unsafe for neonates and has been condemned by some authors. Gastric inflation, mucosal dehydration, and distal tracheal or bronchial seeding by the papilloma virus are all considerations. One major drawback is the relative difficulty in administering volatile anesthesia of a precise amount with this technique. Also, the addition of a vaporizer to the system is cumbersome. For this reason

TABLE 4.4. *Comparison of Different Modes of High-Frequency Ventilation*

	HFPPV	HFJV	HFOV True Oscillators	HFOV Flow Interrupters
Delivery system	Conventional infant ventilator	High-pressure, source-regulator injector	Pistons, diaphragms	Rotating ball valves
Frequency range	60–150 bpm Tidal volume ↓ as frequency ↑	100–900 bpm ≥ Anatomic dead space	400–2400 bpm < Anatomic dead space	400–2400 bpm < Anatomic dead space

From Mammel MC, Boros SJ: High frequency ventilation. In Goldsmith JP, Karotkin EH (eds): *Assisted Ventilation of the Neonate*. Philadelphia, Saunders, 1988, p 191, with permission.

HFPPV = high-frequency positive pressure ventilation; HFJV = high-frequency jet ventilation; HFOV = high-frequency oscillatory ventilation.

intravenous anesthesia is generally used, usually consisting of a barbiturate/benzodiazepine and a narcotic. The newer sedative-hypnotic propofol combined with alfentanil has also been used, but only in adults.[42] Neuromuscular blockade is usually required and can be accomplished with an intermediate-acting agent such as atracurium or vecuronium. The new short-acting nondepolarizing muscle relaxant mivicurium may prove to be useful for this procedure.

High-Frequency Ventilation

High-frequency ventilation has been reported,[43] but not specifically in children. The three main types of high-frequency ventilators are classified according to ventilating pattern as providing high-frequency jet ventilation (HFJV), high-frequency positive pressure ventilation (HFPPV), and high-frequency oscillatory ventilation (HFOV) (Table 4.4).

High-frequency jet ventilation and high-frequency positive pressure ventilation have been accomplished via nasopharyngeal catheter or by insufflation through a needle attached to a straight-blade laryngoscope. A typical rate is between 60 and 150 breaths per minute with an inspiratory time of 25 to 33% of the ventilatory cycle. Unobstructed exhalation is important for this procedure to prevent air trapping.

Advantages of these techniques include minimal equipment in the surgical field, relative immobility of the vocal cords, and the fact that these types of ventilation can be superimposed on spontaneous breathing if muscle relaxants are not used. Drawbacks are air entrainment, the inability to deliver 100% O_2, marginal ventilatory reserve capacity,[43] and distal propulsion of surgical debris. Ventilation may also be affected during instrumentation of the larynx. As during jet ventilation, an intravenous anesthetic is usually used for this technique.

Apneic Anesthesia

The apneic technique of anesthesia[44,45] is used following a standard induction as described previously. After induction the trachea is intubated and positive pressure ventilation begun. The endotracheal tube is changed to a smaller one if no leak is present at less than 20 cm H_2O airway pressure. This is to help reduce the risk of postoperative tracheal edema, which might occur with a too large endotracheal tube.

The patient is positioned and the suspension laryngoscope is placed. Neuromuscular blockade is accomplished with an intermediate-acting relaxant such as vecuronium or atracurium. Intermittent doses of succinylcholine or a continuous succinylcholine infusion could also be used, but the length of the procedure and the absence of cardiovascular side effects make the intermediate-acting agents ideal. Adequacy of blockade is confirmed with a transcutaneous nerve stimulator, usually placed over the ulnar nerve.

Oxygenation is monitored with pulse oximetry and by transcutaneous oxygen monitoring. Pulse oximetry is critical for the safe employment of the apneic technique. When the laser has been properly positioned the patient is ventilated with 100% O_2 until the highest possible reading of the oximeter is attained. The endotracheal tube is removed and the surgery begun. At the first sign of arterial oxygen desaturation, the surgeon replaces the endotracheal tube through the suspended laryngoscope. End-tidal CO_2 is measured after reinsertion of the endotracheal tube. Positive pressure ventilation is resumed until the end-tidal CO_2 tension is at or around 35 torr and the oximeter again reads the highest attainable number. The cycle is then repeated. Most operations require the use of only one or two cycles.

A cycle of 2 or 3 minutes may be employed if the child is older than 2 years.[46] If the child is as young as 3 months, the cycle time may be 90 seconds.[45] The crucial factor is to resume ventilation at the *first sign* of arterial desaturation, even if the reading drops only from 99 or 100% to 97 to 98%. The arterial saturation will be lower by the time ventilation can be resumed.

The rate of change in arterial carbon dioxide and oxygen tensions has recently been studied.[46] In adults, carbon dioxide typically increases by 6 to 8 mmHg in the first minute and by 3 mmHg/min thereafter. Children have a higher metabolic rate. Predictably, carbon dioxide production will increase by 10 to 12 mmHg in the first minute, but the rise in arterial carbon dioxide thereafter is approximately 3 mmHg/min (Fig. 4.9). Arterial oxygen tension also drops faster in the first minute of apnea than in the succeeding minutes.

The apneic technique affords the advantage of a very still operating field without vocal cord motion or a cluttered airway, thus providing ideal operating conditions. The absence of an endotracheal tube precludes an endotracheal tube fire. The distal seeding of papilloma virus during the actual operation is minimal, although the times of reintubation and positive pressure ventilation may present such a risk. Barotrauma, pneumothorax, and pneumomediastinum are not a consideration with this technique.

The apneic method also has disadvantages. Arterial blood gas tensions change during surgery, necessitating intermittent reinsertion of the endotracheal tube with consequent interruption of the surgery. The placement of a tube may traumatize the trachea, although this risk can be minimized by using a small endotracheal tube placed carefully just through the glottis on each occasion.

Contraindications to this technique are reduced relative oxygen availability related to anemia or cyanotic heart disease or an increase in oxygen consumption related to hyperthermia or hyperthyroidism.

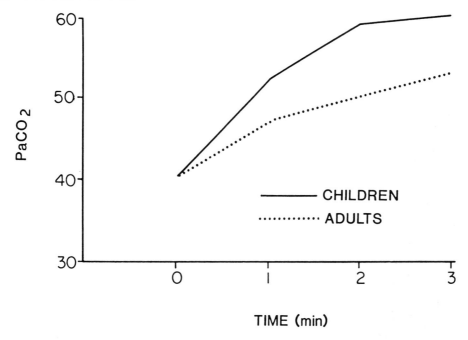

Figure 4.9.   Rise in arterial carbon dioxide during apnea in children vs adults. (Data from Eger EI, Severinghaus JW: The rate of rise of $paCO_2$ in the apneic anesthetized patient. *Anesthesiology* 22:419–425, 1961; and Emhardt JD, Weisberger EC, Dierdorf, et al: The rise of arterial carbon dioxide during apnea in children. *Anesthesiology* 69:A779, 1988. With permission.)

EMERGENCE FROM ANESTHESIA AND POSTOPERATIVE CONSIDERATIONS

The patient will emerge from anesthesia with an airway that is less obstructed than at induction. Even so, children who are intubated should be fairly awake before extubation to avert laryngospasm. An alternative is to administer 2% lidocaine (2 mg/kg) intravenously before extubation. If muscle relaxants were used, the patient should show sustained tetanus at 50 to 100 Hz stimulation or relaxation should be reversed with an anticholinesterase–anticholinergic.

Humified oxygen should be administered during recovery from anesthesia. One attractive feature of the laser is the relative absence of postoperative edema. Nevertheless, some patients experience a fair amount of subglottic edema, especially those with tracheal pathology. Dexamethasone (0.25 to 0.5 mg/kg) can reduce this edema; it is best given at the start of the procedure because of its delayed effect. Nebulized racemic epinephrine (0.5 ml in 2.5 ml normal saline) might also be required for postoperative tracheal edema. Patients who require this treatment should be observed postoperatively for at least 3 hours to ensure that obstructive symptoms do not occur.

Most microlaryngeal laser procedures can be done on an outpatient basis. Depending on the degree of surgical trauma, however, some patients should be admitted to the hospital for observation. This is a decision that must be made individually.

THE NEONATAL AIRWAY

Neonates sometimes require laser surgery, most commonly for laryngeal web, congenital laryngeal cyst, or hemangioma.[47] Since the presenting signs of these lesions are often stridor or hoarseness, it is important first to rule out abnormalities of the vocal cords by direct observation of anatomy and vocal cord movement. Awake laryngoscopy, often performed with a flexible fiberoptic scope, is well tolerated and is the best method for evaluating vocal cord function. If direct laryngoscopy is performed on an awake patient, reflex bradycardia in response to laryngeal stimulation can be averted by pretreatment with atropine, and preoxygenation may allow a longer laryngoscopy before oxyhemoglobin desaturation ensues.

Preservation of spontaneous ventilation is ideal for these patients, but immature anatomy and physiology make the newborn prone to atelectasis and rapid desaturation with airway obstruction during spontaneous ventilation. The anesthetic technique must therefore be flexible to manage these children safely.

After evaluation of vocal cord function, general anesthesia is induced with oxygen, halothane, and nitrous oxide. The vocal cords are sprayed with lidocaine, and a direct laryngoscope is inserted. Laser excision can begin while the infant spontaneously breathes halothane and oxygen entrained orally through a curved metal adapter or a converted suction catheter placed through the nares into the nasopharynx.

Since the newborn heart is especially sensitive to the myocardial depressant effects of halothane, one must protect against anesthetic overdose by carefully monitoring heart rate and blood pressure. Hypotension may become a problem with the use of the spontaneous ventilation technique, especially if the infant has a congenital heart anomaly. In this case, an adequate depth of volatile anesthesia might not be attainable, and one might consider a muscle relaxant combined with lower levels of volatile agent or an appropriate intravenous anesthetic. Apneic or jet ventilation techniques must then be substituted for spontaneous ventilation. However, jet ventilation is considered by some to be contraindicated in neonates.[24]

Use of a wrapped endotracheal tube is often not possible, because even the smallest tube would obscure the view of the airway. Of course, lesions associated with significant airway obstruction may require a concomitant tracheotomy.

Infants often require short periods of postoperative ventilation until muscle relaxants have been reversed and intravenous agents have been metabolized.

To summarize, anesthetic management of the pediatric airway can be safely accomplished in myriad ways. The techniques used will depend upon the skills and preferences of the individual surgeon and anesthesiologist as well as the availability of materials and equipment in the operating suite. Each patient has unique considerations based on age, maturity, and extent of disease process, and the anesthetic management must be tailored for each. Above all, communication between the anesthesia and surgical teams is essential, and patient safety must be the primary consideration.

4B
Anesthesia: Adult Applications

Mitchel B. Sosis

Potential challenges to the maintenance of patient safety during laser surgery include the following:

1. Combustible materials are often used in the manufacture of endotracheal tubes.
2. The laser, a device with high energy density, may be operated in close proximity to the endotracheal tube.
3. The anesthetic gases employed may increase the combustibility of the endotracheal tube.

Applying a laser to a combustible endotracheal tube such as those constructed of rubber or polyvinyl chloride converts the tube into a veritable blowtorch with the potential for severe airway burns to the patient (Fig. 4.10). The occurrence of such tube fires and their associated morbidity and mortality mandates continuing efforts to find safer techniques and equipment for these procedures. That is the thrust of this chapter, which discusses modifications in usual anesthesia practice and equipment to improve patient safety during laser surgery. The focus is on adult otolaryngologic surgery in proximity to the airway. Properly selected equipment and an informed anesthesiologist, surgeon, and operating room team minimize the risks to patients undergoing laser surgery.

ANESTHETIC MANAGEMENT OF CO_2 LASER

Preoperative Evaluation

All patients should have a thorough medical evaluation before undergoing surgery. Patients who present for laser surgery may have tumors or masses with the potential to compromise the patency of their airways. These patients also often have respira-

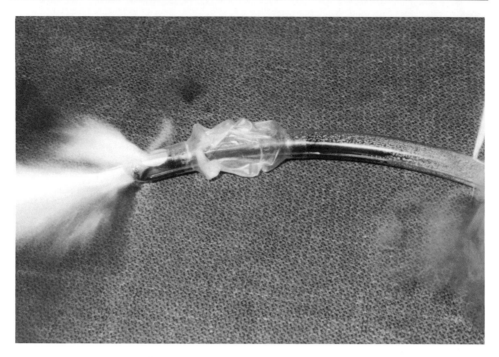

Figure 4.10. Blowtorch fire: A polyvinyl chloride endotracheal tube has been ignited by a CO_2 laser. The site of the laser's impingement is seen at left.

tory compromise of varying degree. Of special concern is the possibility of airway obstruction upon the induction of anesthesia. Airway manipulation such as laryngoscopy may lead to edema or bleeding with consequent airway compromise—even when no history of obstruction has been noted. The anesthetist should carefully examine the patient for abnormalities or potential difficulties in endotracheal intubation. The range of motion of the neck should be observed. Hospital records should be checked to determine whether problems arose during earlier anesthesias.

In patients with significant respiratory impairment, pulmonary function should be measured preoperatively, and arterial blood gas tensions should also be checked. The patient's chart and x-rays should be carefully examined, with particular emphasis on any information regarding airway abnormalities. The surgeon should be consulted about the plans for surgery and the possibility of airway obstruction.

It is important to optimize the patient's physical status before surgery. For example, those receiving aminophylline should have their serum levels checked and the dosages adjusted accordingly. Head and neck surgical procedures may cause hypertension and tachycardia, which are a potent stress to the myocardium.

Adult patients should be kept NPO for 8 hours prior to surgery.

Premedication

If there is a significant risk of airway obstruction, all premedicants except anticholinergics are omitted. Patients who are not at risk for airway obstruction may be premedicated normally without any risk. The anesthesiologist should always visit patients before their operations to explain the procedure and allay fears. Anticholinergic drying agents such as atropine are useful for procedures involving airway manipulation.

Induction of Anesthesia

Patients who are not at risk for airway obstruction may undergo a standard anesthetic induction following preoxygenation with thiopental and succinylcholine if no other contraindication exists. Many patients are at risk for an exaggerated sympathetic response to airway manipulation, and they should receive pharmacologic therapy accordingly.

If the possibility of airway obstruction exists, special precautions should be undertaken when inducing anesthesia. Rapid induction of anesthesia using intravenous agents can be dangerous in a patient with an obstructed airway. It may be safer to allow the patient to spontaneously breathe the anesthetic gas mixture through a mask and by this means achieve the proper depth of anesthesia for intubation.

A variety of airway equipment such as laryngoscope blades, airways, endotracheal tubes, and stylets should be assembled. The techniques of "awake intubation," whereby spontaneous respirations are preserved, and topical anesthesia, possibly along with a superior laryngeal nerve block, should be considered. Transtracheal instillation of local anesthetics should also be considered. A tracheostomy tray should be available. The surgeon should be present during the induction of anesthesia in this group of patients.

Monitoring

In all patients, a noninvasive blood pressure apparatus, electrocardiograph, oxygen analyzer, pulse oximeter, and precordial or esophageal stethoscope should be used during anesthesia. End-tidal CO_2 monitoring is useful for assessing the adequacy of ventilation. An arterial line is helpful in those patients in whom it is desired to obtain arterial blood gas tensions or those in whom a labile blood pressure is expected.

OPERATING ROOM PRECAUTIONS

The eyes of the patient and all operating room personnel should be protected during laser surgery. Paper operating room drapes are hazardous for laser surgery, since once ignited, they are difficult to extinguish and water simply rolls off them.[48] Disposable drapes are treated with fire-retardant chemicals; however, Ott[49] notes that once ignited, they burn quickly. Instead, draping with wet towels that are periodically moistened is recommended.

SPECIAL ANESTHETIC CONSIDERATIONS FOR LASER SURGERY

The standard techniques of anesthesia require no modification for laser procedures if the site of surgery is distant from the airway, such as during gynecologic surgery. However, as mentioned earlier, when the surgical field is near the airway, the possibility of an endotracheal tube fire or explosion necessitates the use of special preventive techniques. One survey of the complications of CO_2 laryngeal surgery found endotracheal fire or explosion to be the most common major complication.[50] Healey and colleagues[51] also found that fires were the most common complication occurring during these cases.

General anesthesia for laser surgery may be conducted with or without an endotracheal tube by techniques such as spontaneous ventilation, venturi jet ventilation, or apneic anesthesia. (See the section on Venturi Jet Ventilation in this chapter.) The selection of an appropriate endotracheal tube for laser surgery is an important one. Commercially available special laser endotracheal tubes are discussed in the section on Special Endotracheal Tubes for Laser Surgery in this chapter. Whether to use a polyvinyl chloride or rubber endotracheal tube for laser surgery is controversial.

Tube Material

Patel and Hicks[5] noted that Rusch red rubber endotracheal tubes could be ignited by a CO_2 laser in 16.5 sec at a power setting of 15 W. A Portex polyvinyl chloride tube was ignited in only 3.7 seconds. They conclude that "red rubber Rusch tubes should be used in preference to PVC [polyvinyl chloride] Portex tubes."[52] In another study of tube combustibility, using a propane torch rather than a laser, Wolf and Simpson[53] observed that polyvinyl chloride endotracheal tubes could be made to burn only when the oxygen concentration was above 26.3%, whereas red rubber tubes would burn above 17.6% oxygen. They summarize their results with the following statement: "When an ignition source is in close proximity to the ETT [endotracheal tube], PVC [polyvinyl chloride] tubes may be preferable to . . . RR [red rubber] tubes. . ."[53] In still another CO_2 laser study using power levels of 5 to 20 W and a duration of up to 1 sec, Myers[54] found that the polyvinyl chloride tubes could be made to burn with 5 W of power and a duration of 0.2 sec in 100% oxygen, but the red rubber endotracheal tubes could not be made to burn under these conditions and were thus preferred.

Esch and Dyer[55] point out that hydrochloric acid, a severe respiratory irritant, is produced by the combustion of polyvinyl chloride. This chemical has been found important in smoke inhalation injuries in fire fighters. Although red rubber tubes produce thick black smoke when burning, they do not appear to release such irritating products of combustion. They are stiffened with nonflammable compounds that reduce their flammability.[56]

Ossoff and colleagues[57] studied injury to the lungs of dogs when polyvinyl chloride, red rubber, or silicone endotracheal tubes were ignited by a CO_2 laser. Black material was noted in the lungs of the dog subjected to a polyvinyl chloride endotracheal tube fire. Midtracheal histologic sections showed acute inflammatory changes along with polymorphonuclear cell infiltration and ulceration. In the dog subjected to the red rubber endotracheal tube fire, only small amounts of carbonaceous material were noted in the trachea. Tissue sections showed a small degree of ulceration and inflammation. These changes were less extensive than those noted with the polyvinyl chloride tube fire. White ash was seen in the entire tracheobronchial tree after the combustion of the silicone tube. Histologic sections, in this case, showed acute inflammatory changes, polymorphonuclear infiltration and mucosal ulceration. Ossoff and coworkers conclude: "This finding should serve to put the final ban on the use of the PVC [polyvinyl chloride] tube for carbon dioxide laser surgery."[57] They also state that until the morbidity associated with the inhalation of the ash from the combustion of silicone has been determined, silicone tubes should not be used for laser surgery.

The shafts of combustible endotracheal tubes, whether polyvinyl chloride or rubber, can be made extremely resistant to the effects of both the CO_2 and Nd:YAG laser by wrapping them with the correct metallic tape. Many reports on this technique did not specify which type of tape to use. Sosis and coworkers,[58,59] in a comparison of metallic foil tapes used to protect combustible endotracheal tubes from the CO_2[58] or Nd:YAG[59] laser, have shown that Radio Shack No. 44-1155 tape, although widely used and even advocated in the medical literature,[60] affords much less adequate protection of polyvinyl chloride or red rubber endotracheal tubes than either 3M (St. Paul, MN) No. 425 aluminum foil tape or Venture (Rockland, MA) copper foil tape. In fact, the latter two tapes prevented combustion when either 70 W of CO_2 or 50 W of Nd:YAG laser power was aimed perpendicularly at wrapped tubes that had 100% oxygen flowing through them, even when the laser's output was continued for 1 minute. The Radio Shack tape, although apparently metallic, has a very thin layer of metal with a thicker layer of combustible Mylar plastic beneath.

Protective-foil self-adhesive tape, $\frac{1}{4}$ inch wide should be wrapped around the endotracheal tube in an overlapping spiral manner, starting just above the cuff (Fig. 4.11) so that no bare areas will be exposed when the tube flexes. Because manufacturers may change the composition of these tapes, each new supply should be tested for combustibility before being used in an operation.[61]

Kinking has been reported when very small endotracheal tubes are wrapped with metallic tape.[62,63] Foil-wrapped tubes may have a rough surface that could traumatize tissue, and the reflection of the laser beam from this tape could cause injury to the patient or operating room personnel.[64] The foil-wrapped tubes may be gas-sterilized prior to use without affecting their combustibility.

Foil wrapping provides an inexpensive, effective means of protecting the shafts of combustible endotracheal tubes. It should be noted, however, that these tubes can be ignited by sparks or the heat generated by adjacent burning materials.[65] The foil tapes are not manufactured for medical applications, and the manufacturers therefore cannot be held responsible for any problems with these products. They also have no approval from the U.S. Food and Drug Administration, although they are widely used and advocated in the literature.[58,59]

Another effective method of protecting the shafts of combustible endotracheal tubes is the use of the Laser-Guard (Americal Corp., Mystic, CT). This product, available in three sizes, consists of a layer of silver foil with a layer of adhesive on

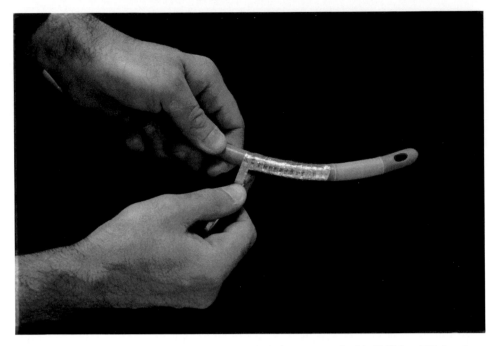

Figure 4.11.   A red rubber endotracheal tube is being wrapped with 3M No. 425 aluminum tape to protect it from the laser.

one side and a coating of sponge on the other side. It can be applied more quickly to the endotracheal tube than the $\frac{1}{4}$-inch tapes described above. Wetting the sponge layer allows it to act as a heat sink. Silver is used because it has a high thermal conductivity. Sosis and coworkers[66] tested the Laser-Guard and found that it effectively protected the shafts of polyvinyl chloride endotracheal tubes from the CO_2 laser operating at 70 W and directed perpendicularly at the wrapped tube for 1 minute. Although the sponge layer was destroyed at the site of the laser's impingement, the silver foil layer was undamaged. These investigators also showed that a reflected laser beam is less likely to cause damage with the Laser-Guard than with foil-wrapped tubes.[64]

The cuffs of foil-wrapped endotracheal tubes are still vulnerable to the effects of the laser even when the shafts have been protected. In fact, because of their thin walls, cuffs are more likely to ignite than shafts. Lasers can perforate tube cuffs at extremely low laser power levels. Perforation renders positive pressure ventilation difficult and increases the risk of combustion because the enhanced fraction of oxygen often used in these cases floods the oropharynx. For these reasons, the cuff should be filled with saline to provide a signal that perforation has occurred. Sosis and coworkers[67] have shown that saline significantly reduces, but does not eliminate, the risk of an endotracheal tube fire when the cuff is struck by a CO_2 laser. In their investigation, an endotracheal tube fire was started in all five tubes that had air-filled cuffs when a CO_2 laser set at 50 W was directed at the cuffs. In contrast, only one of five endotracheal tubes whose cuffs were filled with saline could be set on fire. As a further precaution, wet packing or pledgets should cover the cuff, and these must be moistened periodically.

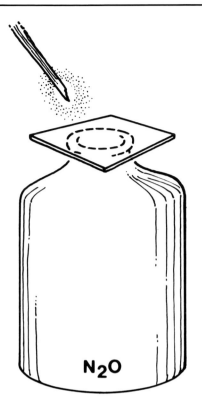
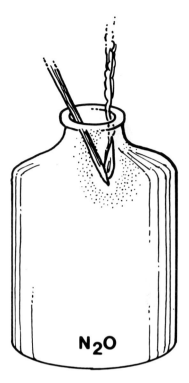

Figure 4.12. A glowing wooden splint thrust into nitrous oxide will burst into flames, demonstrating that nitrous oxide supports combustion. (Reproduced with permission: In Stoelting RK (ed): *Advances in Anesthesia,* vol. 6. Chicago, Year Book Medical Publishers, 1989, p 186.)

The anesthetic gases used can profoundly influence combustibility. Nitrous oxide should not be considered an inert gas in laser airway surgery (Fig. 4.12). Although it cannot support life, it can readily decompose into oxygen, nitrogen, and energy as

$$N_2O = N_2 + \tfrac{1}{2}O_2 + \text{energy}.$$

In an experiment analogous to one with oxygen, a glowing match, when thrust into nitrous oxide, will burst into flame. MacIntosh and colleagues[68] note that, although the decomposition of 1 mole of nitrous oxide leads to the liberation of a 2:1 mixture of nitrogen and oxygen, combustion will be supported more readily than expected from a $66\tfrac{2}{3}\%$ nitrogen, $33\tfrac{1}{3}\%$ oxygen mixture due to the heat liberated in this exothermic reaction. In fact, it has been found that nitrous oxide supports combustion to approximately the same extent as oxygen.

The minimum fraction of oxygen that will provide a satisfactory patient oxygen saturation, as determined by pulse oximetry, should be used in endoscopic surgery employing lasers. The remainder of the inspired gas mixture should consist of nitrogen or helium, not nitrous oxide. Helium may be preferable to nitrogen because its higher thermal conductivity. Pashayan and Gravenstein[69] have suggested that helium will retard combustion better than nitrogen will. Its low viscosity may

TABLE 4.5. *Lower Limit of Flammability (%)*

Isoflurane	7.0
Enflurane	5.75
Halothane	5.75

From Leonard PF: The lower limits of flammability of halothane, enflurane and isoflurane. *Anesth Analg* 34:238–239, 1975.

also promote the flow of gases past a partial obstruction. However, Simpson and Wolf[70] found no difference in flammability when comparing $N_2:O_2$ mixtures to $He:O_2$ mixtures. Whether helium, nitrogen, or air is used, it is desirable to have an anesthesia machine capable of delivering these gases in the operating suite used for laser endoscopic surgery.

Leonard[71] has noted that the lower limits for combustibility of halothane, enflurane, and isoflurane are 4.75, 5.75, and 7.0%, respectively (Table 4.5). Consequently, the concentrations of these agents normally used during clinical anesthesia will not promote combustion.

In a survey of patients undergoing laser resection of central airway lesions, Perera and Mallon[72] note a high incidence of tachycardia and hypertension in these cases. These conditions impose a potent stress on the myocardium that may lead to a myocardial infarction. Perera and Mallon advocate the use of inhalational anesthetics such as enflurane to blunt these responses. In addition, beta blockers such as propranolol, sodium nitroprusside, nitroglycerine, or labetalol may also be useful in normalizing hemodynamic parameters.

Nebulized lidocaine may be useful in blunting the sympathetic response to airway instrumentation. Perera and Mallon[72] also note that delayed extubation is more common following intravenous anesthetics than following inhaled anesthetics.

Muscle relaxants are considered necessary in laser airway, since patient immobility is essential.

A video display of the surgical field enables all members of the operating room team to note the progression of surgery and the state of the airway. In particular, the anesthesiologist can watch the surgery and make sure the endotracheal tube or cuff has not been struck by the laser.

In Nd:YAG surgery of central airway lesions, the surgical and anesthetic techniques must be modified for patient safety. Dumon and coworkers,[73] reporting on a large number of cases, recommend the use of a rigid bronchoscope for laser treatment of obstructing lesions. Brutinel and associates[74] noted difficulty in ventilating and adequately oxygenating patients during Nd:YAG surgery with a fiberoptic bronchoscope in place. Casey and colleagues[75] reported a case in which both the fiberoptic bronchoscope and the endotracheal tube burned during Nd:YAG laser surgery.

Rontal and coworkers[76] suggest that when peripheral lung lesions are to be treated with a fiberoptic bronchoscope, the flexible bronchoscope be placed within a rigid bronchoscope rather than an endotracheal tube. However, they do mention a case of combustion of the flexible bronchoscope with this technique.[76] Rigid bronchoscopy allows better visualization of the surgical field and improved suctioning. It enables the surgeon to remove fragments of tissue or debris and to apply pressure or epinephrine-soaked pledgets to areas of active bleeding.[74,77] Using power levels below 50 W in short bursts lessens the risk of laser impingement on vital structures. McDougall and Cortese[78] have reported that two patients died during Nd:YAG laser treatment of obstructing airway lesions employing a high power level.

Geffin and colleagues[79] compared the combustibility of conventional clear polyvinyl chloride endotracheal tubes with red rubber or silicone endotracheal tubes exposed to the Nd:YAG laser. They found the clear polyvinyl chloride tubes superior to the other types, but the black printing on these endotracheal tubes ignited more readily than the clear portions of the tube. Even the clear parts of the endotracheal tubes ignited if sufficient power was used. These investigators recommend that completely clear (unmarked) endotracheal tubes be used for Nd:YAG laser surgery.[34]

Sosis and coworkers[80] evaluated a new, totally clear Sheridan endotracheal tube designed for Nd:YAG laser surgery. Although a clean endotracheal tube could not be set on fire with the Nd:YAG laser, it caught fire quickly when blood or mucous was applied. They conclude that this tube is unsuitable for Nd:YAG laser airway surgery. If an endotracheal tube must be used, a red rubber tube wrapped with Venture copper foil metallic tape should be used.[59]

General anesthesia is usually recommended for Nd:YAG treatment of central airway lesions,[73,74] although some investigators advocate the use of topical anesthesia.[81] In a retrospective study of 97 patients undergoing Nd:YAG resection of tracheobronchial tumors, George and coworkers[82] determined that significantly more treatment sessions were needed under local than under general anesthesia. General anesthesia provided better muscle relaxation, control of ventilation, and immobility. Bleeding was also thought to be better controlled under general anesthesia. Those patients receiving local anesthesia could only tolerate procedures of up to 1 hour's duration.

Rontal and associates found local anesthesia preferable to general anesthesia whenever a high-grade obstruction of the airway is known to exist or is highly probable. According to them, spontaneous respirations can be preserved under local anesthesia but rarely under general anesthesia. Ventilation in patients with considerable airway encroachment is therefore more likely to remain adequate under local anesthesia. They select local anesthesia for patients whose middle or lower tracheal lumen is reduced by more than 50% of its cross section, because they believe positive pressure ventilation tends to force blood and debris into the distal respiratory tract with consequent hypercarbia and a higher alveolar–arterial oxygen tension gradient. They claim that it also predisposes to pneumothorax and subcutaneous emphysema.[76]

SPECIAL ENDOTRACHEAL TUBES FOR LASER SURGERY

Norton Endotracheal Tube

The Norton tube[83] (A.V. Mueller, Chicago, IL) (Fig. 4.13) is constructed of spirally wound stainless steel. It is the only commercially available, completely nonflamma-

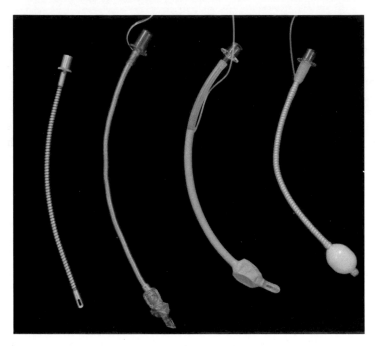

Figure 4.13. From left to right are displayed the Bivona, Xomed, Mallinckrodt, and Norton laser endotracheal tubes.

ble endotracheal tube. It has no cuff. A separate latex cuff, however, may be attached to the tube. Alternatively, the tube may be packed off to create a closed system for positive pressure ventilation.

This tube has a matte or sandblasted finish, rather thick walls, and a somewhat rough exterior.[84] The matte finish should diffuse a reflected laser beam.[83] A 4.8-mm ID Norton endotracheal tube has a wall thickness of 1.3 mm. The large size is a disadvantage, since this tube will obscure the surgeon's view more than would an endotracheal tube with the same internal diameter but with thinner walls. The tube's large size and stiffness may impede surgical exposure and laryngoscope positioning.

Adding an external cuff to this tube introduces flammable material; moreover, the presence of the pilot tube is inconvenient. The sponges or packs that may be used to make a seal are also potentially combustible if they dry out. The tube is not airtight, and difficulty in ventilating a patient has been reported.[85] Even if ventilation is not compromised by the leak, the presence of anesthetic gases increases the possibility of combustion in the surgical field and also contributes to operating room pollution.

The Norton endotracheal tube is reusable and costs $199. It may be autoclaved. The sizes available are 4.0, 4.8, and 6.4 mm ID.

Xomed Laser Shield Endotracheal Tube

The Xomed laser endotracheal tube (Xomed, Jacksonville, FL) (Fig. 4.13) is a silicone tube that has been dipped into a silicone elastomer to which metallic particles have been added. The manufacturer's literature specifies only CO_2 lasers be used, at a power of no more than 25 W in pulsed mode with pulse durations of 0.1 to 0.5 sec and a beam diameter of under 0.8 mm. Xomed also states that no more than 25% oxygen should be used with this tube; a concentration that is too low for some patients presenting for laser surgery. At a laser power of 25 W, 25 pulses of 0.1-sec duration or 5 pulses at 0.5-sec duration perforated the tube, according to the manufacturer. These recommendations are apparently for the shaft of the tube, since the cuff has been shown to be easily punctured by the CO_2 laser.[86] They recommend obtaining informed consent from the patient before using the Xomed tube.

Sosis and Heller,[87] in evaluating the Xomed tube, noted that a blowtorch fire started quickly when a high-powered CO_2 laser was directed perpendicularly at this tube. The fire was more difficult to extinguish than tube fires with polyvinyl chloride or red rubber endotracheal tubes. The Xomed tube fragmented into silica debris and gave off a bright light after laser contact. Similar results were found in an Nd:YAG evaluation of this tube.[88] Sosis and Heller[88] recommend that this tube not be used for laser surgery, since safer equipment is available.

Bivona Laser Endotracheal Tube

The Bivona laser endotracheal tube (Hammond, IN) (Fig. 4.13) has an aluminum core and silicone covering. It has a foam cuff that must have the air or saline filling it aspirated from it before its insertion or removal from the larynx. A large syringe is recommended for this purpose. Its cuff consists of polyurethane foam with a silicone envelope.[89]

Once inserted, the pilot tube can be simply opened to air for it to inflate passively. However, saline is recommended for filling the cuff for laser surgery.[67] The pilot tube runs along the exterior of the tube and is colored black so that it can be positioned away from the laser; damage to it will make deflating the cuff impossible. Trauma to the vocal cords is likely under these circumstances.[90,91]

The external position of the pilot tube and the necessity for active deflation of the cuff are disadvantages. A high incidence of sore throats has been noted with this tube.[92] The tube is nonreusable and costs $80. The manufacturer recommends it only for CO_2 laser use. Sosis and Heller[87] note that an endotracheal tube fire could be started easily when the CO_2 laser operating at high power was applied to this tube. The tube disintegrated into several pieces. Similar results and recommendations were found by Sosis and Heller with the Nd:YAG laser.[88] They do not recommend this tube for laser surgery.

Mallinckrodt Laser-Flex Endotracheal Tube

The Mallinckrodt Laser-Flex endotracheal tube (Fig. 4.13) is constructed from stainless steel. Unlike the Norton tube, its shaft is airtight. It has two cuffs, constructed of combustible polyvinyl chloride. If the proximal one is damaged by the laser, the distal cuff remains to prevent reflux of mixtures containing high levels of O_2. The cuffs can be inflated with two separate pilot tubes which run along the inside of the endotracheal tube. The 15-mm adapter is constructed from polyvinyl chloride.

TABLE 4.6. *Airway Fire Protocol*

1. Stop all anesthetic gases including oxygen.
2. Douse flames with saline.
3. Remove endotracheal tube.
4. Ventilate by mask and bag.
5. Evaluate airway for burns.

Sosis and Heller[87] found that the shaft of this tube was not affected by 70 W of CO_2 laser output lasting 1 minute. They recommend it for use with the CO_2 laser. In another study,[64] they note that this tube presents less danger of a reflected laser beam causing damage than foil-wrapped tubes do. In an evaluation of the Laser-Flex tube with the Nd:YAG laser, however,[88] the same authors found that it could be penetrated by this laser when operated at high power.

This tube is available in 4.5 and 6.0 mm ID sizes. It costs $49 and is nonreusable.

MANAGEMENT OF AN AIRWAY FIRE

Operating room personnel should always be prepared for the possibility of an airway fire during laser endoscopic surgery. In particular, a definite plan of action (Table 4.6) should be rehearsed by all operating room personnel so that rapid action can be taken if a fire occurs.

In the event of an airway fire or explosion, the anesthesiologist should immediately cease the delivery of *all* anesthetic gases *including oxygen*. This can be done by turning off the flow meters or rotometers, disconnecting the common gas outlet, or detaching the endotracheal tube from the anesthesia circuit. The reason for discontinuing these gases is that they usually have a high oxygen fraction, and their interruption alone will often terminate endotracheal tube combustion.

The endotracheal tube should always immediately be removed if an airway fire starts, because it will no longer provide a patent airway. For this reason, the endotracheal tube should not be overzealously taped in place. A container of saline should be available to douse any flames.

Once the endotracheal tube has been removed and the fire extinguished, the patient should be ventilated by bag and mask. At this point the extent of airway damage should be assessed. Doing so may entail fiberoptic bronchoscopy via an endotracheal tube or a rigid bronchoscopy. Extensive burns should be managed with controlled ventilation via endotracheal tube or tracheostomy Antibiotics and steroids should be considered if significant burns have occurred. If the airway burns are minimal, the surgery can proceed.

VENTURI JET VENTILATION

A technique of ventilation not requiring the presence of an endotracheal tube was demonstrated by Sanders in 1967.[93] A catheter or needle is attached to an operating laryngoscope or bronchoscope and connected to a 50 psi oxygen source. A trigger or toggle is pressed to direct a jet of oxygen down the bronchoscope. Satisfactory ventilation of the patient has been achieved by this method.[94]

The pressure delivered to the venturi jet, its diameter, its distance from the laryngeal opening, and the compliance of the patient's lungs define the tidal volume that the patient will receive with this technique. The actual F_iO_2 received by the patient is not 1.0, since room air is entrained along with the oxygen.

The venturi jet technique has the advantage of giving the surgeon excellent exposure to all parts of the airway, since no endotracheal tube is present. The absence of the endotracheal tube also reduces the danger of combustion.

Owing to the entrainment of room air during the venturi technique, 100% oxygen is usually supplied to the catheter. The patient's tidal volume may be 20 times the volume of gas delivered by the venturi jet. A totally intravenous technique of anesthesia is recommended to minimize pollution, since this is an open procedure.

Venturi jet ventilation applies an extremely high pressure to the jetting catheter. A pressure of 50 psi is the equivalent of 3500 cmH_2O. This represents a pressure greatly in excess of those normally applied to the airway. It is for this reason that barotrauma such as pneumothorax or pneumomediastinum have been reported in this technique.[95,96] A further possible hazard is that gastric contents or debris from surgery may be aspirated, since there is no barrier to the passage of foreign materials as there would be with a cuffed endotracheal tube. The jet ventilator must be kept carefully aligned with the larynx, or gastric dilatation and barotrauma may occur. The chest should be continuously examined for bilateral chest wall movement during this mode of ventilation.

Jet techniques involving subglottic position of the venturi catheter have been proposed. Their presumed advantage is that of precluding the jet not reaching the trachea or being misaligned with it. The possibility of laryngospasm makes these techniques unsafe however, since adduction of the vocal cords makes barotrauma from the extremely high pressures very likely.

REFERENCES

1. Keane WM, Atkins JP: CO$_2$ laser surgery of the upper airway. *Surg CLin North Am* 64:955, 1984.
2. Strong MS, Vaughan CW, Healy GB, et al: MACP: Recurrent respiratory papillomatosis. *Ann Otol Rhinol Laryngol* 85:508, 1976.
3. Cote CJ, Todres ID: The pediatric airway. In Ryan JF, Todres ID, Cote CJ, et al (eds): *A Practice of Anesthesia for Infants and Children.* Orlando, FL, Grune and Stratten, 1986, pp 37–38.
4. Crone RK: The respiratory system. In Gregory GA (ed): *Pediatric Anesthesia.* New York, Churchill Livingstone, 1983, pp 43–44.
5. Tharp JA, Lockhart CH: Pediatric anesthesia. In Ballang TJ, Pashley NRT (eds): *Clinical Pediatric Otolaryngology.* St. Louis, Mosby, 1986, p 21.
6. Liu LMP, Goudsouzian NG: Neuromuscular effect of intramuscular succinylcholine in infants. *Anesthesiology* 57:A413, 1982.
7. Cross KW, Flynn DM, Hill JR: Oxygen consumption in normal infants during moderate hypoxia in warm and cool environments. *Pediatrics* 37:565–576, 1966.

8. Friedman WF: Intrinsic physiologic properties of the developing heart. *Prog Cardiovasc Dis* 15:87–111, 1972.

9. Friesen RH, Lichtor JL: Cardiovascular depression during halothane anesthesia in infants: a study of three induction techniques. *Anesth Analg* 61:42–45, 1982.

10. Miller BR, Friesen RH: Oral premedication in infants. *Anesthesiology* 67:A491, 1987.

11. Blitt CD: Monitoring the anesthetized patient. In Barash PG, Cullen BF, Stoelting RK (eds): *Clinical Anesthesia.* London, Lippincott, 1989, p 579.

12. Fanconi S, Doherty P. Edmonds JF, et al: Pulse oximetry in pediatric intensive care. Comparisons with measured saturations and transcutaneous oxygen tensions. *J Pediatr* 107:362–366, 1985.

13. Peabody JL, Gregory GA, Willis MM, et al: Transcutaneous oxygen tension in sick infants. *Am Rev Respir Dis* 118:83, 1978.

14. Gothgen I, Jacobsen E. Transcutaneous oxygen tension measurements. I. Age variation and reproducibility. *Acta Anaesthesiol Scand {Suppl}* 67:71, 1978.

15. Severinghaus JW, Weiskopf RB, Nishimma M, et al: Oxygen electrode errors due to polarographic reduction of halothane. *J Appl Physiol* 31:640, 1971.

16. Dent JG, Netter KJ: Errors in oxygen tension measurement caused by halothane. *Br J Anaesth* 48:195, 1976.

17. Akbery WJ, Nahn CEW, Brooks WM: The polarographic measurement of halothane. *Br J Anaesth* 53:447, 1981.

18. Samra SK: Halothane interference with transcutaneous oxygen monitoring: in vivo and vitro. *Crit Care Med* 11:612–613, 1983.

19. Phillips BL, McQuitty J, Durand DJ: Blood gases: technical aspects and interpretation. In Goldsmith JP, Karotkin EH (eds): Philadelphia, Saunders, 1988, p 221.

20. Cassady G: Transcutaneous monitoring in the newborn infant. *J Pediatr* 103:837, 1983.

21. Wilson RD: Current status of ketamine. *ASA Refresher Courses,* Vol. 1. Philadelphia, Saunders, 1973, pp 157–167.

22. Friesen RH, Lichtor JL: Cardiovascular effects of inhalation induction with isoflurane in infants. *Anesth Analg* 62:411–414, 1983.

23. Watch MF, Forester JE, Connor MT, et al: Minimum alveolar concentration of halothane for tracheal intubation. *Anesthesiology* 69:412–416, 1988.

24. Brummitt WM, Fearon B, Brama I: Anesthesia for laryngeal laser surgery in the infant and child. *Ann Otol* 90:475–477, 1981.

25. Baraka A: Intravenous lidocaine controls extubation laryngospasm in children. *Anesth Analg* 57:506–507, 1978.

26. Wainright AC, Moody RA, Carruth JAS: Anesthetic safety with the carbon dioxide laser. *Anaesthesia* 36:411–415, 1981.

27. Pashayan AG, Gravenstein JS, Cassisi NJ, et al: The helium protocol for laryngotracheal operations with the CO_2 laser: a retrospective review of 532 cases. *Anesthesiology* 68:801–804, 1988.

28. Pashayan AG: Anesthesia for laser surgery. *American Society of Anesthesiologists 1988 Annual Refresher Course Lectures,* 1988, p 124.

29. Talmedge EA: Safe combined general and topical anesthesia for laryngoscopy and bronchoscopy. *South Med J* 66:455–459, 1973.

30. Johans TG, Reichert TJ: An insufflation device for anesthesia during subglottic carbon dioxide laser microsurgery in children. *Anesth Analg* 63:368–370, 1984.

31. Rital L, Seleny F, Holinger LD: Anesthetic management and gas scavenging for laser surgery of infant subglottic stenosis. *Anesthesiology* 58:191–193, 1983.

32. Lawson NW, Rogers D, Seifer A, et al: Intravenous procaine as a supplement to general anesthesia for carbon dioxide laser resection of laryngeal papillomas in children. *Anesth Analg* 58:492–496, 1979.

33. Norton ML, Devos P: New endotracheal tube for laser surgery of the larynx. *Ann Otol Rhinol Laryngol* 87:554–557, 1978.

34. Hirshman CA, Leon D, Porch D, et al: Improved metal endotracheal tube for laser surgery of the airway. *Anesth Analg* 59:789–791, 1980.

35. Sanders R: Two ventilating attachments for bronchoscopes. *Del Med J* 39:170–182, 1967.

36. Lee ST: A ventilating laryngoscope for inhalation anaesthesia and augmented ventilation during laryngoscopic procedures. *Br J Anaesth* 44:874–878, 1972.

37. Scamman FL, McCabe BF: Supraglottic jet ventilation for laser surgery of the larynx in children. *Ann Otol Rhinol Laryngol* 95:142–145, 1986.

38. Hermens JM, Bennett MJ, Hirshman CA: Anesthesia for laser surgery. *Anesth Analg* 62:218–229, 1983.

39. Glenski JA, MacKenzie RA, Maragos NE, et al: Assessing tidal volume and detecting hyperinflation during venturi jet ventilation for microlaryngeal surgery. *Anesthesiology* 63:554–557, 1985.

40. Miyasaka K, Sloan IA, Froese AB: An evaluation of the jet injector (Sanders) technique for bronchoscopy in pediatric patients. *Can Anaesth Soc J* 27:117–124, 1980.

41. Carden E, Galido J: Foot pedal control of jet ventilation during bronchoscopy and microlaryngeal surgery. *Anesth Analg* 54:405–406, 1975.

42. Mayne A, Joucken K, Collard E, et al: Intravenous infusion of propofol for induction and maintenance of anesthesia during endoscopic carbon dioxide laser ENT procedures with high frequency jet ventilation. *Anaesthesia* 43:97–100, 1988.

43. Eng UB, Eriksson I, Sjostrand V: High frequency positive pressure ventilation: a review based upon its use during bronchoscopy and for laryngoscopy and microlaryngeal surgery under general anesthesia. *Anesth Analg* 59:594–603, 1980.

44. Weisberger EC, Miner JD: Apneic anesthesia for improved endoscopic removal of laryngeal pappillomata. *Laryngoscope* 98:693–697, 1988.

45. Cohen SR, Herbert WI, Thompson JW: Anesthesia in management of microlaryngeal laser surgery in children: apneic technique anesthesia. *Laryngoscope* 98:347–348, 1988.

46. Emhardt JD, Weisberger EC, Dierdorf, et al: The rise of arterial carbon dioxide during apnea in children. *Anesthesiology* 69:A779, 1988.

47. Pashley NRT: Congenital anomalies of the upper airway. In Balanky TJ, Pashley NRT (eds): *Clinical Pediatric Otolaryngology,* St. Louis, Mosby, 1986, p 365.

48. Milliken RA, Bizzarri DV: Flammable surgical drapes—a patient and personnel hazard. *Anesth Analg* 64:54–57, 1985.

49. Ott AE: Disposable surgical drapes—a potential fire hazard. *Obstet Gynecol* 61:667–668, 1983.

50. Fried MP: A survey of the complications of laser laryngoscopy. *Arch Otolaryngol* 110:31–34, 1984.

51. Healey GB, Strong MS, Shapshay S, et al: Complications of CO$_2$ laser surgery of the aerodigestive tract: Experience of 4416 cases. *Otolaryngol Head Neck Surg* 92:13–18, 1984.

52. Patel KF, Hicks JN: Prevention of fire hazards associated with use of carbon dioxide lasers. *Anesth Analg* 60:885–888, 1981.

53. Wolf GL, Simpson JI: Flammability of endotracheal tubes in oxygen and nitrous oxide enriched atmosphere. *Anesthesiology* 67:236–239, 1987.

54. Meyers A: Complications of CO_2 laser surgery of the larynx. *Ann Otol Rhinol Laryngol* 90:132–134, 1981.

55. Dyer RF, Esch VH: Polyvinylchloride toxicity in fires. *JAMA* 235:393–397, 1976.

56. Boyd CH: A fire in the mouth. *Anaesthesia* 24:441–446, 1969.

57. Ossoff RH, Duncavage JA, Eisenman TS, et al: Comparison of tracheal damage from laser-ignited endotracheal tube fires. *Ann Otol Rhinol Laryngol* 92:333–336, 1983.

58. Sosis MB: Evaluation of five metallic tapes for protection of endotracheal tubes during CO_2 laser surgery. *Anesth Analg* 68:392–393, 1989.

59. Sosis M, Dillon F, Heller S: A comparison of metallic tapes for protection of endotracheal tubes during Nd:YAG laser surgery. *Anesth Analg* 68:S270, 1989.

60. Lim RY, Kenney CL: Precautions and safety in carbon dioxide laser surgery. *Otolaryngol Head Neck Surg* 95:239–241, 1986.

61. Cork RC: Anesthesia for otolaryngologic surgery involving use of a laser. In Brown BR Jr (ed): *Anesthesia and ENT Surgery*. Philadelphia, Davis, 1987, pp 127–140.

62. Patil V, Stehling LC, Zauder HL: A modified endotracheal tube for laser microsurgery. *Anesthesiology* 51:571, 1979.

63. Kaeder CS, Hirshman CA: Acute airway obstruction: a complication of aluminum tape wrapping of tracheal tubes in laser surgery. *Can Anaesth Soc J* 26:138–139, 1979.

64. Sosis M, Dillon F, Heller S: Hazards of CO_2 laser reflection from laser resistant endotracheal tubes. *Anesthesiology* 71:A444, 1989.

65. Hirshman CA, Smith J: Indirect ignition of the endotracheal tube during carbon dioxide laser surgery. *Arch Otolaryngol* 106:639–641, 1980.

66. Sosis M, Dillon F, Heller S: Prevention of CO_2 laser-induced endotracheal tube fires with the Laser Guard Protective Coating. *Anesthesiology* 71:A419, 1989.

67. Sosis M, Dillon F, Heller S: Saline filled cuffs help prevent laser induced polyvinylchloride endotracheal tube fires. *Anesthesiology* 71:A421, 1989.

68. MacIntosh R, Mushin WW, Epstein HG: *Physics for the Anaesthetist*. Oxford, Blackwell, 1963, pp 353–357.

69. Pashayan AG, Gravenstein JS: Helium retards endotracheal tube fires from carbon dioxide lasers. *Anesthesiology* 62:274–277, 1985.

70. Simpson JI, Wolf GL: Helium does not reduce endotracheal tube flammability. *Anesth Analg* 68:S266, 1989.

71. Leonard PF: The lower limits of flammability of halothane, enflurane and isoflurane. *Anesth Analg* 54:238–240, 1975.

72. Perera ER, Mallon JS: General anaesthetic management for laser resection of central airway lesions in 85 procedures. *Can J Anaesth* 34:383–387, 1985.

73. Dumon JF, Shapshay S, Buorcereau J, et al: Principles for safety in application of neodymium-YAG laser in bronchology. *Chest* 86:163–168, 1984.

74. Brutinel WM, McDougall JC, Cortese DA: Bronchoscopic therapy with neodymium: yttrium-aluminum-garnet laser during intravenous anesthesia. *Chest* 84:518–521, 1983.

75. Casey KR, Fairfax WR, Smith SJ, et al: Intratracheal fire ignited by the Nd:YAG laser during treatment of tracheal stenosis. *Chest* 84:295–296, 1983.

76. Rontal M, Rontal E, Wenokur ME, et al: Anesthetic management for tracheobronchial laser surgery. *Ann Otol Rhinol Laryngol* 95:556–560, 1986.

77. Vourc'h G, Fischler M, Personne C, et al: Anesthetic management during Nd:YAG laser resection for major tracheobronchial obstructing tumors. *Anesthesiology* 61:636–637, 1984.

78. McDougall JC, Cortese DA: Neodymium:YAG laser therapy of malignant airway obstruction: a preliminary report. *Mayo Clin Proc* 58:35–39, 1983.

79. Geffin B, Shapshay SM, Bellack GS, et al: Flammability of endotracheal tubes during Nd:YAG laser application in the airway. *Anesthesiology* 65:511–515, 1986.

80. Sosis M, Dillon F, Heller S: Hazards of a new clear unmarked polyvinylchloride endotracheal tube designed for use with the Nd-YAG laser. *Anesthesiology* 71:A420, 1989.

81. Sia RL, Van Overbeck JJM, Rashkowski OM: Three years' anaesthetic experience with the Groningen Nd:YAG laser coagulation technique. *Anaesthesia* 40:904–906, 1985.

82. George PJM, Garrett CPO, Nixon C, et al: Laser treatment for tracheobronchial tumors: local or general anesthesia. *Thorax* 42:656–660, 1987.

83. Norton ML, DeVos P: New endotracheal tube for laser surgery of the larynx. *Ann Otol Rhinol Laryngol* 87:554–557, 1978.

84. Skaredoff MN, Poppers PJ: Beware of sharp edges in metal endotracheal tubes. *Anesthesiology* 58:595, 1983.

85. Sosis M: Report of a large air leak during surgery with a Norton tube. *Anesthesiology Review* 16:39–41, 1989.

86. Hayes DM, Gaba DM, Goode RL: Incendiary characteristics of a new laser-resistant endotracheal tube. *Otolaryngology* 95:37–40, 1986.

87. Sosis M, Heller S: A comparison of special endotracheal tubes for use with the CO_2 laser. *Anesthesiology* 69:A251, 1988.

88. Sosis M, Heller S: A comparison of special endotracheal tubes for use with the Nd:YAG laser. *Anesth Analg* 68:S271, 1989.

89. Kamen JM, Wilkinson CJ: A new low pressure cuff for endotracheal tubes. *Anesthesiology* 34:482–485, 1971.

90. Birkhan HJ, Heifetz M: "Uninflatable" inflatable cuffs. *Anesthesiology* 26:578, 1965.

91. Hedden M, Smith RBF, Torpey DJ: Complications of metal spiral embedded latex endotracheal tubes. *Anesth Analg* 51:859–862, 1972.

92. Loeser EA, Machin R, Colley J, et al: Postoperative sore throat—importance of endotracheal tube conformity versus cuff design. *Anesthesiology* 49:430–432, 1978.

93. Sanders RD: Two ventilating attachments for bronchoscopes. *Del Med J* 39:170–192, 1967.

94. Norton ML, Strong MS, Vaughan CW, et al: Endotracheal intubation and venturi (jet) ventilation for laser microsurgery of the larynx. *Ann Otol Rhinol Laryngol* 85:656–663, 1976.

95. O'Sullivan TJ, Healy GB: Complications of venturi jet ventilation during microlaryngeal surgery. *Arch Otolaryngol* 111:127–131, 1985.

96. Oliverio R, Ruder CB, Fermon C, et al: Pneumothorax secondary to ball-valve obstruction during jet ventilation. *Anesthesiology* 51:255–256, 1979.

5
Lasers in Dermatology

C. William Hanke
Melissa W. Lee

Leon Goldman, M.D., professor of dermatology at the University of Cincinnati, began working with lasers in the early 1960s. Dr. Goldman established the laser laboratory at the University of Cincinnati in 1961 dedicating it to the development of lasers in dermatology. He applied many types of lasers to dermatologic disease and discussed his findings in several medical journals and books. The research protocols he wrote and the new techniques he developed rapidly spread throughout the specialty of dermatology as well as to others.

Many other physicians have continued research in laser dermatology, including John A. Parrish, Kenneth A. Arndt, Philip L. Bailin, Rox Anderson, Elizabeth McBurney, Barbara A. Gilchrist, Jerome M. Garden, Ronald G. Wheeland, Gary J. Brauner, John L. Ratz, Laurence M. David, Alan Schiftman, Oon TiAn Tan, and Roy Geronemus. Currently, more than 15% of dermatologists use lasers. The CO_2 type is the most commonly employed. The argon laser and the tunable dye laser are being used more and more frequently.

CARBON DIOXIDE LASER

The carbon dioxide laser is the type most widely used for cutaneous surgery. The CO_2 laser emits light at a wavelength of 10,600 nm, which is in the invisible infrared portion of the electromagnetic spectrum.[1] The laser energy is absorbed by the skin in a completely nonspecific manner. Cellular disruption occurs after rapid heating of intracellular water, which is converted to steam at 100°C.[2] The energy is converted to heat within the skin to a depth of 0.1 mm[1]. Because the tissue destruction is rapid, surrounding tissue damage and thermal coagulation are minimal.

The CO_2 laser is unique because it can be used in two different modes of operation. In the focused mode the beam becomes an excisional instrument. Lymphatic and blood vessels up to 0.5 mm in diameter are sealed by the laser, resulting in virtually bloodless surgery.[3] Peripheral nerve endings are also sealed, leading to less postoperative pain.[1] In the defocused mode the CO_2 beam vaporizes tissue. This technique allows the surgeon to destroy very thin, controlled layers of tissue.[3] Disorders in which the CO_2 laser has been used are discussed in the following sections.

Rhinophyma

In the treatment of rhinophyma, the CO_2 laser is used in both modes.[4] First, the cutting mode is used to remove bulk tumor. In this mode the CO_2 laser is set at 15 to 20 W, with a power density of 50,000 to 75,000 W/cm^2, and a spot size of 0.1 to 0.2 mm in diameter. Fine contouring of the nose is then performed with the laser in the vaporization mode. In this mode the CO_2 laser has a power setting of 4 to 5 W, a spot size of 1 to 2 mm in diameter, and a power density of 150 to 500 W/cm^2. The advantages of this technique are minimal blood loss and postoperative pain, and rapid healing. In one series, 12 patients were treated with the CO_2 laser. One patient experienced hypertrophic scarring, which was on the side of the nose.[4] An intralesional application of 20 mg/cc triamcinolone was satisfactory in treating the scar.

Another technique for treating rhinophyma was used by Eisen et al,[5] who employed the Shaw scalpel for bulk tumor removal and the CO_2 laser and dermabrader for contouring. Rapid hemostasis and minimal tissue damage are advantages of the Shaw scalpel. The blade temperature of 150°C seals the larger vessels. Color plates 1 to 3 illustrate a patient with rhinophyma who was treated with the CO_2 laser.

Keloids

Kantor et al[6] used the CO_2 laser for the excision of earlobe keloids. Sixteen patients with earlobe keloids were treated with a focused beam followed by intralesional steroids. Carbon dioxide laser power densities of 200 to 2500 W/cm^2 were used. There were no recurrences. In four patients hypertrophic scarring developed but improved with one or two additional intralesional steroid injections.

Actinic Cheilitis

The CO_2 laser was used to treat 13 patients with chronic actinic cheilitis of the lower lip.[7] Ten patients were treated with the conventional continuous wave CO_2 laser. The parameters were a power setting of 3 to 5 W, a 2-mm spot size, and a power density of 100 to 160 W/cm^2. For additional passes over the lip, laser pulses of 0.05 to 0.1 sec per pulse were employed. In three patients, the superpulsed CO_2 laser was used at 3 to 5 W of power, a pulse duration of 200 to 300 μsec, a 2-mm spot size and a power density of 75 to 125 W/cm^2. After an average followup of 11 months, no recurrences developed. Focal linear scarring occurred in ten patients. One patient experienced hypertrophic scarring and two developed hyperesthesia.

David[8] treated eight patients with actinic cheilitis using the CO_2 laser at a power setting of 15 W, a 3-mm spot size, and a power density of approximately 167 W/cm^2. No recurrences were found after an average followup of 34 months. There was no postoperative scarring, and a normal lip contour was preserved in each patient.

Color Plates

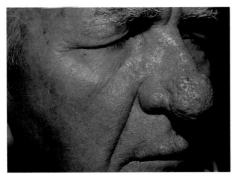

Plate 5.1. A 62-year-old man with rhinophyma involving distal third of nose.

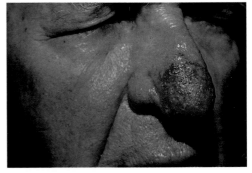

Plate 5.2. Same patient as Plate 5.1, immediately following CO_2 laser vaporization of the rhinophyma.

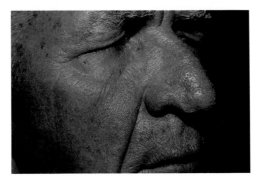

Plate 5.3. Same patient as Plate 5.1, six weeks postoperatively. Nose has healed, with improved contour.

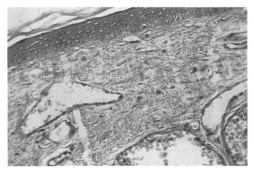

Plate 5.4. Dilated upper dermal blood vessels in punch-biopsy specimen from previously untreated port-wine hemangioma (Hematoxylin and eosin × 100).

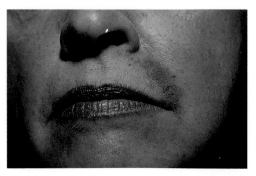

Plate 5.5. A 36-year-old woman with pink macular port-wine hemangioma involving left upper lip.

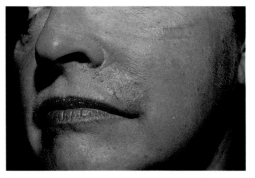

Plate 5.6. Minimal grey char on skin surface immediately following argon laser photocoagulation.

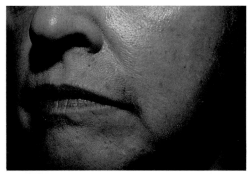

Plate 5.7. Hemangioma exhibits fading six months after single argon laser treatment.

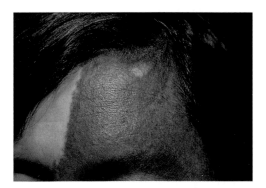

Plate 5.8. A 27-year-old woman with Sturge-Weber syndrome has port-wine hemangioma on left forehead. White test area near frontal hairline shows fading eight weeks following argon laser photocoagulation.

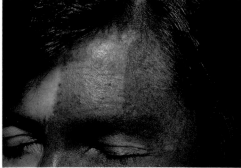

Plate 5.9. Medial half of hemangioma shows fading eight weeks after argon laser photocoagulation. Maximal fading may take 12 months.

Tattoos

Eleven patients with 15 tattoos underwent treatment with the CO_2 laser[9] using 15 to 25 W, a 2-mm spot size, a power density of 478 to 796 W/cm^2, and a pulse duration of 0.05 or 0.1 sec. The patients were comfortable during and after treatment, and pigment was removed completely. The results for all patients were satisfactory or excellent. The CO_2 laser method of tattoo removal was thought to be an improvement over other methods.

A study performed by Groot et al[10] compared the CO_2 laser and the infrared coagulator in removing tattoos. Postoperative pain, healing time, scarring tendency, and residual pigment were investigated. Seven patients with tattoos were treated with both the CO_2 laser and the infrared coagulator. The laser settings included 20 W, 2-mm spot size, 500 W/cm^2 power density, and a defocused beam. The infrared coagulator was used with the tip placed on the skin and a pulse duration of 1.25 sec. The cosmetic results of the two techniques were shown to be equivalent. The main advantage of the infrared coagulator is easily manageable, rapidly healing wounds. Total pigment removal in a single treatment is the chief advantage of the CO_2 laser; however, scarring commonly develops.

Another method for removing tattoos uses 50% urea in hydrophilic ointment as a postoperative dressing in combination with the CO_2 laser. Ruiz-Esparza et al[11] treated 12 patients with 17 decorative tattoos using this chemo-laser technique. The CO_2 laser was adjusted to a continuous vaporization mode with a power output of 10 to 15 W. Over 95% of the pigment in the treated areas was removed in 16 of the 17 tattoos. This method resulted in flat, supple skin with minimal texture alteration. This chemo-laser technique can be used to avoid hypertrophic scarring.

Port-wine Hemangiomas

Port-wine hemangiomas were treated in 37 patients with the CO_2 laser.[12] The power setting was 15 to 25 W, the spot size 2 mm, and the power densities 478 to 796 W/cm^2. The pulse duration was 0.05 to 0.1 sec. Postsurgical results were good to excellent in 21 patients and fair to poor in 10 patients. Three patients were lost to followup, and three developed scars.

Basal Cell Carcinoma

Adams and Price[13] studied the clinical and histologic effects of treating basal cell carcinoma with the CO_2 laser. Eighteen patients with 24 basal cell carcinomas were treated. The laser settings included a power setting of 0 to 25 W, pulse durations of 0.1, 0.2, 0.5, and 1.0 sec, a spot size of 2 mm, and a power density of 0 to 625 W/cm^2. Before the lesions were treated with the CO_2 laser, a 1-mm punch biopsy was taken to confirm the diagnosis and to ascertain the depth of the basal cell carcinoma. None of the lesions was greater than 2 mm in depth. The lesions were treated without overlapping the sites of impact.

A bland ointment was applied to the wound after treatment with the CO_2 laser. After 1 week, biopsies were done, and five were positive for basal cell carcinoma. Between 3 and 12 months following treatment, an additional seven were found to contain basal cell carcinoma. All malignant lesions were excised by conventional surgery. In summary, of the 24 lesions treated with the CO_2 laser, 12 showed incomplete destruction of the basal cell carcinoma. The applied power, duration of exposure, and depth of invasion of the malignancies did not predictably significantly correlate with the complete or incomplete destruction of the lesions.

Wheeland et al[14] used the CO_2 laser technique in treating 52 patients with 370 superficial basal cell carcinomas. High-risk areas (eg, the central face, embryonal fusion plates, or postauricular areas) were not treated with this technique, which combined traditional curettage with CO_2 laser vaporization instead of the more conventional electrocautery. The laser parameters were a spot size of 1 to 2 mm, a power setting of 4 to 5 W, and a power density of 160 to 510 W/cm^2. The lesion's margins were marked and the area was anesthetized. After vaporization the area was examined for persistent tumor. The lesion was then curetted using the standard technique, with the areas of persistent tumor separating readily. This resulted in a small amount of bleeding. If the treatment site still had tumor present clinically, the vaporization/curettage procedure was repeated until the area appeared clear of tumor.

After treatment a thin layer of polymyxin B sulfate–bacitracin zinc ointment was applied to the wound, followed by a nonadherent sterile pad and an appropriate absorbent dressing. The dressing was held in place by paper adhesive tape. Postoperatively, the patient was instructed to clean the wound twice a day with 3% hydrogen peroxide, followed by an application of polymyxin B sulfate–bacitracin zinc oinment.

After a followup period of 6 to 65 months, no evidence of recurrent tumor was detected. Advantages of this technique include minimal bleeding and postoperative pain, rapid healing, and good cosmetic results with little scarring.

Trichoepithelioma

One patient with trichoepitheliomas was treated by Sawchuk and Heald[15] with CO_2 laser excision and vaporizatiopn. The vaporization mode was used for exposing and debulking the tumors. The dermal remnants of the tumors were destroyed and the lesions sculpted with the excisional mode. A power setting of 5 to 15 W was utilized. After eight months, there were no recurrences. Some scarring occurred when larger lesions were treated; however, the results were acceptable to the patient.

Wheeland et al[16] used different techniques to treat three patients with multiple trichoepitheliomas employing only the vaporization mode. Multiple lesions in the external ear canal were vaporized in one patient using the following parameters: 15 to 25 W, a defocused 2-mm beam, and a continuous wave. There was no tumor regrowth after ten months.

A patient with numerous translucent, firm papules in the paranasal and periorbital areas was treated using 10 to 15 W, a defocused 2-mm beam, and a power density of 100 to 125 W/cm^2.[16] After one year there was no evidence of recurrence. Results were acceptable, with minimal scarring and slight epidermal atrophy.

Another patient with trichoepitheliomas around the nose was treated with the CO_2 laser.[16] The parameters used were 4 to 10 W, a defocused 2-mm beam, and a power density of 30 to 100 W/cm^2. After 6 weeks of followup there was no recurrence or evidence of scarring.

Fleming and Brody[17] treated one patient with multiple trichoepitheliomas using only the excision mode. The laser settings used were 17 W, a pulse duration of 1.0 sec, and a focused 1-mm beam. After 4 months the patient experienced recurrence around the eye.

Epidermal Nevi

Over a five-year period, fifteen patients with epidermal nevi were treated with CO_2 laser vaporization.[18] A continuous wave and a defocused 2-mm beam were used for all patients. Most of the patients were treated with a power setting of 5 W, a power density of 160 W/cm^2. Three patients were lost to followup. Of the remaining 12, eight had acceptable results. Two patients experienced recurrence and 2 patients had hypertrophic scarring.

Lentigines

The CO_2 laser was used to treat 146 solar lentigines in five patients.[19] The lentigines were irradiated at energy fluences of 3.0, 3.7, and 4.4 J/cm^2. The CO_2 laser was set at a pulse duration of 0.1 sec and a 4.5-mm spot size. After 6 weeks 12 lesions had cleared completely, 81 lightened substantially, and 28 remained unchanged. Atrophic change occurred in two patients. The results demonstrated that lesions can be lightened without substantial scarring.

Multiple Dermal Cylindromas

One patient with 70 dermal cylindromas was treated successfully with CO_2 laser vaporization.[20] The following parameters were used: 8 W, 1-mm spot size, power density of 1020 W/cm^2, and continuous wave. The cylindromas extruded from the dermis after unroofing with the laser. Postoperative pain was minimal, and complete healing occurred in 2 to 3 weeks with minimal scarring.

Xanthelasma Palpebrarum

The CO_2 laser was used to treat six patients with xanthelasma of the eyelids.[21] The laser was set at a 1-mm spot size and 10 W. The power density was 1,000 W/cm^2. After 4 years there were no recurrences, and satisfactory results were acheived without significant scarring.

Cutaneous Benign Neurofibromas

Four patients with cutaneous neurofibromas were treated with the CO_2 laser in the vaporization mode, with a 2.0-mm spot size, a power setting of 4.0 to 6.0 W, and a power density of 160 W/cm^2[22]. After 20 months the recurrence rate was less than 3% (a total of 483 tumors). The cosmetic results were good to excellent.

Blepharoplasty

A paired study was used to compare the CO_2 laser versus standard cold steel surgery and electrocautery on 13 patients undergoing blepharoplasty.[23] Cold steel surgery and electrocautery were used on one eye, while the CO_2 laser was used on the opposite eye. The CO_2 laser settings were 7 to 10 W, 0.2-mm spot size, a 17,500 W/cm^2 to 25,000 W/cm^2 power density, and continuous wave. Less postoperative ecchymosis and edema occurred when the CO_2 laser was used. Operating time was reduced and no bleeding occurred. Cosmetic results and scarring were compared at 3 hr, 5 days, and 30 days. No cosmetic differences were seen between the eye treated with the laser and the eye treated with cold steel surgery.

Blue Rubber Bleb Nevus

A patient with extensive cutaneous and visceral manifestations of the blue rubber bleb nevus syndrome was treated with the CO_2 laser.[24] Minimal blood loss, no recurrence, and good cosmetic results after 4 years of followup were reported. No laser parameters were given.

Scalp Reduction Surgery

Wheeland and Bailin[25] performed scalp reduction surgery with the CO_2 laser in the excisional mode. During the surgery there was virtually no bleeding. Because the laser seals the lymphatics and nerve endings, and tissue swelling and postoperative pain are reduced. The following laser parameters were employed: a power setting of 15 to 25 W, continuous wave, a beam diameter of 0.1 mm, and a power density of 50,000 to 70,000 W/cm^2.

Revision of Skin Grafts

The CO_2 laser was used to revise hypertrophy following full-thickness skin grafting.[26] The laser parameters were 5 W, a 2-mm beam diameter, a continuous wave, and a power density of 160 W/cm^2. After 6 months the graft showed a normal contour, good texture, and slight residual erythema.

Mohs Micrographic Surgery

The CO_2 laser can be used to excise thin layers of tissue during Mohs micrographic surgery (MMS).

This chemosurgical technique for skin cancer was developed by Frederic E. Mohs.[27] The original fixed-tissue technique used a zinc chloride fixative paste, which was applied to the cancer and left on overnight. The cancer was excised on the following day without bleeding or the need for local anesthesia. The excised tissue specimens were color coded, and a tissue map was drawn. Horizontal frozen sections were prepared and examined. If the frozen sections showed residual tumor microscopically, the procedure was repeated.

The chemosurgical technique was extremely time-consuming. Mohs in 1953 and Tromovitch in the late 1960s modified it by eliminating the zinc chloride paste and using local anesthesia.[27] The fresh-tissue technique reduced treatment time from several days to several hours. Reconstruction could be done immediately. MMS achieves a higher cure rate for skin cancer than any other method with maximum preservation of normal tissue.

When the CO_2 laser is used for Mohs micrographic surgery, the advantages of the fixed-tissue and fresh-tissue techniques are combined.[28] Like the fixed-tissue technique, the CO_2 laser provides nearly perfect hemostasis and clear visualization of the operative field. Lymphatics are sealed, and bone can be removed with the laser. The CO_2 laser also has the advantages of the fresh-tissue technique: rapid work pace, minimal pain and inflammation, minimal tissue destruction, and no histologic distortion. Surgical reconstruction can be performed immediately.[28] The disadvantages of the CO_2 laser in this situation as in others include high purchase price and the large size of the laser apparatus.[28]

THE ARGON LASER

The argon laser is commonly used to treat vascular disorders as well as pigmented conditions of the skin and mucous membranes. The argon laser emits a blue-green light at more than one wavelength. Peak emissions occur at 448 nm (blue) and 514 nm (green).[1] These peaks coincide with the absorption spectrum of the target-tissue chromophores, hemoglobin, and melanin.[2] The blue-green light interacts with the strongly pigmented lesions at the red end of the electromagnetic spectrum. The argon laser light passes into the skin to approximately 1 mm, reaching the upper dermis, which contains the highly pigmented areas. The laser light is converted to heat, that coagulates the protein in the pigmented areas of the upper dermis.[3] The end result is a blanching or lightening of the abnormally pigmented area. The normal skin structures are largely undamaged.[3] A number of disorders that have been treated with the argon laser are discussed in the following sections.

Port-wine Hemangiomas

Port-wine hemangiomas can be treated under local anesthesia, although general anesthesia may be required for extensive lesions. One-centimeter spot tests are often performed at different power settings to determine the best treatment parameters. In one study the argon laser was used to treat 130 patients with port-wine hemangiomas.[29] The spot size used was 1 mm, and the power density was 100 to 250 W/cm^2. The power varied between 1.0 and 2.5 W, depending upon the brightness of the lesion. The darker the lesion, the greater the power used. The most consistently used pulse duration was 0.2 sec. After a followup period of 24 months, 79 patients had excellent (total lightening without scar) or good (marked lightening without scar) results, and 34 patients had poor (limited change) results. Seventeen patients experienced significant scarring.

Finley et al[30] treated 28 patients with port-wine hemangiomas and studied the healing process after treatment with the argon laser. Biopsies were performed before and after treatment. The laser settings were 2 W, 1.0-mm spot size, a power density of 200 W/cm^2, and pulse duration of 0.2 sec. Investigators concluded that the paucity of erythrocytes typically seen in the smaller, newly formed dermal blood vessels following argon laser treatment are thought responsible for the lightening of the port-wine hemangiomas.

Another technique for treating port-wine hemangiomas with the argon laser was described by Rotteleur et al.[31] During a 12-month period one hundred and twenty-three patients were treated with a robotized hand piece was equipped with a scanning mechanism and a microprocessor control. The procedure was rapid, easily performed, and reproducible. The laser settings were up to 10 W, a 1-mm spot size, and a power density of up to 1,000 W/cm^2. The "point by point" (pulse) technique is slow and takes at least 47 min to treat a hemangioma measuring 6 cm × 8 cm. The "painting" (continuous) technique takes 9 min to treat a hemangioma measuring 6 cm × 8 cm and requires anesthesia. The results using the robotized hand piece showed no hypertrophic scarring and took 10 min to treat a 6 cm × 8 cm area.

Landthaler et al[32] used argon-laser treatment in 176 adult patients 18 years or older, with port-wine hemangiomas. The parameters were 1.9 to 2.6 W, pulse duration of 0.3 sec, spot size of 2 mm, and power density of 60 to 83 W/cm^2. Approximately 70% of the patients experienced excellent or good results. Laser therapy was discontinued if scar formation or insufficient lightening occurred.

A patient with a mixed nodular cavernous and port-wine hemangioma of the face was treated with both the ruby and argon lasers.[33] The pulsed ruby laser was set at 55 to 75 J/cm^2, 3.0 μsec pulses, and 2.1 cm^2 treatment sites. The argon laser was set at a power setting of 1 to 3 W, a spot size of 1.5 to 3.5 mm and a power density of approximately 25 W to 44 W/cm^2. Substantial cosmetic improvement was achieved, with no deep scarring and no secondary telangiectatic reactions or chronic radiation changes. Plates 4–9 illustrate port-wine hemangiomas treated with the argon laser.

Capillary Cavernous Hemangiomas

Apfelberg et al[29] treated 14 patients with capillary cavernous hemangiomas. The laser spot size was 1 mm. Power setting was 1 to 2.5 W and the power density was 100 to 250 W/cm^2. The darker the lesion, the greater the power required. After 29 months, 11 patients experienced excellent or good results, and three patients experienced poor results. No scarring occurred in any of the patients.

Telangiectasia

The argon laser was used to treat 33 patients with telangiectasia.[29] The laser spot size was 1 mm. Power varied between 1 and 2.5 W, and the power density was 100 to 250 W/cm^2. The pulse duration was 0.2 sec. After 30 months, 32 patients experienced excellent-to-good results; one patient experienced a poor result.

Apfelberg et al[34] treated four patients with hereditary hemorrhagic telangiectasia. The spot size was 2 mm, and the power was 1.5 watts, and the power density was 37.5 W/cm^2. The treatment was palliative and did not prevent future bleeding. The frequency and amount of bleeding, however, was reduced. The laser treatments were repeated at 3- to 6-month intervals.

In another study, four patients with telangiectasia were treated using a spot size of 0.02 cm or 0.1 cm and a pulse duration 0.2 sec.[35] The power ranged from 0.1 to 2.0 W, with a power density of 3.93 to 78.6 W/cm^2. Of two patients with lesions in the nasolabial fold area, one experienced atrophy in the treatment site 2 months later, and the telangiectases were still visible. The other patients had fair results with vessels slightly less visible. One patient was treated in the facial area had a 50% resolution after one treatment, with no adverse effects. Another patient with unilateral facial nevoid telangiectasia had complete ablation of all telangiectases in the treated areas after 9 months.

In 92 patients with telangiectasia,[32] the laser parameters were 1.4 to 1.8 W, pulse duration of 0.3 sec, spot size of 1 mm, and power density of 180 to 230 W/cm^2. Eighty-four of the 92 patients experienced excellent-to-good results. Temporary hyperpigmentation occurred in a few patients.

The argon laser was used to treat one patient with diffuse erythema and multiple minute ectatic vessels.[35] The laser settings were 0.2 sec pulse duration, 0.1 to 2.0 Watts, with a power density of 3.93 to 78.6 W/cm^2 using the 0.02-cm spot size, and 7.31 to 146 W/cm^2 using the 0.1-cm spot size. The test site showed no erythema or visible ectasia 5 months following therapy. Slight hypopigmentation and epidermal atrophy occurred.

Kaposi's Sarcoma

In a 62-year-old white male patient with Kaposi's sarcoma, four cutaneous papules were treated with the argon laser.[36] A 2-mm spot size, a power setting of 4 W, a 0.5 sec pulse, and a power density of 130 W/cm^2 were utilized for the procedure. Gradual disappearance of all the treated lesions occurred. For the next 2 years, on a 3- to 4-month cycle, argon laser photocoagulation was used to treat new lesions. After 5 years, no recurrence or appreciable scarring was evident.

Seborrheic Keratoses

Three patients with seborrheic keratoses were treated with the argon laser.[29] The laser settings were 1 to 2.5 W, 1-mm spot size, pulse duration of 0.2 sec, and a power density of 100 to 250 W/cm^2. After 6 to 9 months, satisfactory resolution of the lesions occurred. No scarring or recurrences were reported.

Pyogenic Granuloma

Pyogenic granulomas in three patients were treated with the argon laser.[29] The laser parameters included a 1-mm spot size, 1.0 to 2.5 W, a 0.2 sec pulse duration, and a power density of 100 to 250 W/cm^2. Satisfactory resolution of the lesions occurred. No scarring or recurrences were observed after 6 to 9 months.

Seven patients with pyogenic granulomas were treated by Apfelberg et al.[34] The parameters were 1- to 5-mm spot size, 1.0 to 4.5 Watts, a power density of 4 to

450 W/cm^2, and continuous wave. Five of the patients had good results, with the lesions completely disappearing and no recurrence or residual scarring. Two patients had recurrences within 2 weeks.

Spider Nevi

The argon laser was used to treat 15 patients with spider nevi.[32] The parameters were 1.9 to 2.6 W, pulse duration of 0.3 sec, spot size of 0.5 mm, and power density of 970 to 1320 W/cm^2. The results were good for all patients.

Nevi

Four patients with pigmented nevi were treated with the argon laser.[29] The laser settings were 1.0 to 2.5 W, a 1-mm spot size, a pulse duration of 0.2 sec and a power density of 100 to 250 W/cm^2. After 6- to 9-months, no scarring or recurrences were noted. Satisfactory resolution of the lesions occurred in all patients.

Landthaler[32] treated three patients with epidermal nevi. The treatment parameters included 4.0 W, pulse duration of 0.4 sec, spot size of 2 mm, and power density of 127 W/cm^2. Results were good in all patients. The argon laser was used to treat three additional patients with epidermal nevi.[31] The parameters were a power setting of 4.0 W, a pulse duration of 0.4 sec, a spot size of 2 mm, and a power density of 127 W/cm^2. The argon laser was used to remove pigmented localized epidermal nevi in two additional patients, with no recurrence in one patient after 12 months. A patient with a verrucous nevus improved but experienced recurrence after 12 months.

Venous Lakes

Venous lakes in the perioral area were treated with the argon laser in nine patients.[34] The laser parameters were set at 1- to 5-mm spot size, 1 to 4.5 Watts, a power density of 4 to 480 W/cm^2 and continuous wave. The lesions were permanently removed with no scarring.

Landthaler et al[32] successfully treated 24 patients with venous lakes, using 2.6 W, a pulse duration of 0.3 sec, a spot size of 2 mm, and a power density of 65 W/cm^2.

Senile Hemangiomas

Seven patients with 25 senile hemangiomas were treated with the argon laser.[34] The parameters were 1 to 4.5 W, 1- to 5-mm spot size, a power density of 4 to 480 W/cm^2, and continuous wave. Total blanching of the lesions occurred, and no recurrences were reported.

Landthaler[32] successfully treated ten patients with cherry angiomas, using 1.9 to 2.6 W, pulse duration of 0.3 sec, spot size of 0.5 mm, and power density of 970 to 1320 W/cm^2.

Arndt[35] treated two patients with cherry angiomas. The laser parameters were a

0.2 sec pulse and 0.1 to 2.0 W, with a power density of 3.93 to 78.6 W/cm^2 using a 0.02-cm spot size, and 7.31 to 146 W/cm^2 using a 0.1-cm spot size. The results were excellent. The minimal power required for effectiveness was 0.5 to 0.7 W.

Spider Ectasia

Spider ectasia was treated in seven patients.[85] A pulse duration of 0.2 sec was used. The power ranged from 0.1 to 2.0 W, with a power density of 3.93 to 78.6 W/cm^2 using a 0.02-cm spot size, and 7.31 to 146 W/cm^2 using a 0.1-cm spot size. The results were good to excellent, with no recurrences or atrophy.

Angiofibroma

Six patients with angiofibromas were treated using the argon laser.[32] The settings were 1.9 to 2.6 W, a pulse duration of 0.3 sec, a spot size of 2 mm, and a power density of 60 W/cm^2. The cosmetic results were good in all patients.

A patient with angiofibromas on the face and nose was treated.[35] The power ranged from 0.1 to 2.0 Watts, with a power density of 3.93 to 78.6 W/cm^2 using a 0.02-cm spot size, and 7.31 to 146 W/cm^2 using a 0.1-cm spot size. The pulse duration was 0.2 sec. The results were excellent.

Lymphangiomas

The argon laser was employed in treating eight patients with lymphangiomas, using 2.6 to 3.0 W, pulse duration of 0.2 to 0.5 sec, 2-mm spot size, and power density of 83 to 96 W/cm.[32] Regression occurred in all patients, but with some scar formation. Three to four months following treatment, recurrence of pseudovesicles developed in all patients.

Tattoos

One hundred and thirteen patients with tattoos were treated with the argon laser, using 4.0 W, pulse duration of 0.3 sec, spot size 0.5 mm, and power density of 2040 W/cm^2.[32] Twenty of the patients completed treatment, and 16 patients were still undergoing therapy. Seventy-seven patients did not return following the laser test patch because of poor results. The disadvantages of the argon laser for tattoo removal include scar formation with the same configuration as the tattoo, formation of keloids, and multiple repeat treatments for extensive tattoos. Therefore, it is not an ideal treatment for this purpose.

Verrucae

Landthaler et al[32] treated verrucae, in five patients, using 4.0 W, a pulse duration of 0.8 sec, a 0.5-mm spot size, and a power density of 2040 W/cm^2. Very high power densities were needed to vaporize the verrucae. One patient experienced a recurrence; four were treated successfully.

Xanthelasma

Five patients with xanthelasma of the eyelids were treated with the argon laser, using 2.6 W, a pulse duration of 0.3 sec, a spot size of 2 mm, and a power density of 83 W/cm^2.[32] A nonspecific, superficial coagulating effect of the argon laser was employed to remove these nonvascular, nonpigmented lesions. All patients were successfully treated.

Keloids

Five patients with keloids were treated with the argon laser, using 4.0 W, a pulse duration of 0.3 sec, a spot size of 2 mm, and a power density of 127 W/cm^2.[32] Followup showed no improvement.

PULSED TUNABLE DYE LASER

The pulsed tunable dye laser is used in treating cutaneous vascular lesions because of its highly specific effect on blood vessels in the upper dermis. The laser contains a fluorescent dye, rhodamine 6 G, which emits yellow light at 577 nm.[1] Using different dyes causes changes in the wavelength.[3] The 577 nm wavelength allows a laser penetration of 3 mm, which is ideal for selective absorption by intravascular oxyhemoglobin in the superficial dermis. The three absorption peaks of the target oxyhemoglobin are 415, 544, and 577 nm.[4]

In addition to the specific wavelength, a specific pulse duration of 360 μsec is used. This matches the thermal relaxation time for dermal blood vessels.[5] Thermal energy from laser exposure remains in the absorbing structure for a limited amount of time. If the exposure time is greater than the time necessary for the heated target structure to cool (the thermal relaxation time), the heat will spread to the surrounding tissue. If laser-exposure time is less than that needed to cool it, the target structure will remain much hotter than the surrounding area. Consequently, specific laser-induced blood vessel damage may be increased if the period of exposure to laser energy is within the thermal relaxation time of the target blood vessels. Therefore, diffuse, nonspecific thermal necrosis and scarring are avoided with the pulsed dye laser.

Port-wine Hemangiomas

The pulsed tunable dye laser (577 nm wavelength) theoretically appears to be a good instrument for port-wine hemangiomas because of its selectivity for cutaneous microvessels with minimal damage to surrounding tissue.[37] The CO_2 and argon lasers produce more epidermal damage. Three volunteers with port-wine hemangiomas had test areas treated with the CO_2, argon, and tunable dye lasers. The argon laser was used in a focused mode, with a 1-mm diameter spot size, a power density of 150 W/cm^2, and continuous wave. The CO_2 laser was used with a power density of 150 W/cm^2, a 2-mm diameter spot size, and continuous wave. The flashlamp–pumped tunable dye laser was used at 577 nm with rhodamine 575 dye, a 1-mm diameter spot size, and a pulse duration of 360 μsec.

After one year of followup, the tunable dye laser–treated areas appeared normal, with no scarring or abnormal pigmentation. The areas treated with the CO_2 and argon lasers showed atrophy, hypopigmentation, and an alteration of surface skin markings. This preliminary study concluded that at least some port-wine hemangiomas can be treated effectively, without scarring, using the tunable dye laser.

Garden et al[38] treated fifty-two patients with port-wine hemangiomas using the tunable dye laser at 577 nm.[38] Seventy-three percent of the patients treated using a 360 μsec pulse duration had an overall color fading of 50% or greater. Twenty-seven percent had fading of less than 50%. After multiple treatment sessions at the same site, no sclerosis or scarring was seen. The anatomic location, color of the lesion, and age of the patient were not related to the outcome.

Morelli et al[39] treated ten patients with port-wine hemangiomas using the tunable dye laser at 577 nm. The laser parameters used were a 3-mm spot size, an energy fluence of 70 J/cm^2, and a pulse duration of 300 μsec. After 6 weeks, the areas were treated again to achieve complete clearance. Four to six weeks after the second treatment normal skin color returned to the treated areas, and no hypertrophic scarring developed.

Glassberg et al[40] treated 28 patients with port-wine hemangiomas with the tunable dye laser at 577 nm. A 5-mm diameter spot size, and an energy fluence of 5.50 to 7.50 J/cm^2 was used on all patients. Of the 28 patients treated, 27 experienced fading of the port-wine hemangiomas. Ten patients had excellent results, with 75% fading. Eleven patients had good results, with 50% to 57% fading. Six patients had fair results, with 25% to 50% fading. One patient had minimal fading to none. Limited areas of hyperpigmentation developed in five patients. Minimal scarring developed in one patient because of an equipment malfunction.

In another study the flashlamp-pulsed tunable dye laser was employed to treat 35 children ranging in age from 3 months to 14 years.[41] The laser was used at a wavelength of 577 nm, a pulse duration of 360 μsec, a 5-mm diameter spot size, and 6 J/cm^2 exposure. The port-wine hemangioma were cleared completely in the test areas in 32 patients (91.4%). No scarring was observed. An average of 6.5 treatments was required to clear the port-wine hemangiomas. Thirty-three of the 35 patients had normal skin color and texture after treatment. Isolated superficial depressed scars 5 mm in diameter occurred in two of the 35 children treated. The patients who experienced scarring had accidentally traumatized the area within 24 hr following laser treatment. Twenty of the 35 patients experienced hyperpigmentation, which cleared in 3 to 4 months. The pulsed tunable dye laser appears to reduce the risk of inducing hypertrophic scarring compared with the argon laser in treating vascular lesions in children.

Finally, the argon-pumped, continuous tunable dye laser at 577 nm was used to treat single blood vessels within port-wine hemangiomas.[42] A 0.1-mm beam of light under 8× magnification was used for treatment. Excellent results were reported. Adverse effects such as textural change, permanent pigmentary abnormality, or hypertrophic scarring were not seen.

TABLE 5.1. *Cutaneous Disorders Treated With Laser Surgery Not Covered in This Chapter*

Disorder	Spot size (nm)	Power W	Power density (W/cm²)
CO₂ laser			
Acne keloidalis nuchae[61]	. . .	. . .	130–150
Angiofibroma[49]	2	5	160
Angiolymphoid hyperplasia[47]	2	4	127
Blastomycosis-like pyoderma[52]	. . .	8	. . .
Bowenoid papulosis & Bowen's disease[68]	1.5	13	414–736
Chromomycosis[57]	0.1	15	. . .
Circumscribed plaque psoriasis[48]	2	5–6	160–200
Familial benign chronic pemphigus[59]	1	8	1020
Granuloma annulare[51]	. . .	10–14	. . .
Granuloma faciale[60]	0.5	5	638
Hereditary multiple glomus tumors[67]	2	4	127.4
Linear porokeratosis[53]	0.3	. . .	5700–8600
Linear porokeratosis[54]	0.17	5	2941
Lymphangioma circumscriptum[55]	2	15–25	480–780
Lymphangioma circumscriptum[56]	2	5	159
Multiple eruptive vellus hair cysts[58]	2	5	160
Nodular primary localized cutaneous amyloidosis[62]	2	4	130
Syringoma[50]	2	5	159
Syringoma[17]	. . .	10	. . .
Argon laser			
Acne rosacea[34]	1–5	1–4.5	. . .
Acne rosacea[35]	0.2–1.0	0.1–2.0	3.93–146
Angiokeratoma[64]	1	1–3.5	4.45–127
Angiokeratoma[32]	0.5	1.9–2.6	970–1320
Angioma serpiginosum[32]	0.5	1.9–2.6	970–1320
Bowenoid papulosis & Bowen's disease[68]	2	3	95
Granuloma faciale[63]	1–5	0.6–1.8	. . .
Hereditary multiple glomus tumors[61]	2	. . .	63.7
Lymphocytoma[66]	2	3.5	111
Nevus of Ota (oculodermal melanocytosis)[34]	1–5	1–4.5	. . .
Postsolar poikiloderma[65]	5	2	10
Syringoma[32]	2	2.6	83
Nd:YAG laser			
Bowenoid papulosis & Bowen's disease[68]	2	20	637

Nd:YAG LASER

The Nd:YAG laser emits light from a stimulated crystal at the near-infrared portion of the electromagnetic spectrum at a wavelength of 1060 nm.[2] The tissue-laser interaction is different from other lasers—the laser light is absorbed by proteins instead of water or chromaphores. This causes energy from the laser to scatter, causing a zonal area of destruction.[2] The laser can penetrate deep into the dermis and coagulate vessels up to 4 mm in diameter. The coagulating effect makes this laser extremely useful in achieving hemostasis.[2] Deep angiomas and angiomas with large vascular channels have been effectively treated with the Nd:YAG laser.

Research continues in using this laser for treating fibrotic diseases such as keloids. The Nd:YAG laser has been shown to inhibit fibroblasts in tissue culture. Laser welding for skin incisions is also being investigated.[2] The laser is able to produce a protein coagulum that seals the incised wound. The following dermatologic disorders have been treated with the Nd:YAG laser.

Vascular Lesions

The Nd:YAG laser was used to treat three patients with nodular port-wine hemangiomas, one patient with macrocheilia resulting from a hypertrophic hemangioma, and one patient with capillary hemangioma.[43] The energy fluence was 400 to 1600 J/cm^2 with a power density of 800 to 1600 W/cm^2. Lesions were lightened and flattened after a few treatments; however, scars formed in two patients. After two years, the patient with the macrocheilia was stable. After 18 months and five treatments, the capillary hemangioma had regressed significantly.

Shapshay et al[44] treated hemangiomas of the head and neck. Sixteen patients (adult and pediatric) were treated for hypertrophic port-wine hemangiomas, cavernous hemangiomas, capillary hemangiomas, and mixed hemangiomas. The parameters used were 0.5 to 0.7 sec exposure time and 20 to 30 W. Fourteen of the 16 patients experienced excellent results, and two patients had good results. The mean followup time was 18 months.

Skin Closure

In a comparison study, 6-mm skin incisions were made on the backs of hairless mice.[45] An incision closed by laser welding with the Nd:YAG laser was designated as the experimental wound, and an incision closed with interrupted 5-0 polypropylene sutures was designated as the control wound. The Nd:YAG laser settings were 1.0 W, continuous wave, 1-mm spot size, and 50 W/cm^2 power density. Rapid healing was seen in the laser-welded wounds. Throughout the healing process the tensile strength remained the same for both the control and experimental wounds. The control group showed higher levels of collagen-specific mRNA than the laser group showed. The results imply that laser welding is advantageous because of its nontactile, sterile nature. Also no foreign material is introduced into the wound and cosmetic results can be excellent.

Three different lasers were used to close cutaneous wounds:[46] the CO_2, argon, and Nd:YAG. A spot size of 0.02 cm², a power setting of 1.0 W, and a power density of 5000 W/cm² were used. The laser-welded closure of cutaneous wounds was successful with all three lasers.

Miscellaneous disorders not described in this chapter are covered in Table 5.1.

REFERENCES

1. Bailin PL: Lasers in dermatology—1985. *J Dermatol Surg Oncol* 11:328–334, 1985.
2. Wheeland RG: *Lasers in Skin Disease.* New York, Thieme, 1988, pp 7–137.
3. Ratz JL: *Lasers in Cutaneous Medicine and Surgery.* Chicago, Year Book, 1986, pp 22–111.
4. Wheeland RG, Bailin PL, Ratz JL: Combined carbon dioxide laser excision and vaporization in the treatment of rhinophyma. *J Dermatol Surg Oncol* 13:172–177, 1987.
5. Eisen RF, Katz AE, Bohigian RK, et al: Surgical treatment of rhinophyma with the Shaw scalpel. *Arch Dermatol* 122:307–309, 1986.
6. Kantor GR, Wheeland RG, Bailin PL, et al: Treatment of earlobe keloids with carbon dioxide laser excision: a report of 16 cases. *J Dermatol Surg Oncol* 11:1063–1067, 1985.
7. Dufresne RG Jr, Garrett AB, Bailin PL, et al: Carbon dioxide laser treatment of chronic actinic cheilitis. *J Am Acad Dermatol* 19:876–878, 1988.
8. David LM: Laser vermillion ablation for actinic cheilitis. *J Dermatol Surg Oncol* 11: 605–608, 1985.
9. Bailin PL, Ratz JL, Levine HL: Removal of tattoos by CO_2 laser. *J Dermatol Surg Oncol* 6:997–1001, 1980.
10. Groot DW, Arlette JP, Johnston PA: Comparison of the infrared coagulator and the carbon dioxide laser in the removal of decorative tattoos. *J Am Acad Dermatol* 15:518–522, 1986.
11. Ruiz-Esparza J, Goldman MP, Fitzpatrick RE: Tattoo removal with minimal scarring: the chemo-laser technique. *J Dermatol Surg Oncol* 14:1372–1376, 1988.
12. Ratz JL, Bailin PL, Levine HL: CO_2 laser treatment of port-wine stains: a preliminary report. *J Dermatol Surg Oncol* 8:1039–1044, 1982.
13. Adams EL, Price NM: Treatment of basal cell carcinomas with a carbon dioxide laser. *J Dermatol Surg Oncol* 5:803–806, 1979.
14. Wheeland RG, Bailin PL, Ratz JL, et al: Carbon dioxide laser vaporization and curettage in the treatment of large multiple superficial basal cell carcinomas. *J Dermatol Surg Oncol* 13:119–125, 1987.
15. Sawchuk WS, Heald PW: CO_2 laser treatment of trichoepithelioma with focused and defocused beam. *J Dermatol Surg Oncol* 10:905–907, 1984.
16. Wheeland RG, Bailin PL, Kronberg E: Carbon dioxide laser vaporization for the treatment of multiple trichoepithelioma. *J Dermatol Surg Oncol* 10:470–475, 1984.
17. Fleming MG, Brody N: A new technique for laser treatment of cutaneous tumors. *J Dermatol Surg Oncol* 12:1170–1175, 1986.
18. Ratz JL, Bailin PL, Wheeland RG: Carbon dioxide laser treatment of epidermal nevi. *J Dermatol Surg Oncol* 12:567–570, 1986.
19. Dover JS, Smoller BR, Stern RS, et al: Low-fluence of carbon dioxide laser irradiation of lentigines. *Arch Dermatol* 124:1219–1224, 1988.

20. Stoner MF, Hobbs ER: Treatment of multiple dermal cylindromas with the carbon dioxide laser. *J Dermatol Surg Oncol* 14:1263–1267, 1988.

21. Apfelberg DB, Maser MR, Lash H, et al: Treatment of xanthelasma palpebrarum with the carbon dioxide laser. *J Dermatol Surg Oncol* 13:149–151, 1987.

22. Roenigk RK, Ratz JL: CO_2 laser treatment of cutaneous neurofibromas. *J Dermatol Surg Oncol* 13:187–190, 1987.

23. David LM, Sanders G: CO_2 laser blepharoplasty: a comparison of cold steel and electrocautery. *J Dermatol Surg Oncol* 13:110–114, 1987.

24. Olsen TG, Milroy SK, Goldman L, et al: Laser surgery for blue rubber bleb nevus. *Arch Dermatol* 115:81–82, 1979.

25. Wheeland RG, Bailin PL: Scalp reduction surgery with the carbon dioxide laser. *J Dermatol Surg Oncol* 10:565–569, 1984.

26. Wheeland RG: Revision of full thickness skin grafts using the carbon dioxide laser. *J Dermatol Surg Oncol* 14:130–134, 1988.

27. Cottel WI, Bailin PL, Albom MJ, et al: Essentials of Mohs' micrographic surgery. *J Dermatol Surg Oncol* 14:11–13, 1988.

28. Bailin PL, Ratz JL, Lutz-Nagy L: CO_2 laser modification of Mohs' surgery. *J Dermatol Surg Oncol* 7:621–623, 1981.

29. Apfelberg DB, Maser MR, Lash H: Extended clinical use of the argon laser for cutaneous lesions. *Arch Dermatol* 115:719–721, 1979.

30. Finley JL, Barsky SH, Geer DE, et al: Healing of port-wine stains after argon laser therapy. *Arch Dermatol* 117:486–489, 1981.

31. Rotteleur G, Mordon S, Buys B, et al: Robotized scanning laser handpiece for the treatment of portwine stains and other angiodysplasias. *Lasers Surg Med* 8:283–287, 1988.

32. Landthaler M, Haina D, Waidelich W, et al: A three-year experience with the argon laser in dermatotherapy. *J Dermatol Surg Oncol* 10:456–461, 1984.

33. Goldman L, Dreffer R: Laser treatment of extensive mixed cavernous and portwine stains. *Arch Dermatol* 113:504–505, 1977.

34. Apfelberg DB, Maser MR, Lash H, et al: Expanded role of the argon laser in plastic surgery. *J Dermatol Surg Oncol* 9:145–151, 1983.

35. Arndt KA: Argon laser therapy of small cutaneous vascular lesions. *Arch Dermatol* 118:220–224, 1982.

36. Wheeland RG, Bailin PL, Norris MJ: Argon laser photocoagulative therapy of Kaposi's sarcoma: a clinical and histologic evaluation. *J Dermatol Surg Oncol* 11:1180–1185, 1985.

37. Tan OT, Carney JM, Margolis R, et al: Histologic responses of portwine stains treated by argon, carbon dioxide and tunable dye lasers. *Arch Dermatol* 122:1016–1022, 1986.

38. Garden JM, Polla LL, Tan OT: The treatment of portwine stains by the pulsed dye laser. *Arch Dermatol* 124:889–896, 1988.

39. Morelli JG, Tan OT, Garden J, et al: Tunable dye laser (577) treatment of portwine stains. *Lasers Surg Med* 6:94–99, 1986.

40. Glassberg E, Lask GP, Tan OT, et al: The flashlamp-pumped 577 nm pulsed tunable dye laser: clinical efficacy and in vitro studies. *J Dermatol Surg Oncol* 14:1200–1208, 1988.

41. Tan OT, Sherwood K, Gilchrist BA: Treatment of children with portwine stains using the flashlamp-pulsed tunable dye laser. *New Engl J Med* 320:416–421, 1989.

42. Scheibner A, Wheeland RG: Argon-pumped tunable dye laser therapy for facial port-

wine stain hemangiomas in adults: a new technique using small spot size and minimal power. *J Dermatol Surg Oncol* 15:277–282, 1989.

43. Landthaler M, Haina D, Brunner R, et al: Neodymium-YAG laser therapy for vascular lesions. *J Am Acad Dermatol* 14:107–117, 1986.

44. Shapshay SM, David LM, Zeitels S: Neodymium-YAG laser photocoagulation of hemangiomas of the head and neck. *Laryngoscope* 97:323–330, 1987.

45. Abergel RP, Lyons RF, White RA, et al: Skin closure by Nd:YAG laser welding. *J Am Acad Dermatol* 14:810–814, 1986.

46. Abergel RP, Lyons R, Dwyer R, et al: Use of lasers for closure of cutaneous wounds: experience with Nd:YAG, argon, and CO_2 lasers. *J Dermatol Surg Oncol* 12:1181–1185, 1986.

47. Hobbs ER, Bailin PL, Ratz JL, et al: Treatment of angiolymphoid hyperplasia of the external ear with carbon dioxide laser. *J Am Acad Dermatol* 19:345–349, 1988.

48. Bekassy Z, Astedt B: Carbon dioxide laser vaporization of plaque psoriasis. *Br J Dermatol* 14:489–492, 1986.

49. Wheeland RG, Bailin PL, Kantor GR, et al: Treatment of adenoma sebaceum with carbon dioxide laser vaporization. *J Dermatol Surg Oncol* 11:861–864, 1985.

50. Wheeland RG, Bailin PL, Reynolds OD, et al: Carbon dioxide (CO_2) laser vaporization of multiple facial syringomas. *J Dermatol Surg Oncol* 12:225–228, 1986.

51. Rouilleault P: CO_2 laser and granuloma annulare. *J Dermatol Surg Oncol* 14:120, 1988.

52. Sawchuk WS, Heald PW: Resident's corner: blastomycosis-like pyoderma—report of a case responsive to combination therapy utilizing minocycline and carbon dioxide laser debridement. *J Dermatol Surg Oncol* 12:1041–1044, 1986.

53. Hunziker T, Bayard W: Carbon dioxide laser in the treatment of porokeratosis. *J Am Acad Dermatol* 16:625, 1987.

54. Barnett JH: Linear porokeratosis: treatment with the carbon dioxide laser. *J Am Acad Dermatol* 14:902–904, 1986.

55. Bailin PL, Kantor GR, Wheeland RG: Carbon dioxide laser vaporization of lymphangioma circumscriptum. *J Am Acad Dermatol* 14:257–262, 1986.

56. Eliezri YD, Sklar JA: Lymphangioma circumscriptum: review and evaluation of carbon dioxide laser vaporization. *J Dermatol Surg Oncol* 14:357–364, 1988.

57. Kuttner BJ, Siegle RJ: Treatment of chromocycosis with a CO_2 laser. *J Dermatol Surg Oncol* 12:965–968, 1986.

58. Huerter CJ, Wheeland RG: Multiple eruptive vellus hair cysts treated with carbon dioxide laser vaporization. *J Dermatol Surg Oncol* 13:260–263, 1987.

59. Don PC, Carney PS, et al: Carbon dioxide laser abrasion: a new approach to management of familial benign chronic pemphigus (Hailey-Hailey disease). *J Dermatol Surg Oncol* 13:1187–1194, 1987.

60. Wheeland RG, Ashley JR, Smith DA, et al: Carbon dioxide laser treatment of granuloma faciale. *J Dermatol Surg Oncol* 10:730–733, 1984.

61. Kantor GR, Ratz JL, Wheeland RG: Treatment of acne keloidalis nuchae with carbon dioxide laser. *J Am Acad Dermatol* 14:263–267, 1986.

62. Truhan AP, Garden JM, Roenigk HH Jr: Nodular primary localized cutaneous amyloidosis: immunohistochemical evaluation and treatment with carbon dioxide laser. *J Am Acad Dermatol* 14:1058–1062, 1986.

63. Apfelberg DB, Druker D, Maser MR, et al: Granuloma faciale treatment with the argon laser. *Arch Dermatol* 119:575–576, 1983.

64. Hobbs ER, Ratz JL: Argon laser treatment of angiokeratomas. *J Dermatol Surg Oncol* 13:1319–1320, 1987.

65. Goldman L, Bauman WE: Laser test treatment for postsolar poikiloderma. *Arch Dermatol* 120:578–579, 1984.

66. Wheeland RG, Kantor GR, Bailin PL, et al: Role of the argon laser in the treatment of lymphocytoma cutis. *J Am Acad Dermatol* 14:267–272, 1986.

67. Barnes L, Estes SA: Laser treatment of hereditary multiple glomus tumors. *J Dermatol Surg Oncol* 12:912–915, 1986.

68. Landthaler M, Haina D, Brunner R, et al: Laser therapy of bowenoid papulosis and Bowen's disease. *J Dermatol Surg Oncol* 12:1253–1257, 1986.

6

Rhinology and Surgery of the Paranasal Sinuses

James A. Stankiewicz

Laser surgery in the nose and paranasal sinuses is becoming increasingly popular among head and neck surgeons because improved laser delivery systems permit better visualization and exposure. Initially, the carbon dioxide (CO_2) laser was used for the majority of endonasal procedures, but the Nd:YAG, argon, and KTP/532 lasers have also been found useful, and the indications for laser surgery continue to expand. Although the laser is not always better than nonlaser or traditional techniques, it is an adjunctive tool that expands the alternatives of treatment.

INSTRUMENTATION AND TECHNIQUE

The CO_2 laser can be used either hand-held or microscopically. Several authors have adapted otologic instruments such as an ear speculum and Shea speculum holder to allow for microscopic intranasal laser surgery (Fig. 6.1).[1]

As with any laser surgery, the face, body, and endotracheal tube are protected with wet drapes and all skin is covered. A slit can be cut in a surgical towel to allow the speculum to be inserted. The towel is, of course, kept moist. The nasal speculum should be kept moist, especially in the continuous mode, to avoid overheating and a nasal burn. The ala must be protected, especially if the hand-held laser is used. The eyes are protected with moist sponges or goggles. To aid smoke removal, a laser smoke evacuation unit should be used instead of standard suction.

The patient's head is positioned without the use of a donut or rolled sheets, making it easier to adjust the head during surgery. One surgeon recommends using wet cotton work gloves to avoid laser damage to the hands.[1]

Any bony structure will turn an intensely bright white when the laser strikes it. Repeated impacts can cause eye pain, and there is a possibility of eye damage. Any

Acknowledgment: My thanks to Julie O'Keefe for her help in the preparation of this manuscript.

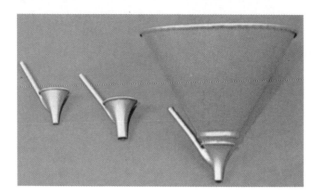

Figure 6.1. Suction specula for carbon dioxide laser nasal surgery. (Printed with permission: Selkin S: Pitfalls in intranasal laser surgery and how to avoid them. *Arch Otolaryngol Head Neck Surg* 112:285–289, 1986. © 1986, American Medical Association.)

work on septal cartilage should preserve perichondrium on the opposite side to avoid a septal perforation.

The Nd:YAG, argon, and KTP/532 lasers require special glasses to avoid eye injury. Glasses are much easier than goggles to use with the microscope or telescope. The Nd:YAG fiber has a metal tip that prevents it from bending easily. Thus, it cannot be used in smaller curved carriers, which can be inconvenient. The fiber should be backed off 1 to 2 cm from the lesion. The contact tip need be used only if cutting is necessary. Unless the lesion is particularly vascular, the CO_2 laser might work better for excision. Special carriers to hold the Nd:YAG fiber can be made from otologic-suction or suction-irrigation units (Figs. 6.2 and 6.3).

Endoscopic telescopes are very helpful in removal or coagulation of intranasal pathology. The microscope is also helpful, but hands and instruments tend to obstruct the field of vision. A second suction/smoke evacuator placed in the nose or attached to the carrier helps clear smoke from the operative area.

The argon and KTP/532 lasers can cauterize vessels up to 1 mm in diameter. These lasers at low power settings can vaporize submucosal vessels without epithelial or mucosal damage. Higher power settings can cause damage however. The Nd:YAG can cauterize vessels up to 1.5 mm in diameter with deep absorption, making it useful for vascular lesions in the nose and nasopharynx.

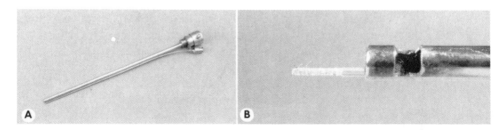

Figure 6.2. KTP/532 endoscopic sheath. (Printed with permission: Levine H: Endoscopy and the KTP/532 laser for nasal sinus disease. *Ann Otol Rhinol Laryngol* 98:46–51, 1989. © 1989, Annals Publishing Company.)

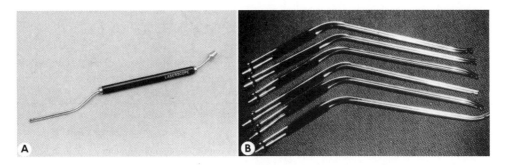

Figure 6.3. Suction hand pieces with channels for laser fiber and smoke evacuation. (Printed with permission): Levine H: Endoscopy and the KTP/532 laser for nasal sinus disease. *Ann Otol Rhinol Laryngol* 98:46–51, 1989. © 1989, Annals Publishing Company.)

SPECIFIC CLINICAL ENTITIES

Rhinophyma

Rhinophyma, occurs as the end stage of acne rosacea. The nose becomes enlarged and often unsightly as sebaceous glands and fibrous tissue proliferate. The CO_2 laser can be used to ablate rhinophyma in a bloodless field. Roenigk[2] uses the carbon dioxide laser in a defocused mode to vaporize skin.

The skin is painted preoperatively with gentian violet. Local anesthesia is injected as for a rhinoplasty. The handpiece focused to 0.5 mm spot size is used in continuous mode. It is retracted about 1.5 inches from the nose, with the power setting at 3 to 7 W. to provide the depth of penetration desired. If a microscope (400-mm lens) is used, the power is set at 10 to 50 W.

The skin is vaporized in layers. All hypertrophic tissue receives one pass and then the nose is sculpted. Charred debris is removed at each pass. Vaporization is continued only so long as sebaceous pores are visualized. If vaporization continues until the pores are obliterated, healing is prolonged and unacceptable scarring occurs (Fig. 6.4). Shapshay and coworkers[3] recommend leaving an intact rim of skin around the nares to prevent stenosis.

The nose is debulked and then contoured. An index finger "milks out" sebum from the sebaceous ducts to the point where sebum is barely expressible; this point represents the dissection limit.

Postoperatively, antibiotic oinment is placed. Antibiotics are not given. Pain is minimal. Reepithelialization occurs from the skin margins and appendages of the sebaceous pores and takes 3 to 4 weeks. During healing, the wound is cleansed with dilute hydrogen peroxide, and antibiotic oinment is applied to the nasal surface. The skin is red for several months, and the patient must be instructed to avoid exposure to the sun.

Complications are minimal and mainly related to prolonged healing or scarring from too aggressive laser surgery.

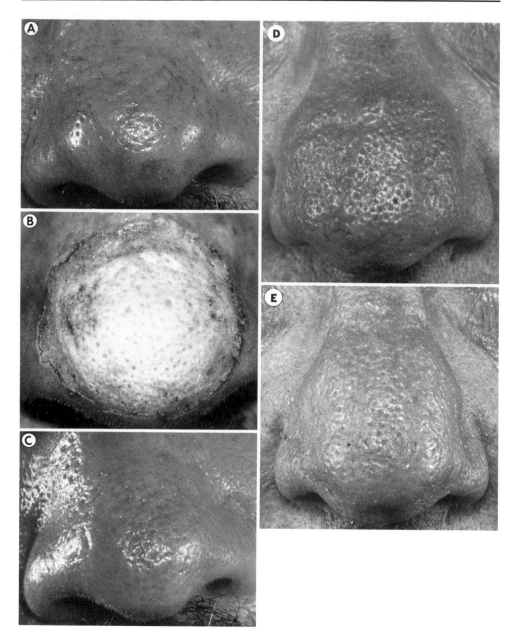

Figure 6.4. Results of carbon dioxide laser treatment of rhinophyma in two patients. Case 1 A,B,C: (*A*) preoperatively; (*B*) immediate postoperatively; (*C*) 2 months postoperatively. Case 2 D,E: (*D*) preoperative appearance; (*E*) 2 months postoperatively. (Printed with permission: Roenigk R: Carbon dioxide vaporization for treatment of rhinophyma. *Mayo Clin Proc* 62:676–680, 1987.)

Hypertrophic Turbinates

When nasal turbinate hypertrophy is obstructive and unresponsive to medical therapy, including allergy evaluation and management, it may be necessary to perform a partial turbinate resection. The laser is ideal for this, and either a CO_2 or a KTP/532 laser may be used. Cryotherapy is an alternative to laser turbinectomy and may be tried prior to turbinate resection. It is important to gauge whether the turbinate in an individual patient is hypertrophic secondary to soft tissue engorgement or bony hypertrophy. The treatment for bony hypertrophy is submucous resection. The laser is helpful only with soft tissue hypertrophy.

The nose is prepared as previously described and a nasal/otologic speculum is inserted. Visualization is better and the chance of inadvertent injury is less if the microscope is used.

The CO_2 laser is set at 10 to 15 W and a 0.1-sec duration in pulsed mode or a continuous mode can be used. The whole turbinate is not removed; only the medial anterior portion is vaporized. The lateral subturbinate mucosa is avoided to spare the nasolacrimal duct. Also avoided is the superior turbinate mucosa.[1] Vaporizing too posteriorly may cause a synechia. A white flash of light indicates turbinate bone and is the limit of vaporization. Continued vaporization may lead to turbinate bone necrosis or may injure the surgeon's eyes.[1]

Furitake and colleagues[4] used the CO_2 laser in 140 patients with allergic rhinitis; 1 year after surgery 48% had excellent results and an additional 29% had good results. Fibrous proliferation and scar formation were noted histopathologically in the superficial layer of submucosa. The mucosa healed within 2 months after surgery.

The KTP/532 or argon laser is used in an intermediate power setting 5 to 8 W and a midrange slightly defocused spot size (0.6 to 1.0 mm).[5] According to Levine,[5] the surface is vaporized and coagulated to include the anterior one half to two thirds of the inferior turbinate, crosshatching the mucosa from anterior to posterior and then superior to inferior. If the middle turbinate is involved, it is also photocoagulated (Fig. 6.5). The flexible fiber facilitates photocoagulation. Endoscopy also greatly aids in visualization and specific photocoagulation.

Polypoid mucosal changes or mulberrylike turbinates require higher wattage (9 to 12 Watts). Levine's 32 patients treated with the KTP/532 laser have all done well at 1 year.

Complications have to do with overenthusiastic laser photocoagulation. Synechia(e), bone necrosis and sequestration with infection, and injury to the nasolacrimal duct may occur.

Hereditary Telangiectasia (Osler-Weber-Rendu)

Treatment for the vascular disorder known as hereditary telangiectasia is difficult, and no single treatment method is curative. Bleeding originates from subepithelial thin-walled, vascular lesions that burst easily and cause profound epistaxis. Numerous techniques of cautery, whether it be electrocautery, cryotherapy, or laser cautery, have been used, with only temporary control of epistaxis. Abnormal vessels

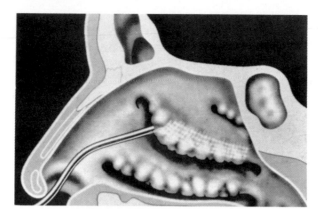

Figure 6.5.   KTP/532 laser crosshatching of turbinates. (Printed with permission: Levine H: Endoscopy and the KTP/532 laser for nasal sinus disease. *Ann Otol Rhinol Laryngol* 98:46–51, 1989. © 1989, Annals Publishing Company.)

in the anterior part of the nasal cavity are accessible to laser treatment. By using an endoscope, the surgeon can reach some telangiectasias located more posteriorly; even so, some posterior telangiectasias are obviously left untreated. Laser cautery of the anterior lesions seems to be very effective, however, probably because bleeding in these lesions is related to drying and changes in humidity. Even though not all the telangiectasia are treated, a bloodless procedure performed under a local anesthesia may provide welcome relief lasting months to years to many patients.

The CO_2 laser has been tried with varied results. The procedure can be performed under local anesthesia if the lesions are anterior. Otherwise, general anesthesia is necessary. The microscope is used at 400 mm. Laser power at 5 W is applied for 0.1-sec in a single burst or in pulses. Continuous mode is avoided to prevent nasal septal injury and perforation. The power setting of 5 W averts bleeding and excessive septal injury. Telangiectasia will form at other sites and can be treated as necessary. Simpson and coworkers[6] reported nine patients who experienced 4 to 18 months of relief from epistaxis.

The Nd:YAG laser can be used under a local anesthetic at 1- to 2-cm fiber distance from the lesion. A microscope or endoscope may be used. Low power settings (20 to 30 W) are used to avoid deep penetration into the septum. Exposure is set at a 0.2- to 0.5-sec range. The fiber can be placed into an ear suction irrigator or a straight tube carrier to aid in handling (Figs. 6.6, 6.7, and 6.8). Parkin and Dixon[7] treated patients with a great reduction in epistaxis. Five patients had not been helped by earlier nonlaser surgery. Shapshay and coworkers[8,9] treated 19 patients (15 successfully), with no epistaxis in a 6- to 9-month follow-up.

The argon and KTP/532 lasers have also been used for telangiectasia. The argon laser with selective absorption may leave overlying tissue intact without cartilage injury. However, reported control of epistaxis has been no better than with other lasers. Levine used the KTP/532 in 11 patients at 4- to 6-W power density and large spot size (0.8 to 2 mm) to gain effective coagulation.[5] The laser beam is

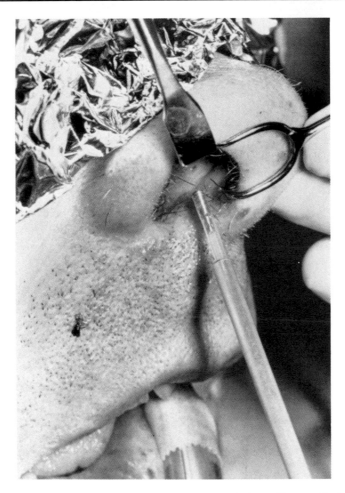

Figure 6.6. Intraoperative photograph showing Nd:YAG laser fiber applied to nasal cavity. (Printed with permission: Kluger P, et al: Neodymium:YAG laser intranasal photocoagulation in hereditary hemorrhagic telangiectasia: an update report. *Laryngoscope* 97:1397–1401, 1987,)

moved in a circular fashion around the edges of the lesion, approaching the central vessel or vascular stalk last. Bilateral treatment of lesions on the same anatomic septal area was avoided. Local anesthesia is preferred. A variety of fiber carriers for the KTP/532 are becoming available to enhance nasal use.

Follow-up of 3 to 16 months has shown a marked decrease in the severity and frequency of epistaxis.

Complications associated with any of the lasers are minimal and include septal perforation, synechia(e), and epistaxis. Patients requiring many repeated transfusions, or those having septal perforation, do not respond well to laser photocoagulation.

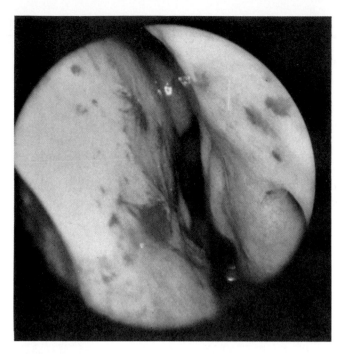

Figure 6.7. Preoperative photograph showing multiple telangiectasia. (Printed with permission: Kluger P, et al: Neodymium:YAG laser intranasal photocoagulation in hereditary hemorrhagic telangiectasia: an update report. *Laryngoscope* 97:1397–1401, 1987.)

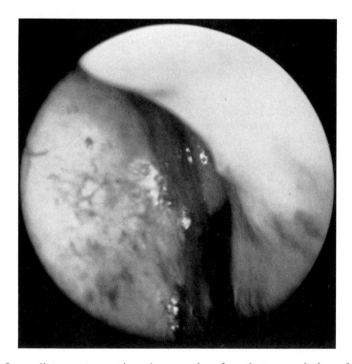

Figure 6.8. Immediate postoperative photography after photocoagulation of nasal septal telangiectasia. Note blanching effect and lack of crusting. (Printed with permission: Kluger P, et al: Neodymium:YAG laser intranasal photocoagulation in hereditary hemorrhagic telangiectasia: an update report. *Laryngoscope* 97:1397–1401, 1987.)

Choanal Atresia

Many surgical treatments for choanal atresia have been tried. At present, the transpalatal correction is probably the most reliable operation, but it is much more complex than endonasal repair. The areas of difficulty, especially if bony stenosis is present, are the bony septum and the hard palate, which are difficult to approach intranasally. Fortunately, repair can be accomplished endonasally in over 70% if preoperative preparation and the operation is carefully planned.[10]

The main concerns in deciding whether to use the laser are (1) whether the atresia is bony or membranous and (2) the thickness of the atresia plate. A preoperative CT scan can determine the nature of the atresia and help in selecting cases most suited to laser surgery.[1] If the atresia is membranous, the CO_2 laser with microscope may be used.

The patient's face is completely covered with wet towels. The internal nares are viewed with an otology speculum in a Shea holder. A wet sponge is placed in the nasopharynx. Otology instruments and suction devices are employed.

The laser is set to a power of 10 to 20 W in pulsed or continuous mode (0.1- to 0.2-sec duration). Flaps are raised, if possible, and the stenosis is vaporized to an adequate lumen size. The surgeon should try to remove the posterior bony septum to enhance healing. Leaving a raw surface around the surgical wound fosters restenosis, the major complication of this surgery.

Stenting is placed for 8 to 12 weeks, but Healy reports that laser surgery reduces edema and scarring, allowing stenting time to be reduced to 2 to 3 weeks.[12] Stenting for too long may actually contribute to restenosis.[13] Illum[14] reported nine cases in which choanal atresia was treated with the CO_2 laser. Success was achieved in six of the patients. Stenting was not used.[14] Muntz[15] noted that septal deviation, enlarged inferior turbinates, a high arched palate, and craniofacial anomalies impede surgical correction.

No reports of treatment of choanal atresia with KTP/532, argon, or Nd:YAG lasers are available at present.

As already mentioned, the main complication of this surgery is restenosis. Bleeding and infection are minimal.

Nasal Polypectomy

The laser can be used to perform polypectomy, but it is very tedious. Conventional and endoscopic techniques are probably more efficient and effective. Sometimes, however, control of bleeding is of paramount concern: in patients with underlying bleeding disorders, in cases of long-term steroid use, and in patients who have had many polypectomies. For these patients, laser polypectomy may be beneficial.

The laser provides no advantage in delaying polyp regrowth. Selkin[1] found that the CO_2 laser offers no major reduction in intraoperative and postoperative bleeding. Levine[5] suggests that the KTP/532 laser, while not helpful in totally removing polyps, can be beneficial as a debulker before and during ethmoidectomy. Special benefit is noted for removal of choanal polyps in patients with a bleeding diathesis. Both authors note that higher power densities are required to remove polyps. The surgeon should also be wary of using the laser near a potentially dehiscent lamina papyracea. Heat transferred intraorbitally may damage the medial rectus muscle or the optic nerve.

The CO_2 laser is used through the microscope with power density at 15 to 25 W. Pulsed or continuous mode can be used. The polyp is grasped in a suction tip or forceps to put it on tension. The laser is used to remove the lesion as close to its roots as possible.

The KTP/532 is used at high wattage (9 to 12 W) with a small spot size (0.4 to 0.8 mm).[5] The sinus endoscopes are used to visualize the polyps. Once polyps are debulked, intranasal ethmoidectomy is performed.

Postoperative care is as with standard polypectomy, although extensive packing is normally not required.

Chronic Sinusitis

The laser is of tremendous benefit in sinus surgery. The release of postoperative nasal synechiae or synechiae due to sarcoidosis can be handled with the laser.[5] Flexible-fiber lasers such as the KTP/532, argon, or Nd:YAG are easier to manipulate, and visualization is usually better through an endoscope. Polyps in the maxillary sinus may be debulked through the natural antrostomy with a sinus endoscope and flexible-fiber laser. The KTP/532 seems to be the most effective laser for this purpose.[5] Lenz and associates[16] noted that antrostomies could be made with the argon laser, but no one else has reported this use. The concha bullosa middle turbinate, which can contribute to the patient's sinus problems, can be opened with the KTP/532 and the endoscope. Higher power (9 to 12 W) with a small spot size is used to incise the turbinate. The turbinate tissue can then be vaporized or removed with endoscopic equipment.

Miscellaneous

Simple nasal papilloma, pyogenic granuloma, and hemangioma can easily be handled with the CO_2 or KTP/532 laser. Complete excision is possible. The CO_2 laser is used through the microscope and the KTP/532 with the endoscope. Carbon dioxide power settings are 10 to 15 W and KTP/532 are 5 to 10 W. Local wound care suffices nicely after the operation.

Vidian neurectomy with the carbon dioxide laser was reported by Williams,[17] who believed it offered advantages over conventional techniques. The laser was used to make a window in the superior posterior maxillary sinus walls. The Vidian canal was identified and its contents vaporized with a defocused beam. Patients had less pain, edema, and hyperesthesia than with conventional surgery. The reader is referred to Williams' article[17] for anatomic and technical details. No complications occurred.

Palliative treatment of recurrent skull base tumors can be performed with the CO_2 laser through the maxillectomy cavity.[18] The laser is used first to debulk the tumor and then to heat the bone of the skull base to destroy occult areas of tumor. No intracranial tumor extension should be apparent preoperatively. Cerebrospinal fluid leakage may occur from overheating of the skull base bone.

REFERENCES

1. Selkin S: Pitfalls in intranasal laser surgery and how to avoid them. *Arch Otolaryngol Head Neck Surg* 112:285–289, 1986.

2. Roenigk R: Carbon dioxide vaporization for treatment of rhinophyma. *Mayo Clin Proc* 62:676–680, 1987.

3. Shapshay S, et al: Removal of rhinophyma with the carbon dioxide laser. *Arch Otolaryngol* 106:257–259, 1980.

4. Furitake T, Yamashita T, Tomoda K, et al: Laser surgery for allergic rhinitis. *Arch Otolaryngol* 112:1280–1282, 1986.

5. Levine H: Endoscopy and the KTP/532 laser for nasal sinus disease. *Ann Otol Rhinol Laryngol* 98:46–51, 1989.

6. Simpson G, Shapshay S, Vaughan C: Rhinologic laser surgery. *Otolaryngol Clin North Am* 16:829–837, 1983.

7. Parkin J, Dixon J: Laser photocoagulation in hereditary hemorrhagic telangiectasia. *Otolaryngol Head Neck Surg* 89:204–208, 1981.

8. Shapshay S, Oliver P: Treatment of hereditary hemorrhagic telangiectasia by Nd:YAG laser photocoagulation. *Laryngoscope* 94:1554–1556, 1984.

9. Kluger P, Shapshay S, Hybels R: Neodymium:YAG laser intranasal photocoagulation in hereditary hemorrhagic telangiectasia: an update report. *Laryngoscope* 97:1397–1401, 1987.

10. Healy G, McGill T, Jako G, et al: Management of choanal atresia with the carbon dioxide laser. *Ann Otol Rhinol Laryngol* 87:658–662, 1978.

11. Crockett D, Healy G, McGill T: Computed tomography in the evaluation of choanal atresia in infants and children. *Laryngoscope* 97:174–183, 1987.

12. Crockett D, Healy G, McGill T: Benign lesions of the nose, oral cavity, and oropharynx in children: excision by carbon dioxide laser. *Ann Otol Rhinol Laryngol* 94:489–493, 1985.

13. Crockett D, Strasnick B: Lasers in pediatric otolaryngology. *Otolaryngol Clin North Am* 22:607–619, 1989.

14. Illum P: Congenital choanal atresia treated by laser surgery. *Rhinology* 24:205–209, 1986.

15. Muntz H: Pitfalls to laser correction of choanal atresia. *Ann Otol Rhinol Laryngol* 96:43–46, 1987.

16. Lenz H, Euhler J, Schafer G: Production of a nasoantral window with argon laser. *J Maxillofac Surg* 5:314–317, 1977.

17. Williams J: Laser Vidian neurectomy. *Ann Otol Rhinol Laryngol* 92:281–283, 1983.

18. Rontal M, Rontal E: Treatment of recurrent carcinoma at the base of the skull with the carbon dioxide laser. *Laryngoscope* 93:1261–1265, 1983.

7A
Diseases of the Oral Cavity and Pharynx: Benign Diseases

Daniel P. Akin

The oral cavity is easily accessible for application of the laser. A list of some benign oral pathologic entities that have been treated with the laser includes hemangioma,[1,2] pyogenic granuloma,[3] gingival and other dental-related problems,[4-6] ranula,[7] papilloma,[7] fibroma,[7] and pharyngeal pouch.[7] Lasers have also been used in excision of portions of Waldeyer's ring (i.e., palatine tonsillectomy),[8-11] and in lingual tonsillectomy,[12] adenoidectomy,[8,13] and palatal pharyngoplasty.[14] The CO_2, argon, KTP, and Nd:YAG lasers have been employed.

The wavelength of these lasers determines their application for specific problems because it affects absorption and penetration. In brief, the CO_2 laser is absorbed by water, the argon and KTP lasers are color-sensitive to hemoglobin and melanin, and Nd:YAG laser is color- and water-insensitive. The Nd:YAG laser has the greatest tissue penetration potential.

The CO_2 laser has the greatest number of applications in head and neck surgery, including the oral cavity and nasopharynx. Its therapeutic advantages include more precise resection of tissue, reduced trauma to the tissue bed, better control of bleeding, reduced postoperative pain, and quicker healing.[7-9]

The CO_2 laser has enjoyed fairly widespread acceptance in papilloma removal. Again, precision and depth of penetration are key factors in this application.

Application of the CO_2 laser on Waldeyer's ring has been controversial, but there seems to be little question of its benefits for excision of the lingual tonsils.[12] Here, no other technique compares with the laser's control of tissue removal and reduction in swelling, which is needed to minimize dificulties in swallowing and breathing.

The removal of palatine tonsils with the laser has been met with much skepticism.[15] Traditional approaches to this procedure have been well developed and tested by time.[16] The bulkiness and cost of laser equipment, have understandably affected surgeons' enthusiasm about the technique's advantages. Surgery training programs emphasize that good exposure and light are crucial to performing good surgery. The laser, coupled with the operating microscope, maximizes these factors in tonsillectomy and adenoidectomy.

TONSILLECTOMY AND ADENOIDECTOMY

The patient is placed in the supine position with the surgeon at the head of the table. The anesthesiologist and surgical nurse are situated at each side of the surgeon, with the anesthesiologist toward the patient's feet. When possible, a ceiling-mounted microscope is preferable, but if none is available, a floor microscope can be positioned at the head of the table and to one side of the physician. The technique for a right-handed surgeon is most effective with the laser placed to the right and behind the surgeon.

The endotracheal tube that is used should be either stainless steel or red rubber wrapped with aluminum foil. (See Chapter 3B regarding safety precautions.) Aluminum foil is also placed over the patient's upper teeth to avoid dental injury. The patient's mouth is kept open with a Crowe-Davis mouth gag. A Mayo stand is brought over the chest and the mouth gag is hooked to this stand. The endotracheal tube is secured by both the gag and (Plastopore) tape that is easily torn for quick tube removal in case of an endotracheal tube fire. Anesthesia tends to use[9] heavier tape. The eyes are protected with moist pads that are secured in position by a towel head wrap.

A small red rubber catheter (8–10 Fr., Davol® #9410) is passed through the right nostril and pulled through the mouth to retract the palate. A larger whistle-tip catheter (Davol® #10815) is passed through the opposite nostril and positioned with the tip just at the posterior aspect of the vomer bone for suction of the plume. These red rubber catheters may be flammable in an oxygen-rich environment. The entire head is wrapped with a moistened towel. A wet Mericel sponge is placed in the hypopharynx as a laser backstop. Institution of these vital protective measures takes about 1 minute.

Tonsil removal is then started. The surgeon is positioned on the side opposite the tonsil being removed, with the microscope adjusted to float easily along. A 300-mm lens is used. The CO_2 laser is set on 15 W with a spot size of 1 mm. An Allis clamp is used to grasp the apex of the capsule of the superior pole, and medial traction is applied.

Cutting with the laser is begun superiorly, hugging the tonsil capsule and cutting in layers to deliver the superior pole. Care is taken to avoid making deep holes or cutting through the tonsil capsule. Keeping the field dry is mandatory to maximize the laser's advantages. An assistant, who also has binocular microscopic vision through an observation arm, uses a suction catheter unit to control and remove any blood not controlled with the laser. The dissection proceeds from superior to inferior, delivering the tonsil with the anterior and posterior tonsillar arches intact.

After the dissection of the upper one half of the tonsil is completed the lower portion is removed as follows. Regarding the right tonsil the Allis clamp used to grasp the tonsil is rotated in a way that exposes and places tension on the lower portion of the posterior pillar. The right tonsil is also rotated in a counter clockwise direction when looking from the head of the table above the patient. This places the tonsillar tissue immediately behind the line of dissection in position to absorb any slightly errant laser impacts thus increasing safety. Removal of the left tonsil is completed in a similar fashion except that rotation is in a clockwise direction viewed from the head of the table.

One hand of the surgeon is on the joystick of the microscopic laser attachment and the other is used to apply medial traction. Again, it is very important to stay in the tonsillar capsule plane to perform the dissection efficiently and with minimum need for further electrocautery. The amount of electrocautery used correlates with the severity of postoperative pain.[9,10,17]

Good visualization at the tonsillar plane allows identification of major vessels before they are cut or injured. With this approach and the aforementioned precautions, blood loss is usually less than 1 to 3 ml. Larger vessels can be either electrocauterized or constricted with the periphery of the laser beam before cutting them. The latter maneuver comes with practice. Any tonsillar tissue left can be vaporized if complete dissection in the tonsillar plane is difficult to achieve.

Adenoidal resection is performed with the use of a front-surfaced mirror, which is placed in the oropharynx to visualize the nasopharynx. The angle of the mirror is adjusted to maximize the view of the choanal area. The surgeon is seated directly at the head of the table. Using 20 W continuous mode, the laser beam is reflected off the mirror onto the adenoids, allowing the surgeon to sculpture the adenoid tissue present. A rim of tissue is left at the level of the palate, in all cases, to eliminate the possibility of velopharyngeal incompetence. This approach also permits the removal of adenoidal tissue in a patient with submucous cleft of the soft palate.

All of the adenoidal tissues between the torus tubarious bilaterally and the vomerine bone anteriorly are vaporized. Rolling the tissue away from the torus virtually eliminates the possibility of injury to this structure. Adenoidal tissue can also be "chased" into the posterior nose beyond the end of the vomer bone. With this technique, visualization is excellent and blood loss is minimal. Incidentally, this exposure can be used in excision of other pathologic entities such as choanal atresia and nasopharyngeal tumors.

At the completion of the tonsillectomy and adenoidectomy, the red rubber suction and traction catheters are removed, and the mouth gag is then closed and taken from the mouth. The patient is awakened and taken to the recovery room. After 1 to 2 hours, the patient is taking fluids and is discharged. The patient is usually seen in 5 days, at which time a regular diet is resumed and return to work or school is permitted.

DISCUSSION

In experience at the Akins Medical Center involving over 1000 patients,[13] the following clinical observations have been made. Laser tonsillectomy with or without adenoidectomy had the following advantages:

Less postoperative pain
Quicker healing

Minimal blood loss (1–2 ml)

Less operative time (approximately 10 min)

An outpatient procedure for more than 99% of patients

Postoperative bleeding in less than 2.0% of cases

No complications due to the laser.

No transfusions were required.

The routine use of the CO_2 laser for the tonsillectomy and adenoidectomy is gaining acceptance. It is no longer reserved for special cases such as patients with bleeding disorders.

The high cost of the laser has been a concern. Recovery of such surcharges from insurance companies has been difficult. However, the cost of laser technology can be controlled by the physician if approached aggressively. In the above series, no surcharge for laser use was applied. Instead, the laser cost was recovered through increased efficiency for the surgeon and more effective use of operating room time. As hospitals become more cost-conscious and efficient, the laser tonsillectomy and adenoidectomy will become more attractive.

Appropriate endotracheal tube selection and tissue protection make the use of the laser safe (see Chapter 3). Again, no complications attributable to the laser occurred in the above series. Care must be taken to avoid impacting the teeth with the laser as tattooing of the enamel may result.

We observed less postoperative pain than with traditional techniques. Reports in the literature support this observation.[9,10,11,13] Alternative techniques such as dissection with electrocautery certainly reduce bleeding but cause increased pain and scarring.[17]

Although the KTP laser has been tried in tonsillectomy,[15,18-21] it has a greater depth of burn than the CO_2 laser and may cause more postoperative pain.

VASCULAR LESIONS OF THE ORAL CAVITY

Hemangiomas in the oral cavity are readily accessible to the laser,[1] as exemplified in the following case presentations.

A 39-year-old white male presented with a large cavernous hemangioma of the tongue. It was causing bleeding when he ate and was pushing his teeth out of normal alignment. Before laser therapy was considered, the patient was offered the alternatives of conventional hemiglossectomy or continuing "to live with it."

The Nd:YAG laser was selected because its depth of penetration would provide better coagulation. The laser was set at 11 W, a total of 1759 joules was delivered in 5-sec pulses. The operation was accomplished under general anesthesia and lasted approximately 15 minutes. No blood was lost. One week after surgery the patient's tongue appeared relatively normal.

A 33-year-old white female with a hemangioma of the oral cavity had bleeding every time she brushed her teeth. The argon laser was selected because it is well absorbed by red tissues. One treatment resolved the bleeding.

REFERENCES

1. Apfelberg DB, et al: Benefits of the CO_2 laser in oral hemangioma excision. *Plast Reconstr Surg* 75:46–50, 1985.

2. Dixon JA, et al: Laser photocoagulation of vascular malformations of the tongue. *Laryngoscope* 96:537–541, 1986.

3. Modica LA: Pyogenic granuloma of the tongue treated by carbon dioxide laser. *JAGS* 36:1036–1038, 1988.

4. Hylton RP: Use of CO_2 laser for gingivectomy in a patient with Sturge-Weber disease complicated by dilantin hyperplasia. *J Oral Maxillofac Surg* 44:646–648, 1986.

5. Abt E: Removal of benign intraoral masses using the CO_2 laser. *J Am Dent Assoc Clin Tech* 115:729–731, 1987.

6. Pick RM, et al: Use of the CO_2 laser in soft tissue dental surgery. *Lasers Surg Med* 7:207–213, 1987.

7. Evans R, et al: A review of carbon dioxide laser surgery in the oral cavity and pharynx. *J Laryngol Otol* 100:69–77, 1986.

8. Martinez SA, Akin DP: Laser tonsillectomy and adenoidectomy. *Otolaryngol Clin North Am* 20:371–376, 1987.

9. Barron J: Tonsillectomy with the CO_2 laser. *Int Laser Surg Cong 1* Chicago, June 1984.

10. Paulson M: Late effects of tonsillectomy. *Int Laser Surg Cong 1* Chicago, June 1984.

11. Lipman SP: CO_2 laser tonsillectomy. *Int Laser Surg Cong 2* Nashville, TN, June 1988.

12. Krespi YP: Endoscopic laser lingual tonsillectomy. *Int Laser Surg Cong 2* Nashville, TN, June 1988.

13. Akin DP, McDaniel AB: CO_2 laser tonsillectomy and adenoidectomy. *Int Laser Surg Cong 2* Nashville, TN, June 1988.

14. Lipman SP: Laser palatal pharyngoplasty. *Int Laser Surg Cong 2* Nashville, TN, June 1988.

15. Stevens MH: Laser surgery of tonsils, adenoid and pharynx. *Otolaryngol Clin North Am* 23:43–47, 1990.

16. Kornblut AD: A traditional approach to surgery of the tonsils and adenoids. *Otolaryngol Clin North Am* 20:349–364, 1987.

17. Mann D: Some like it hot. *Laryngoscope* 94:677–679, 1984.

18. Strunk YP: Laser versus cold steel. *Int Laser Surg Cong 2* Nashville, TN, June 1988.

19. Hightower D: KTP laser tonsillectomy, *Int Laser Surg Cong 2* Nashville, TN, June 1988.

20. Oas RE, Jr., Bartels JP: KTP-532 Laser Tonsillectomy; a comparison with standard technique. *Laryngoscope,* 100:385–388, 1990.

21. Linden B, et al: Morbidity and pediatric tonsillectomy. *Laryngoscope,* 100:120–124.

7B
Diseases of the Oral Cavity and Pharynx: Malignant Lesions

Sharon Collins

Laser excision of selected cancers of the oral cavity and oropharynx has become an accepted surgical practice. Although press reports have encouraged a public belief that the laser has magical curative properties, it is primarily a cutting tool for excision of pathologic tissues.

Early use of the laser in cancer therapy was restricted mainly to excision of small and superficial lesions for which cure could be expected with single modality treatment. Since then, indications for use of the CO_2 laser in cancer surgery have been extended to include its use in treatment of larger primary tumors as a component of multimodality head and neck cancer treatment. It has been used in cases requiring comcomitant neck dissection or reconstruction of the primary site.

The early experience in cancer treatment showed that laser excision yielded results comparable to those attained with standard surgical techniques. No wound-healing complications occurred that were attributable to laser use.[1,2] A high rate of serious complications encountered in one recent series,[3] however, was attributed primarily to the addition of postoperative radiotherapy. This matter is discussed in detail later in this chapter.

This chapter first addresses some general considerations pertaining to laser surgery, including wound healing and relevant laser physics. A discussion of technique expresses preferences based on nearly 200 laser excisions of cancers in the oral cavity, oropharynx, and pharynx. In controversial areas contrasting viewpoints will also be presented. The major portion of the technique section is a description which applies to all sites in the mouth and throat, followed by specific details relevant to the individual sites. In conclusion, this chapter will review cancer treatment and complication results.

GENERAL CONSIDERATIONS

Any lesion suitable for a *transoral* approach should be removed with the laser rather than with "cold steel." Damage to adjacent tissue is limited to a few cells, and a burn is not created. Consequently, products of acute inflammation do not accumulate, resulting in less edema and less painful stimulation of nerve endings. The fibrin coagulum that forms over the open wound provides a biologic "dressing" that also decreases pain. With negligible swelling, a tracheotomy is seldom required. These factors shorten the patient's hospital stay, thereby improving the cost effectiveness of treatment.

Because vessels less than 0.5 mm in diameter are sealed during dissection, bleeding is reduced and visualization of tissue is excellent. Small lymphatics are similarly sealed and scattered cells are vaporized and nonviable, affording the laser at least a theoretical advantage in resecting cancers.[4] Since experimental laser defects heal with little collagen formation and the wounds contain few myofibroblasts, there is said to be less contracture and scarring than after scalpel or electrocautery excision—an advantage in the mouth, where preservation of function depends on maintaining mobility after tissue excision. Subsequent examination for local recurrence would also be made easier. Clinically, there seems to be little objective difference in the amount of scar which results from a mucosal laser wound which heals by secondary intention and a traditional surgical wound.

Wound-Healing Principles

The healing process following laser excision differs in many respects from that following conventional surgical excision because of the difference in the instrument used to make the cut. Certain aspects of laser physics are relevant here.

The CO_2 laser beam's wavelength of 10.6 μm is absorbed by water. Intracellular and extracellular fluid vaporizes, and cell membranes rupture. The amount of tissue destruction and depth of penetration depend on two factors: power density and duration of exposure (see also Chapter 2). Power density (the effective penetrating power of the laser beam at the tissue surface) is determined by the spot size and by the power setting on the console (0 to 50 W). The spot size, in turn, depends on the focal length of the converging lens through which the laser beam passes, either in the handpiece (125 mm) or in the operating microscope (300 to 400 mm). To reduce tissue damage, it is desirable to *increase* power density and *decrease* contact time with tissue. This is accomplished by using a low wattage, a concentrated spot size, and a short focal length (handpiece rather than micromanipulator). With a shorter tissue-contact time, fewer pathologic artifacts confuse margin interpretation and wounds heal better. Laser manufacturers state that the intermittent repetitive pulse mode is best for the tissue.

Comparative histologic studies of wound healing in the mouth following CO_2 laser versus conventional surgical excision have been carried out.[5,6] With the laser, vaporized cellular particles are deposited as a carbonized layer on the wound surface, and within 24 hours formation of a fibrinous coagulum begins with a buff-colored base that is thickest after 7 days. The acute inflammatory reaction reaches its maximum after 4 days and is only mild. Epithelial cell migration is apparent at 4 days and continues until completed at 28 days. In contrast, surgically excised areas contract considerably and have rolled margins that flatten with time. Laser-treated wounds exhibit little contraction, and their edges are level with the adjacent tissue. Few myofibroblasts are present beneath the lasered surface, in contrast to large numbers in the "surgical steel" sites.

Myofibroblasts are thought to be the effectors of wound contraction.[7,8] In the surgical sites, myofibroblasts align parallel to the surface so that contraction in the longitudinal axis reduces the size of the defects. The few myofibroblasts in the lasered area lack orientation; thus their contraction has little effect on the overall dimensions of the defect. The reason why few myofibroblasts occur in superficial laser wounds is unknown, although their paucity may be related to the relatively minor degree of tissue irritation.

Laser wounds of the oral mucosa seem slower to reepithelialize than those made with a scalpel.[5,6] Epithelial migration occurs *over* the surface coagulum, whereas in a scalpel wound it occurs *between* the coagulum and the underlying granulation tissue. Reepithelialization clinically begins after 1 to 2 weeks and is complete by 4 to 6 weeks. The absence of wound contraction may account for the apparent delay in complete reepithelialization when compared with scalpel defects, because the surface area to be covered is greater. Resection of a large bulk of soft tissue, such as in a partial glossectomy, is associated with slightly greater wound contraction and some scarring.

Many surgeons believe that for floor of mouth lesions, using the laser instead of the knife or electrocautery has the advantage of avoiding stenosis of the submandibular ducts, which can cause obstructive problems requiring later submandibular gland excision. Although one clinical investigation found no difference in duct stenosis between the three techniques,[9] experiments have shown that transecting the orifices of the submandibular ducts with laser produces no evidence of obstruction to salivary flow.[6] Histologically, there was no stenosis of the ducts, and the epithelium of the floor of mouth and duct orificies regenerated completely, without narrowing or distortion of the opening. Sections of the submandibular glands confirmed that no obstructive changes had occurred. (Transection of the parotid ducts can be performed with even more impunity, since they tend to stay open to the surface even when transected with a knife, if not included in a suture line.)

Penetration of the CO_2 laser beam into tissue depends on the concentration of water in the cellular and extracellular compartments. Cortical bone and tooth enamel contain very little water, and charring from laser contact may result in permanent damage and tattooing. It should be remembered that the CO_2 laser is primarily an instrument used for soft tissue excisions in the head and neck, and care must be taken when using it for removal of soft tissue over the mandible. Damaging underlying cortical bone usually causes chronic inflammation of the soft tissue, delayed healing, and subsequent bone necrosis with sequestration of devitalized fragments.[6] Similarly, wounding the teeth with the CO_2 laser beam creates craters involving the enamel and dentine, and there may be damage to and degeneration of the tooth pulps even after a short laser impact. If burned, tooth enamel can be restored with composite filling materials using the acid-etch technique.

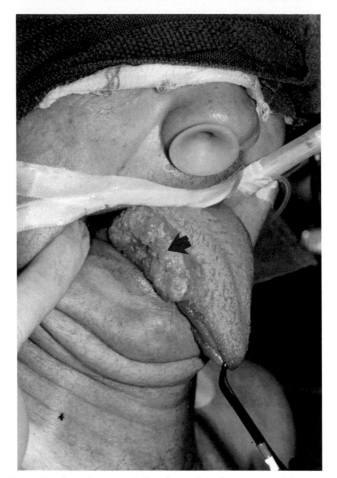

Figure 7.1. Lesion characteristics favorable for transoral laser excision.

Assessing Suitability of Cases for
Laser Excision

When the laser was first used for excision of oral cavity cancers, only superficial lesions covering a relatively small area were considered suitable. The size, thickness, and histology of the lesion (squamous or salivary gland tumors) are not the primary factors determining whether or not the laser can be used. Rather, the major determinant is whether or not exposure of the tumor is adequate through the open mouth. All margins around the tumor must be directly visible or palpable when exposed with suitable retraction (Fig. 7.1). If the lesion is not freely accessible through the open mouth, cancer control and wound healing will be disappointing, and even disastrous. This is especially true for lesions that are partially or completely submucosal (as after failure of radiotherapy with curative intent) where the extent is more difficult to assess than for exophytic lesions with clearly demarcated raised borders.

Although many small benign or premalignant lesions in the mouth can be easily excised with a scalpel under local anesthesia, the CO_2 laser has the advantages discussed above. Although a general anesthetic is usually required, no needles for injection of local anesthesia need be placed in the area of a possibly malignant tumor. The potential for spreading and seeding cancer is consequently reduced. Also, excessive bleeding may be a problem with sharp dissection, especially in such a vascular area as the mouth. Bleeding can hinder accurate excision, particularly of large superficial patches of leukoplakia where unnecessary removal of the underlying muscle will promote scar contracture.

Excisional biopsy of suspicious (premalignant) lesions of the mouth (or symptomatic benign lesions—e.g., lichen planus) is well addressed with the laser because of the absence of associated morbidity and scarring. For these reasons also, excisional biopsies can be repeated over time with relative impunity in patients with chronic, recurrent lesions of the mouth.[10-12]

As is well known, the incidence of malignant transformation in leukoplakia ranges from 0.13 to 6%. Although low, this represents a likelihood of developing oral cancer that is 50 to 100 times greater than in the normal population. Lesions with a red velvety component (erythroplasia) have 17 times the incidence of malignant transformation that is found with pure white lesions, and "speckled" (mixed red and white) areas have the same prognosis as their red counterpart. Leukoplakia in the floor of mouth and ventral surface of the tongue is an area at relatively high risk for malignant transformation.[13,14]

Two other types of lesions that have a low incidence of malignant transformation are chronic hyperplastic candidiasis (candidal leukoplakia) and lichen planus, which appears as a lacelike network of raised white striae on the buccal mucosa or dorsum of the tongue. These lesions are usually asymptomatic, although the atrophic and erosive forms may be painful. The rare malignant transformation is usually seen with the atrophic types.

Treatment of these latter two lesions usually includes topical medications—antifungals for *Candida,* and corticosteroids for lichen planus. Persistent discomfort and resistance to long-term therapy with topical medications constitute indications for surgery. The CO_2 laser is probably not suitable for vaporizing erosive lichen planus or candidal leukoplakia because these lesions recur rapidly. Several patients in the extensive experience of Frame's group[15] did report, however, that their mouths were less painful after laser therapy.

Patients with leukoplakia in the mouth often have generalized instability of the oral epithelium with dysplastic changes in the healthy-appearing mucosa adjacent to a white patch. Apparent recurrences may originate in the new epithelium that migrates from the periphery to cover the wound.

Patients with widespread mucosal changes may be reasonably approached with the premise that only the most suspicious or symptomatic area should be excised. Attempting to remove every millimeter of abnormal tissue does not prevent recurrence and can enhance scar contracture. A better approach is limited excision combined with close follow-up by a single observer who is familiar with the appearance of the patient's mouth and alert to suspicious changes.

For the same reasons, the laser is uniquely advantageous in handling certain types of malignant situations. For example, patients with "field cancerization" ("condemned" mucosa) develop *multiple* primaries in the mucosa of the upper aerodigestive tract over time.[16] In this situation, structure and function can be optimized by progressive "whittling" with the laser, with radiotherapy held in reserve. Many patients with this situation are amenable to repeated transoral laser excision of the sequential primary cancers that occur over time.

Similarly, patients who present with *simultaneous* primaries in the head and neck sometimes have multiple small superficial lesions suitable for laser excision. Here, scalpel operations might impose functional deficits and could require a larger operation to afford adequate exposure and control of the airway.

It should be remembered that the laser is to be used only for excision of soft tissue. Lesions can approach and even involve attached mucosa overlying bone, but lesions requiring excision of bone for adequate cancer removal are not suitably approached with the laser since exposed bone frequently does not remucosalize and tends to remain devitalized and sequestered, causing wound-healing problems and delaying postoperative radiotherapy. Whenever possible, the periosteum should be left intact over the mandible or maxilla by lasering through the overlying soft tissue and using a Freer elevator to elevate the soft tissue off the bone in the extraperiosteal plane. When absolutely necessary, it is possible to remove small areas of periosteum with the laser, but this is safe only when adjacent soft tissue can be mobilized to cover the defect. Undermining at cancer margins always risks implanting neoplastic cells in a wider area.

Tumors fixed to periosteum over a large surface should be approached with a standard surgical technique that includes some type of bone excision—either marginal mandibulectomy; inner table mandibulectomy;[17] or exposure via cheek flap, mandibular "swing,"[18] or composite resection.

Thickness of a neoplasm is not an absolute contraindication to laser excision but tumors that penetrate soft tissue deeply are generally not suitable. Examples would include tumors in the muscular sling of the floor of mouth, in the pterygoid area, or deep in the posterior oral cavity (as demonstrated by the clinical signs of trismus and/or tongue tethering). Although laser excision is technically possible, such lesions tend to involve additional areas such as the mandible or the neck, where excision by standard techniques is more appropriate. Their removal leaves a large defect that generally requires reconstruction. Similarly, tumors extending from the primary site into the neck by direct continuity should be approached with a standard *en bloc* operation. In the context of standard surgical techniques more extensive than transoral excisions, there is no advantage to using the laser to do the soft tissue work. It is more time-consuming and has no additional advantages over scalpel and scissor techniques.

Defects suitable for laser excision are those that require virtually no reconstruction. The use of skin grafts in such instances is controversial. Some surgeons prefer to resurface large tongue defects with skin grafts so that less time is required for reepithelialization. A technique in which the mucosal margins of the defect are partially closed down on the wound (see below) converts large defects into relatively small ones and obviates this problem. Skin grafts do not always "take" reliably over bone, although the chances are higher over maxillary than mandibular bone. If a skin graft is used it can be "quilted" onto the wound, or a small tie-over bolster can be applied. Using a skin graft is undesirable in that it constitutes an extra surface that can contract. Also, enhanced scarring and extra tissue covering the bed interferes to some extent with palpation for recurrence.

Fisher and Frame[6] believe skin grafting is contraindicated in laser wounds of the oral cavity because the use of the laser leaves a surface that in itself interferes with graft survival. In their experiments, skin grafts failed.

If the soft tissue defect is of sufficient magnitude to require major soft tissue reconstruction, a transoral approach is not appropriate. For deep lesions that require large margins and leave large defects, the laser may offer no significant difference in morbidity as compared with standard surgical techniques. As with any other technique, it can be difficult to assess the deep margin and as much clinical experience with head and neck cancer excision is necessary when using the laser as when standard techniques are employed.

Controversy also surrounds the use of the laser to excise recurrent cancers where surgery and/or irradiation has been previously employed. Dedo's[1] philosophy is that wide local excision after radiotherapy can be curative and that failure does not greatly lessen the chance of salvage with composite resection. He feels that if the recurrent lesion is small and localized, wide local excision may be tried with more radical treatment being immediately undertaken if the cancer recurs, and that the use of the laser minimizes healing problems in an irradiated field.

Conversely, Strong[2] states that laser management of irradiation failures is fraught with danger. The specimen may demonstrate free margins, but because tumors do not shrink concentrically after radiotherapy[18] (or after chemotherapy),[19] "skip" areas of tumorfree tissue may create the illusion that the cancer has been completely excised, when the margins are really biologically positive.

Although there is no absolute contraindication to excising carefully selected small recurrent cancers with the laser, the situation should be approached with great caution. Such tumors have already selected themselves into a biologically aggressive category by resisting cure by the initial treatment (assuming it was appropriate). The visible and palpable tumor may only be the tip of the iceberg, and the surgeon should assume that all adjacent scar tissue is contaminated with cancer. Tumor margins are more difficult to assess than with a previously untreated cancer. Also, one cannot reliably salvage a second recurrence, even with close follow-up. In short, the situation of a recurrence is probably best handled with standard surgical techniques. Surgeons who desire to attempt laser excision should have firsthand knowledge of the preradiation (or prechemotherapy) extent of the lesion, and the original margins should be excised.

Vaporization Versus Excision

As a basic principle, it is better to excise rather than destroy (vaporize) a lesion whose histologic nature is uncertain. Cancerous lesions should *always* be excised so that the specimen and its margins are available for pathologic examination. If a lesion is to be vaporized, it is important that a biopsy be obtained, either preoperatively or from the most suspicious area at the time of laser treatment.

Highly keratinized lesions are resistant to vaporization because of their low water content. They are therefore best excised because surface vaporization may not completely eradicate the basal layers, and regrowth is likely. Excision allows the surgeon to remove the entire affected area of epithelium and some of the underlying connective tissue. Investigations of malignant lesions have indicated that the subepithelial tissues may play a role in the induction of leukoplakia,[20] so eliminating this deeper layer may reduce the risk that such lesions will recur.

Handpiece Versus Microslad®

Dissection can be carried out with the handpiece or under magnified control using the "joystick" and a laser coupling attachment on the operating microscope (Microslad®). The primary reason for choosing one or the other relates to the principle of laser physics that spot size is directly related to focal length. The short focal length of the handpiece produces a much smaller spot size—a prime determinant of the power density, which is one of the two major determinants of depth of penetration and amount of tissue destruction.

For example, using the Sharplan 733 handpiece with a 125-mm fixed focal length generates a 0.2-mm spot size which, at 10 W continuous power, yields a power density of 26,322 W/cm^2. By contrast, the longer focal 300-mm length of the Microslad® setup yields a more diffuse spot size (0.6 mm) which, results in a power density of only 3529 W/cm^2. The development of new smaller microspot sizes for the microscope adaptation will soon decrease the difference in power density between the two techniques.

The small spot size achieved with the short focal length of the handpiece is preferable for fine dissection and deep excisional biopsies. For example, if a large tongue tumor is being resected using the laser as a knife, the powerful narrow beam obtained with the handpiece is ideal. Conversely, a larger spot size is ideal for surface vaporization because the area can be treated more rapidly.

The surgeon's personal preference is another major determinant of whether a handpiece or the Microslad® is used. The surgeon may find the use of the operating microscope cumbersome and therefore use the handpiece for resection in the oral cavity, oropharynx, and pharynx. Those who prefer the microscope cite the advantage of enhanced tissue detail, affording better definition of abnormal mucosal anatomy than the unassisted eye (although loupes can improve visualization). When the laser microscope is used for lesions in the mouth, a 300-mm lens is best. It allows the instrument to be sufficiently far away from the tissue surface for unimpeded use of retractors and instruments, yet gives a fairly small spot size (0.6 mm). For dissection in the posterior part of the tongue and the pharynx, the microslad® with a 400-mm lens is frequently necessary because of the extra distance involved. The spot size here is 0.8 mm.

A major objection to the use of microscope technology relates to the lower power density associated with the long focal length and diffuse spot size. To enhance power density to achieve a reasonable cutting power and reduce tissue contact time, wattage must be correspondingly raised. The final result is a lasered area covered with much vaporized tissue char that increases tissue damage, complicates would healing, and compromises the ability of the pathologist to evaluate margins on the excised specimen. These problems exist with the machines currently in widespread use, but, as noted, will lessen as new microspot technology becomes more widely distributed.

The handpiece beam with its smaller spot size has a greater power density than the microscope beam. It has the disadvantage that dissection is not under magnified control. However, excision with the handpiece is more rapid. Surveillance for subtle mucosal abnormalities can be improved by use of toluidine blue (Table 7.1) with close visual observation. Palpation allows detection of very small cords of tumor tissue. On the other hand, when accurate dissection rather than a powerful beam

TABLE 7.1. *Technique for Application of Toluidine Blue Dye*

1. Rinse mouth with water twice, for about 20 seconds each time, to remove debris.
2. Rinse mouth well with 1% acetic acid for 20 seconds to remove ropy saliva.
3. Gently dry areas with gauze; do not abrade tissue.
4. Apply 1% toluidine blue solution to the lesion and swab high-risk areas.
5. Rinse with acetic acid (approximately 150 ml) for 1 minute to clear excess stain.
6. Rinse with water.

is required (such as for surface leukoplakia), the magnified image with the operating microscope allows more accurate control, with minimal damage to deeper tissues.

TECHNIQUE

Preoperative Evaluation

The anatomy of patients with large tongues, short, fat necks, and "deep throats" sometimes precludes adequate exposure of the lesion, even with the patient anesthetized and retractors in use. These unfavorable features of individual anatomy, when combined with a tumor in the posterior oral cavity or oropharynx, sometimes mitigate against adequate transoral excision with the laser.

Likely candidates for laser excision can usually be identified in the office by evaluating the individual's anatomy (Fig. 7.2) and the lesion characteristics enumerated above. Surgeons experienced with head and neck cancer can adequately map and biopsy oral and oropharyngeal and some pharyngeal cancers in the clinic. A separate staging procedure under general anesthesia is not required.[21] Panendoscopy can be performed at the beginning of the definitive operation to confirm the initial impression. Likely candidates should be asked to sign permission for a laser procedure. Those whose anatomy is questionable so that final determination of suitability can be made only with relaxation under general anesthesia should also sign permission for an appropriate standard surgical technique (usually a mandibular swing—sometimes marginal mandibulectomy, inner table mandibulectomy, or a "pull-through" procedure). Surgeons who only occasionally treat head and neck cancers or those inexperienced in evaluation of lesions for transoral excision are well advised to assess the exact situation at a separate staging procedure. This can often be performed in the outpatient surgicenter.

Biopsy is performed in the office, taking tissue from a central area of the lesion. Tumors are mapped by vision and palpation—not with biopsies at the periphery, which can interfere with evaluation of margins at the time of definitive surgery because of the induced inflammatory response. The purpose of a biopsy is to diagnose the pathology present. So, one samples tissue in an area that is most likely to give the diagnosis.

Defining the extent of mucosal lesions is enhanced in the oral cavity, oropharynx, and pharynx by topical application of toluidine (tolonium) blue dye. The mechanism of action of toluidine blue is unknown. It is a metachromatic dye used as a nuclear

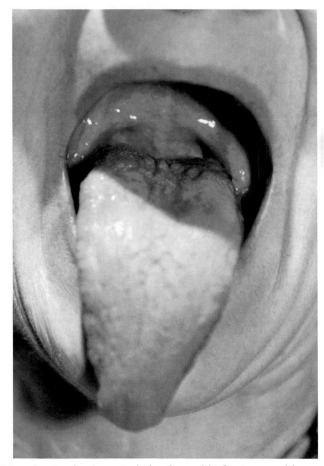

Figure 7.2. Anatomic characteristics favorable for transoral laser excision.

stain, and presumably works because there is quantitatively more nucleic acid in dysplastic and malignant cells than in normal ones, although Strong and coworkers[22] suggest that diffusion through three to four layers of haphazardly arranged tumor cells allows for deeper penetration of the dye.

Typically, there is differential uptake in leukoplakia and erythroplasia, and hyperkeratotic lesions do not take up the dye. The overall accuracy of the technique (specificity and sensitivity for determining malignant lesions) is 90%. The most common error results from the dye being taken up by ulcerated, benign red lesions, so toluidine blue is not a good screening agent. Of note is the fact that tongue papillae always take up the dye, possible because of increased protein synthesis in this tissue.

Although toluidine blue is applied to the oral cavity, oropharynx, and pharynx, the extent of the lesion and resection margins, as defined by the dye, is seldom significantly different from what can be appreciated in the undyed tissue by gross visualization and palpation of the lesion. Occasionally, otherwise unrecognized, discontinuous areas of dye uptake are identified.

The technique used is described in standard references.[23] The mouth is first

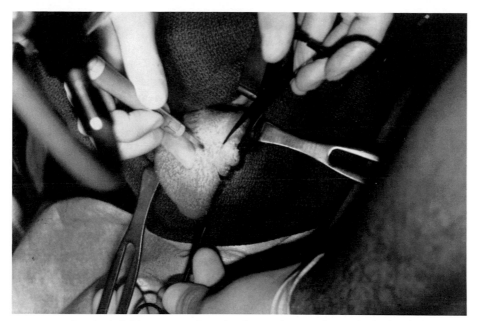

Figure 7.3. Surgical field—appropriate draping and retraction. The lesion is being outlined with the laser handpiece.

cleansed with acetic acid, then dye is applied. A second acetic acid wash is then performed (Table 7.1). Following this, the entire mouth and throat are irrigated with normal saline so that the mucosa is not left in contact with acetic acid, no matter how dilute, during the remainder of the procedure.

Intraoperative Technique

General safety precautions are outlined elsewhere (see Chapter 3). The eyes are protected with ointment and overlaid with sponges wetted with saline. Towel drapes are placed over the patient's face, soaked with room-temperature water (Fig. 7.3). Extremes of temperature can cause facial puffiness and redness.

Laser excisions are performed under general anesthesia to maximize patient comfort and avert unpredictable motion of the patient, which can cause unintended laser burns. Injecting local anesthetic in the vicinity of a cancer is also avoided. In rare instances when there are significant contraindications to general anesthesia, small anteriorly located lesions can be excised under local anesthesia.

For excision of lesions in the oral cavity, nasotracheal intubation is convenient, although not necessary. If the lesion to be excised is in the oropharynx or pharynx, orotracheal intubation is employed, with a Crowe-Davis mouth gag retracting the tube anteriorly. A similar arrangement is convenient for exposure of buccal mucosa lesions. A "laser-safe" endotracheal tube is used for larynx lesions (see Chapters 3 and 4). An ordinary tube can be used for lesions in the mouth and throat, since the laser beam can be easily manipulated to avoid the tube. Similarly, it is not necessary to fill the endotracheal tube's balloon with methylene blue dye, since the laser beam will not be in the vicinity. The advantage of this heretical method is that if it is desired to leave the patient intubated for an observation period postoperatively, the patient need not be reintubated at the end of the procedure.

A moist Kerlix is placed in the throat to prevent aspiration or swallowing of blood, to protect the endotracheal tube, and to enhance exposure in the particular area of the field in which the surgeon is working. For example, pushing the tongue forward from the base props the tongue upward and enhances exposure in the floor of mouth. The pack can also be placed behind the soft palate to protect the posterior pharyngeal wall during oropharynx excisions.

When laser surgery is performed on the tongue, exposure can be enhanced by retracting the tongue with a sharp towel clamp or with sutures. Human assistants are invaluable in retracting the lips and cheeks. A Dingman mouth gag can be quite helpful and is used in an inverted manner, that is, with the blade placed in the palate, which is protected with a gauze sponge, leaving the tongue free for surgical manipulation. The Dedo-Pilling® retractor[11] has been specifically designed to decrease the need for retracting personnel. Assistants also suction blood, assist with hemostasis, and direct the smoke evacuator. If the Crowe-Davis retractor is used, tension is released at 20-minute intervals to allow reperfusion of the tongue circulation. Depending on the size of the lesion, the laser excision can take from 1 minute to 1 hour.

Swelling frequently occurs in the tongue and lips in response to manipulation. In the absence of contraindications to steroids (active tuberculosis, gastric ulcers, diabetes mellitus), Decadron is used intraoperatively (8 to 10 mg IV push) and frequently for one postoperative dose. Postoperatively, cold packs to the lips, as well as oinment, help reduce swelling. A nasopharyngeal airway is sometimes placed at the end of the procedure. If the patient has been properly selected it is rarely necessary to leave the patient intubated or to do a tracheotomy.

The laser is used on 10 to 15 W continuous power. The lesion is first outlined (mucosa incised completely) with a suitable margin—2 mm for benign lesions, 1 cm for malignant lesions. Some operators prefer to outline the lesion on the intermittent pulse mode or to make separate dots. This is not helpful however, and it can lead to somewhat greater tissue destruction. Using the handpiece at 10 to 15 W continuous power leads to rapid, accurate cutting and leaves a negligible amount of char on the specimen and wound bed. Efficiency is enhanced by moving the beam slowly, with constant countertraction. A frequent mistake of the novice is moving the beam too fast, thus necessitating repetition and excessive tissue–laser contact time. As already mentioned, lesions should be excised, not vaporized, for the reasons discussed.

The operator must develop two reflexes in the performance of a laser excision. First, the surgeon must attend to the line of the laser beam from origin to tissue contact point and make sure that nothing intervenes, such as the finger of an assistant, metal instruments, or normal parts of the patient's anatomy. The operator must also be alert to movement on the part of the assistants—specifically, a slipping retractor. If the laser beam strikes a nonblackened instrument being held by an assistant, the heat will be transmitted through the instrument to the assistant or to the patient. A wounded assistant or operator is likely to jump or move, and this can lead to uncontrolled burns to the patient and operating room personnel.

The second reflex relates to the operator's foot. Whenever the laser is not in use,

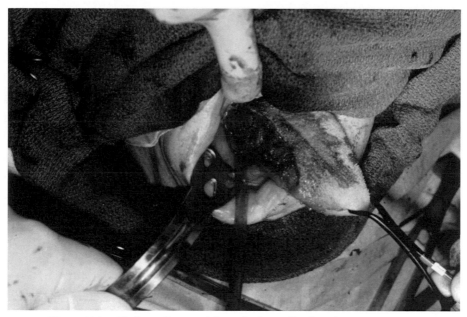

Figure 7.4.   Defect after excision of a lateralized oral tongue cancer.

the operator should remove his or her foot from the pedal box. This obviates the need for the nurse to be constantly turning the machine to "stand-by" or off and facilitates rapid progress.

The area and direction in which lasering is commenced can frequently enhance exposure to the rest of the lesion, thereby facilitating its removal. For example, in patients with floor of mouth lesions who have teeth, releasing the tissue anteriorly from inside the mandibular arch can allow the specimen to be retracted posteriorly out of an obscure sulcus. Similarly, incising the palatoglossal fold (anterior tonsillar pillar) allows lesions in the posterior oral cavity and base of tongue to be brought forward into a more directly accessible field.

After the mucosa has been incised around the desired margins of the lesion, the excision is carried through the underlying soft tissue to a depth appropriate to circumscribe the lesion, including an adequate margin of normal tissue. The lesion is progressively removed in a manner that creates a smooth, saucerlike defect without multiple levels of excision or a ragged base (Fig. 7.4). During the last portion of the excision, the specimen should be manipulated so that the laser beam points into the defect, rather than passing through obliquely to hit adjacent normal structures such as teeth or the inside of the lips or cheeks.

During excision, the laser beam can be defocused to coagulate small blood vessels, although obvious bleeders are best controlled with electrocautery. Even with moderately large arteries, a tie or ligature is rarely necessary.

As the specimen is removed, its orientation is maintained to allow accurate labeling of margins to be submitted for microscopic examination. Margins of excision are determined by vision and palpation during excision.

The defect is flooded with saline and gently wiped with a peanut sponge to remove any carbonized deposits. The deep surface of the specimen is similarly

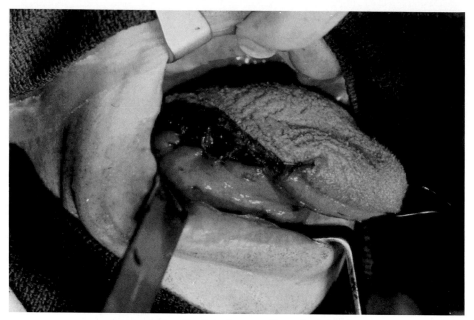

Figure 7.5. Partial closure of surgical defect.

cleansed. This is very important in reducing histologic artifacts and enhancing wound healing.

A few sutures of 3-0 or 2-0 vicryl are generally used to realign the mucosal edges and tack them to the immediately underlying soft tissue to guide reepithelialization in the desired direction. For large defects (e.g., tongue), the wound is closed down to about half its original size to decrease the amount of surface area that must heal by reepithelialization. In general, all wounds are deliberately left open centrally, which brings the deep portion of the defect to the surface and facilitates examination for recurrence (Fig. 7.5). Primary closure is occasionally used in elderly, debilitated patients in whom oral intake must be expedited—usually when the treatment goal is palliation. Similarly, complete primary closure is sometimes best in diabetic patients in whom an open mouth wound could lead to serious infection. Guidelines for reconstruction and managing bone have already been enumerated.

Immediate intraoperative stenting—the need for which can be anticipated preoperatively—can be helpful when the excision has removed apposing mucosal surfaces from a sulcus. Examples include excision of buccal mucosa contiguous with attached mucosa on the outer surface of the alveolar ridge, and removal of mucosa from the inner surface of the mandible or alveolar ridge contiguous with the floor of mouth/ventral tongue. In this context, a stent can be anything that holds the tissue in a sulcus apart until epithelium resurfaces the defect.

A dental roll covered with antibiotic ointment and secured with tie-over sutures is sometimes adequate for small defects. If teeth are present, a prefabricated prosthetic appliance can be attached to the residual teeth. Covering the bare wound diminishes pain and prevents scar contracture during healing if maintained for an adequate period (at least several months). In edentulous patients, a Gunning splint or denture can be secured with circumandibular or circumzygomatic wires or su-

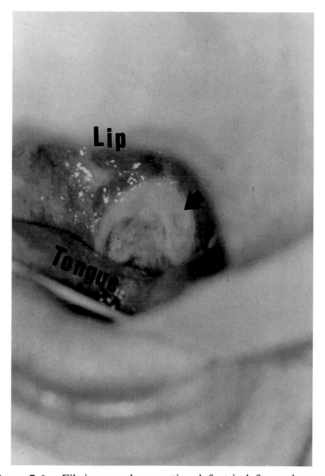

Figure 7.6. Fibrin coagulum coating defect in left oropharynx.

tures. A denuded maxilla is advantageously covered with a denture during healing, which greatly reduces pain.

Postoperative Care

A yellow-white fibrin coagulum quickly coats the wound and nearly obviates pain for the initial 2 to 3 days (Fig. 7.6). the denatured collagen on the surface of the lasered area probably forms an impermeable layer in the immediate postoperative period and reduces the degree of tissue irritation from the oral contents. The patient may experience increased pain from 3 to 14 days postoperatively, and should be thus warned so that a complication is not suspected. Pain experienced is usually adequately controlled with mild oral analgesics.

If the defect is small, patients are allowed to have water and ice chips on the day of surgery. If the excision is large, this may not commence until 1 or 2 days postoperatively. The diet is advanced from clear liquids to full liquids, to a soft diet, as tolerated, according to the pain experienced by the patient and the presence or absence of teeth.

Penicillin is given intravenously during surgery and at 3- to 4-hour intervals during the first 12 postsurgical hours, as long as the patient's intravenous apparatus remains in place. A maintenance dosage of 250 mg of penicillin four times a day is given for approximately 1 week after surgery. With this regimen, infections do not occur.

Depending on the nature of the defect, oral irrigations with salt water can generally be commenced on the first or second postoperative day. The patient uses saltwater mouthwash after meals for the first 5 days so that the surface coagulum is not disturbed. Thereafter, irrigations with half-strength peroxide can be instituted.

When laser excision of the primary tumor is the only operation to be performed, the outpatient center is used for the surgery if the patient's general condition permits. Patients are usually admitted overnight for observation for bleeding, swelling, and airway distress. In healthy patients, discharge can be anticipated the following day, with oral intake having been established. A nasogastric tube is rarely necessary. After small excisions of the buccal mucosa where swelling and/or bleeding are not likely to be problematic, overnight admission may not be necessary.

Treatment may fail if neck dissection or appropriate radiation therapy to the neck is not performed in more extensive lesions, and especially lesions of the tongue, which place the cervical lymphatics at significant risk for metastasis. If a neck dissection is to be performed, the surgery is performed in the hospital. If a neck dissection is indicated, it can be performed at the same sitting, usually without communicating between the primary site and the neck, if the case was properly selected. In the rare event that a communication occurs, a simple means of flap reconstruction should have been planned (transposition flap with available local tissue).

Ancillary maneuvers to decrease postoperative scarring include local steroid injections (Kenalog®, 40 mg at weekly intervals for 1 month), and after initial healing the patient should institute oral exercises to maintain mobility of the lasered area and decrease the scarring tendency. This includes tongue exercises, in which the mouth is opened and the tongue touches the roof of the mouth and is protruded away from the side of a lateralized excision, and/or mouth-opening excercises in the case of an excision involving the retromolar trigone, pterygoid muscles, and buccal mucosa (Fig. 7.7).

Histopathologic Considerations

As with any type of cancer operation, the excision of the primary tumor should remove all gross disease with an adequate margin of normal tissue. Grossly positive margins should never be left *in situ* in the hope that radiotherapy will cure them.

Because extensions more than 1 cm beyond the clinically apparent tumor margin occur in 70% of head and neck mucosal squamous carcinomas,[24] any surgeon can encounter pathology reports of positive margins for surgical cases where the tumor was thought to have been adequately removed. Between the time of removal of the specimen from the patient and processing in the pathology department, the mucosal margins frequently dehydrate and contract down on the tumor. When the margin is then cut, a positive reading can also result—an artifact of this method of

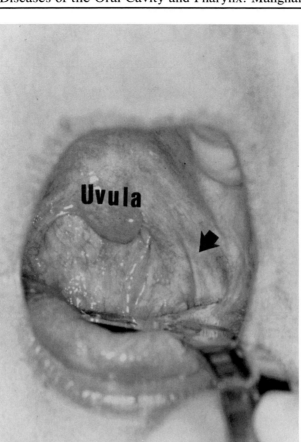

Figure 7.7. Healing of oropharynx defect after 3 to 4 weeks. Note normal mouth opening.

submitting the specimen. This can occur even when the primary tumor is anchored to a substrate to orient it and prevent contraction (Fig. 7.8). To forestall arguments with radiotherapists concerning the need for adjuvant treatment, the surgeon can cut the tumor margins as soon as the specimen is removed from the patient rather than leaving this important task to the pathologist who is unfamiliar with the anatomy. Generally four quadrant mucosal and several deep margins are sampled. Unless suspicious for tumor, these margins are submitted for permanent sectioning and are labeled in a way that will be meaningful at a future date—not merely as anterior, posterior, medial, lateral, and deep, but named by specific anatomic area. This policy applies to *all* excisions, not only when the laser is used.

Suspicious areas that require frozen section examination are handled as with any cancer resection. A frequently suspicious area that is questioned is the sublingual gland. After excision of a floor of mouth lesion, this area can feel firm. This firmness usually represents reactive inflammation and is rarely positive for cancer.

When the laser is used at low power with a small spot size there are almost no burn artifacts, and consequently there is no distortion of the histopathologic tumor–host interface to confuse interpretation of margin adaquacy.

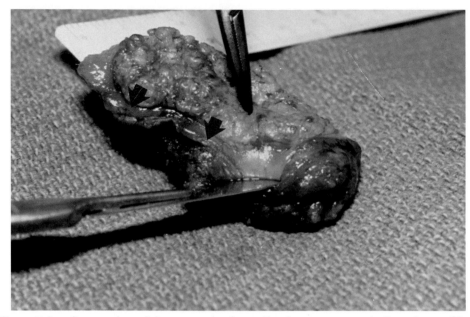

Figure 7.8.   Contraction of tissue margins immediately upon removal of specimen. (Normal margin width at knife, tumor at hemostat, contracting margin at arrow.)

Management of Specific Sites

Oral Cavity

Floor of Mouth. Laser excision of oral cavity lesions can generally be accomplished without the need to transect major sensory nerves in the vicinity. For example, in the floor of mouth, the lingual nerve can usually be preserved, since lesions suitable for transoral excision generally do not penetrate the floor of mouth muscle sling. The plane of dissection frequently exposes the nerve, however, and to decrease postoperative pain and reduce neuromas the surgeon can tack adjacent mucosa over the nerve.

Tongue. For major tongue resections in which the thick dorsal mucosa is cut for a considerable length, leaving such wounds open to heal by secondary intention leads to considerable scar contracture. Scarring is somewhat less with primary closure.

Large tongue resections leave a noticeable defect in the immediate postoperative period. However, because residual tongue muscle hypertrophies, an open defect tends to "fill in." As early as 2 months postoperatively it can be difficult to identify the previous excision site, since normal tongue bulk and contour is generally restored.

Excision of large lateralized oral tongue cancers (hemiglossectomy) can be accomplished by lasering along the midline raphe and coming across the tongue at a right angle for the posterior margin. Such a defect can be closed primarily by suturing the contralateral tongue tip to the posterolateral margin on the side of excision. This creates a somewhat shorter tongue of normal contour and results in very acceptable articulation and swallowing.

Oropharynx

In the oropharynx in particular, variation in individual anatomy will either facilitate or inhibit transoral laser excision, even if characteristics of the lesion are suitable. Patients with long, thin necks are more frequently operable by this route than those with short, fat necks and "deep throats." In the latter, an alternative approach such as mandibular "swing" or exposure through a cheek flap is required.

It is stated in the head and neck cancer literature that tumor tonsillectomy is to be condemned. However, many lesions—even with significant surface extent (T_3)—are suitable for transoral laser excision if the previously enunciated excision criteria have been satisfied. The lesion should be mobile with respect to the ptery-goid muscles, and trismus should be absent. Observing these caveats, excision can generally proceed with preservation of the lingual nerve and inferior alveolar nerve bundle at the lingula, since the plane of excision is along the fascia deep to the tonsillar bed. Dissection at this plane also allows the pterygoid muscles to be pre-served intact with their fascia. Transecting the pterygoids or exposing the mandible in the area of the retromolar trigone can lead to significant complications,[3] as dis-cussed below.

Lesions of the soft palate appropriate for laser excision are most frequently super-ficial, requiring only partial-thickness excision. The uvula can be removed with impunity. However, if excision of a superficial lesion would require creating a large, full-thickness defect with significant functional consequences (velopharyngeal incompetence, nasal regurgitation), radiotherapy is the preferred method of treatment.

Pharynx

In a personal series of nearly 40 cases, it was found that cancers of the posterior pharyngeal wall are usually mobile and do not invade the prevertebral fascia—a necessary prerequisite for transoral excision. If the inferior extent of the lesion can be exposed with the Crowe-Davis mouth gag (facilitated by placing a peanut sponge on a long clamp on the border of the tumor, inferiorly or laterally, and pulling either upward or medially), then the tumor is suitable for transoral laser excision. Such manipulations remove the tumor margin from major lateral submucosal ves-sels and allow excision to proceed in an almost bloodless manner.

The surgeon should use only the laser to excise cancers that are accessible to the handpiece. Using the microscope with a laryngoscope setup in an attempt to trans-orally excise cancers in the folded "nooks and crannies" of the lower hypopharynx is so difficult that the objective of achieving negative margins is unlikely to be met. Therefore one should not use this technique, since the goal is complete excision of the lesion with the intent of achieving local control rather than palliation of painful ulcers, as advocated by some surgeons who consider the prognosis of phar-ynx cancers hopeless.

The mucosal margins of the pharyngeal defect are generally undermined and tacked to the prevertebral fascia. This is particularly important inferiorly and superi-orly, to avoid dissection of secretions into the chest and nasopharyngeal stenosis, respectively. If the prevertebral fascia is intact, a skin graft or dermal graft is not used.

Very few pharynx cancers are suitable for laser excision. Pharyngeal cancers such as those that are hypomobile, implying penetration of the prevertebral fascia, or those that involve the lateral pharyngeal wall, generally require a formal open surgical approach.

CANCER TREATMENT: RESULTS AND COMPLICATIONS

The laser is subject to the same limitations as any other surgical technique used to treat head and neck cancer, namely, the experience and expertise of the surgeon and the treatment plan.

Since 1979, several series have reported techniques and treatment results following transoral laser excision of cancers of the oral cavity and oropharynx. At first, relatively small superficial primary tumors (T_1 and T_2) for which surgical treatment alone was adequate were selected for laser excision. Aggregate results[1,2] show good local control rates and only a few minor complications when the laser was used as the only treatment method.

On the basis of these initial favorable reports, the laser has gradually been used to excise larger lesions as the initial step in planned combination treatment (i.e., for cancers in which postoperative radiotherapy is to be used). To date, only one series has been published reporting cancer treatment results and complications in this context.[3] Local control was comparable to that achieved with standard surgical techniques. Local control (including salvage) was approximately 85% in previously untreated patients and approximately 65% in previously treated patients.

This series included several T_3 tumors. Some patients underwent laser excision followed by planned postoperative radiation. The results, however, indicated an unusually high rate of complications. The Collins series[25] demonstrated that the laser can be used as the first step in planned combination therapy (surgery followed by radiotherapy) with good local control rates *and* a low complication rate.

Both series (Sessions[3] and Collins[25]) are comparable in that postoperative radiotherapy was used in some patients and T_3 lesions were included. In the Collins series, laser excision was selected on the basis of accessibility of the tumor to transoral resection, and the patients were treated with curative intent. Only soft tissue excisions were included. In 58 laser excisions, the overall local control rate was 84%—comparable to series reporting control rates using scalpel techniques. Failure of local control contributed to the death of two patients, although attributing the failure to the use of the laser technology alone is unreasonable. More likely, the outcome represents a deficit in the treatment plan. Neither patient received postoperative radiation because the margins were negative and surgery alone was considered adequate.

In Sessions' series, 11 of the 28 patients (39%) experienced wound-healing complications that caused severe disability. These included exposure of the mandible, trismus and ankylosis, nonhealing wounds, fistula, and nasopharyngeal stenosis. Delayed healing required 4 to 10 months and was managed with repeated office debridements or more major operations. These included excision of a portion of mandible, debridement of infratemporal fossa necrosis via antrostomy, and complex wound closure with multistaged local and distant flaps. Hyperbaric oxygen was also used as an adjunct to help wound healing. (The use of increased oxygenation in a wound likely contaminated with neoplastic cells is of concern with respect to enhancing cancer regrowth.[26]) The 17 complications required 31 operations, and in 3, debilitating trismus persisted despite operations to relieve mandibular ankylosis. Because of decreased mouth opening, none of these patients could chew or wear dentures, and follow-up examination for recurrent cancer was compromised.

The authors attribute these complications to the use of postoperative radiation, since the problem rate was higher in patients who had radiation postoperatively than in those who did not (58% vs 25%). It is not specifically stated whether or not the complication ever caused cancellation or a delay in planned postoperative radiation.

The incidence and type of complications reported by Sessions would be of concern following any type of oral cavity cancer surgery, and as sequelae to laser excision are, in the author's own words, "especially catastrophic."

In the Collins series, a complication was defined as any event altering function (speech, deglutition), resulting in a delay of planned postoperative radiation, or requiring additional surgery. On the basis of this definition, 4 of 53 patients (8%) were designated as developing a complication. Chronic sialoadenitis was seen in two patients, floor of mouth scar formation in one, and hemorrhage in one. These four complications led to five additional operations: two submandibular gland excisions, two laser procedures to release scar, and one tracheotomy. Three of the complications were seen in the 24 floor of mouth procedures, all of which involved transection of the submandibular ducts. All complications occurred less than 6 months after treatment.

The floor of mouth scar formed in a patient with teeth who underwent laser excision deep in the lateral gingivolingual sulcus where a scalpel excision of a T_1 cancer had been performed 4 months previously. Progressive scarring developed with slight tongue tethering, which minimally altered the patient's articulation. This complication was attributed to the laser procedure, although it was undoubtedly aggravated by prior surgery in the operative field. The problem was corrected with two additional laser "releases" in the scarred lateral floor of mouth, as well as local steroid injections and stenting with a prosthesis attached to the teeth. This was the only patient who experienced a detectable alteration of function.

One patient was returned to the operating room 2 days postoperatively for ligation of a bleeding vessel in the lasered tonsil bed (6 months following full-course radiotherapy to the area). A tracheotomy was also performed for airway protection in the event of further bleeding. This was the only tracheotomy in the Collins series.

No patient experienced a complication that delayed or canceled the planned postoperative radiation, and the incidence of complications did not seem to be related to the addition of this treatment method. Postoperative radiation therapy was uniformly begun after 3 weeks of healing, at which time even extensive surface wounds were almost completely healed. None of the patients developed exposed mandible, trismus/ankylosis, nonhealing bone or soft tissue necrosis, fistula, or nasopharyngeal stenosis. Similarly, no healing problems occurred in the nine patients in this series who had previous radiation to the lasered area for a prior head and neck cancer.

Dedo's series[1] is comparable to the Collins series with respect to complications, although there were no T_3 lesions, nor was postoperative radiation employed. Of four patients in whom Wharton's duct was transected, submandibular gland obstruction resulted in two and was managed conservatively. One patient developed limited tongue movement, and two developed mucus retention cysts. Of four patients in whom laser resection included periosteum, three healed well and one developed an oral fistula. Bleeding from the tongue was seen postoperatively in three patients, one of whom required return to the operating room for control.

The source of the problems in Sessions' series[3] seems to be a significant incidence of nonhealing soft tissue ulcers and exposed mandibular bone. Sessions cites the fact that the laser literature shows that wounds from removal of lesions over mandible, including periosteum, heal primarily without difficulty. As indicated earlier in this chapter (see the section on Wound-Healing Principles above), in fact this is not so. There is considerable evidence that lasered bone does not remucosalize, but rather is devitalized and sequestered. Sessions' series provides clinical evidence that exposure of mandibular bone by laser used at a high power density leads to nonhealing wounds.

Sessions' reference to "burn margins" (which precluded pathologic interpretation) suggests that a major cause of the wound-healing problems was the use of an inordinately high power density: tissues were exposed to the Microslad® laser beam used at 50 W continuous power (see the section on Wound-Healing Principles for a discussion of laser physics).

The use of radiotherapy on incompletely healed or partially devitalized wounds cannot be blamed for the poor results, for the reasons cited above. Also, the patients who required radiation were probably those who had the largest tumors and therefore required the more extensive excisions, with a resultant high incidence of wound-healing complications.

The significant differences between the laser technique outlined in this chapter and those used by Sessions account for the absence of wound-healing problems in the Collins series. Recommendations for avoiding complications include selecting cases properly, optimizing laser power density (decreasing contact time with the tissue minimizes tissue destruction and artifacts at the margins), leaving mandibular periosteum intact, and avoiding direct laser contact with bare cortical bone. When postoperative radiotherapy is planned, the operation (laser or scalpel) must be performed in a manner that allows adequate soft tissue coverage of the defect so that bone is not left exposed and susceptible to radionecrosis. Deep apposing sulci denuded of mucosa should be stented. Surgeries involving major bone excision or flap reconstruction should be performed using a standard scalpel technique. In the near future, lasers with microspot sizes will allow laser excisions using microslab setups to be carried out with a much lower power density and a decreased potential for wound-healing problems.

REFERENCES

1. Guerry TL, Silverman S, Jr., Dedo HH: Carbon dioxide laser resection of superficial oral carcinomas: indications, technique and results. *Ann Otol Rhinol Laryngol* 95: 547–555, 1986.

2. Strong MS, Vaughan CW, Shapshay SM, et al: Transoral management of localized carcinoma of the oral cavity using the CO_2 laser. *Laryngoscope* 89:897–905, 1979.

3. Nagorsky MJ, Sessions DG: Laser resection for early oral cavity cancer—results and complications. *Ann Otol Rhinol Laryngol* 96:556–560, 1987.

4. Mihashi S, Jako GJ, Incze J, et al: Laser surgery in otolaryngology—interaction of CO_2 laser and soft tissue. *Ann NY Acad Sci* 267:263–294, 1976.

5. Fisher SE, Frame JW, Browne RM, et al: A comparative histological study of wound healing following CO_2 laser and conventional surgical excision of canine buccal mucosa. *Arch Oral Biol* 28:287–291, 1983.

6. Fisher SE, Frame JW: The effects of the carbon dioxide surgical laser on oral tissues. *Br J Oral Maxillofac Surg* 22:414–425, 1984.

7. Gabbiani G, Ryan GB, Majno G: The presence of modified fibroblasts in granulation tissue and their possible role in wound contraction. *Experientia* 27:549–550, 1971.

8. Montandon D, D'Andiran G, Gabbiani G: The mechanism of wound contraction and epithelialization: clinical and experimental studies. *Clin Plast Surg* 4:325–348, 1977.

9. Mihail R, Zajtchuk JT, Davis RK: Incidence of Wharton's duct stenosis in floor of the mouth cancers excised with scalpel or cautery versus CO_2 laser. *Head Neck Surg* 9:241–243, 1987.

10. Frame JW, Dasgupta AR, Dalton GA: Use of the carbon dioxide laser in the management of premalignant lesions of the oral mucosa. *J Laryngol Otol* 98:1251–1260, 1984.

11. Chu FWK, Silverman S, Jr, Dedo HH: CO_2 laser treatment of oral leukoplakia. *Laryngoscope* 98:125, 1988.

12. Chiesa F, Tradati N, Sala L, et al: Follow-up of oral leukoplakia after carbon dioxide laser surgery. *Arch Otolaryngol Head Neck Surg* 116:177–180, 1990.

13. Pindborg JJ: *Oral Cancer and Precancer*. Bristol, England, Wright, 1980.

14. Mashberg A, Meyers H: Anatomical site and size of 222 early asymptomatic oral squamous cell carcinomas. *Cancer* 37:2149–2153, 1976.

15. Rhys Evans PH, Frame JW: CO_2 laser surgery in the oral cavity. In Carruth JAS, Simpson GI (eds): *Lasers in Otolaryngology*. Chicago, Year Book Medical Publishers, 1988, pp 101–132.

16. Slaughter DO, Southwick HW, Sinejkal W: "Field cancerization" in oral stratified squamous epithelium: clinical implications of multicentric origin. *Cancer* 6:963–968, 1953.

17. Collins SL, Saunders VW Jr: Excision of selected intraoral cancers by use of sagittal inner table mandibulectomy. *Otolaryngol Head Neck Surg* 97:558–566, 1987.

18. Spiro RH, Gerold FP, Strong EW: Mandibular "swing" approach for oral and oropharyngeal tumors. *Head Neck Surg* 3:371–378, 1981.

19. Olofsson J, van Nostrand AWP: Growth and spread of laryngeal and hypopharyngeal carcinoma with reflections on the effect of preoperative irradiation. *Acta Otolaryngol {Suppl}* 308:1, 1973.

20. Norris CM, Jr, Clark JR, Ervin TJ, et al: Pathology of surgery after induction chemotherapy: an analysis of resectability and local regional control. *Laryngoscope* 96:292, 1986.

21. Smith CJ: Connective tissue influence of epithelial malignancy or premalignancy. In MacKenzie IC, Dabelsteen E, Squier CA (eds): *Oral Premalignancy*. Iowa City, University of Iowa Press, 1980.

22. Bastian RW, Collins SL, Kaniff TE, et al: Indirect video laryngoscopy versus direct endoscopy for larynx and pharynx cancer staging. Toward elimination of preliminary direct endoscopy. *Annals of Otorhinolaryngology* 98:693, 1989.

23. Strong MS, Vaughn CO, Incze JS: Toluidine blue in the management of carcinoma of the oral cavity. *Arch Otolaryngol* 87:527–531, 1968.

24. Mashberg A: Final evaluation of tolonium chloride rinse for screening of high risk patients with asymptomatic squamous carcinoma. *Am J Dent Assoc* 106:319–323, 1983.

25. Davidson TM, Haghighi P, Astarita R, et al: Mohs for head and neck mucosal cancer: report on 111 patients. *Laryngoscope* 98:1078, 1988.

26. Collins SL, Mamikunian C: Transoral CO_2 laser excision of oral cavity and oropharynx squamous cancers—treatment results and complications. Submitted for publication in *Laryngoscope*.

27. McMillan J, Calhoun KH, Maden JT, et al: The effect of hyperbaric oxygen on oral mucosa carcinoma. *Laryngoscope* 99:241, 1989.

8A
Lasers in Otology: General Otology

Steven D. Rowley

In the field of otology the challenge of removing all disease, restoring normal function, and avoiding complications is made more difficult because of the small field of surgery and the large number of vital structures in close proximity to the pathology. Over the decades physicians have vigorously pursued any creative technique or newly discovered treatment modality that might allow them to better accomplish these three goals.

HISTORICAL REVIEW

The idea that energy could be used in the ear to accomplish these goals has long fascinated otologists. Prompted by Einstein's theories of quantum physics, Miaman[1] developed the first laser in 1960, using a solid ruby crystal. In 1977 Wilpizeski and associates[2] examined "this new tool" in the field of ear surgery. They had worked to develop a practical microsurgical laser for commercial use and reported damaging the organ of Corti in monkeys by using "excessive power" and 500-μsec bursts of CO_2 laser energy. They also performed myringotomy with argon lasers on normal monkey ears, reporting no evidence of sensorineural hearing loss but noting that tympanic membrane perforations healed in approximately two weeks. They performed middle ear surgery—ossicular amputations, stapes footplate fenestrations, stapedial tenotomy, and crurotomy—with both the argon and CO_2 lasers and were impressed at the usefulness of the CO_2 laser with its increased power.

The first clinical use of lasers in the human ear was described in a 1977 presentation by Escudero.[3] He described tacking temporalis fascia to tympanic membranes for closure of perforations using an argon laser directed through a 100-μm quartz fiber, hand-manipulated under microscopic vision. Bleeding was also able to be stopped remarkably well.

In January 1979 Perkins[4] presented a preliminary report of laser stapedotomy with a microsurgical argon laser of his design. Excellent initial surgical results were obtained in 11 patients. Three months later Goode[5] reported myringotomy with the CO_2 laser in dry temporal bones, cat ears, and human subjects. A 1979 report by Palva[6] suggested that perforation of the stapes footplate with an argon laser provided slightly better results than mechanical perforation.

In 1980 DiBartolomeo[7] expanded the clinical applications of the argon laser in otology in a report of 30 patients who received treatment for external and middle ear diseases. Of these patients, 15 were treated for soft tissue problems and 15 for bony growths of the external ear canal, middle ear ossicle problems, or otosclerosis. DiBartolomeo was able to achieve closure in six of seven previously unhealed traumatic perforations by using the laser beam to spot weld temporalis fascia to the margins of the tympanic membrane. Lysis of middle ear adhesions and myringotomies were performed in other patients, and ear canal osteomas were removed in two. Otosclerosis was corrected in a total of ten patients, including one revision and one case in which a congenital stapedial artery persisted and required laser cauterization.

McGee[8] described even broader application in the use of the argon laser in otosclerosis and chronic ear disease, when he reported over 500 procedures with no laser-related complications. In 100 patients treated with argon laser stapedotomy, the results of this compared favorably with small fenestra stapedectomy performed manually. Although results at six months and one year showed no statistical differences in hearing levels or vestibular status, the procedure was shown to be safe in a large sampling of patients.

Vollrath[9] and Gantz[10] published separate studies that led to some concern about the use of the argon laser for middle ear work. Vollrath showed significant but temporary cochlear microphonic changes in the guinea pig. These changes were believed related to the crackling noise of the melting bone and not to thermal trauma. Gantz reported saccular rupture in three of eight cat ears when the argon beam was passed through the anterior stapes footplate.

Since the mid-1980s an ever-increasing number of articles has described the use of the laser in ear surgery. Arguments persist, however, regarding the safety and efficiency of laser surgery and laser types. This chapter addresses the role of lasers in the treatment of ear diseases and discusses the selection of lasers best suited for treatment of specific diseases.

USES IN GENERAL OTOLOGY

Auricle Procedures

Surgeons have employed the laser in the cutting and cautery modes to remove a multitude of superficial skin lesions that occur in and around the auricle. Because of the large volume of skin lesions seen by dermatologists, owning a laser in a solo or group office setting can save time and money in performing the required excision. Since wound closure is generally not required and dermatologic surgery can be performed in an office setting with local anesthesia and low risk of infection, nonmalignant lesions can be removed easily and quickly.

For larger, deeper, and more aggressive lesions, partial wedge resections or even total auricular resection can be done with the laser in cutting mode. The use of the laser for making skin incisions, with hogs as subjects, indicate that good healing could be obtained. Norris stated that the beginning migration of epithelium was observed much earlier in laser incisions compared with incisions made with a scalpel.[11] At day 30 and at day 90 he found no differences in wound healing between the two types of incisions. Hall[12] measured wound tensile strength after both knife and CO_2 laser–produced incisions and found less tensile strength in the CO_2 laser incision up to day 20, after which the strength in both healing incisions was similar.

The properties of wound closure have also been studied by many investigators. In wounds closed with sutures, staples, or laser, the same standard sigmoid healing curve is seen. That is, tensile strength of the wound is low for the initial 21 days but rather rapidly increases to day 90. Tensile strength appears to be about the same for all methods of closure. There is some evidence that argon lasers produce a higher initial wound tensile strength initially than low-power CO_2 lasers do. By nature, standard or high-power CO_2 lasers are not good biostimulators and produce too much thermal necrosis to be useful for skin incising and bonding.

In 1984 Gillis and associates[13] studied tissue interactions with the argon laser. Central pallor appeared first, followed by blanching of the tissue surrounding the area of impact. Continued application caused epithelial elevation, vesicle formation, and rupture of the vesicle with the appearance of a crater that progressively deepened. There was some lateral spread, giving evidence of thermal damage. The authors concluded that in nonpigmented tissues, laser energy was either transmitted beyond the initial first cell layers to deeper tissues or was scattered laterally. Healed lesions generally were seen by 21 days. The investigators concluded the laser could be controlled by microscopy, but the use of fiberoptic tips caused difficulty in estimating the distance from the tip to the tissues to be treated, thus creating uncertainty about the ultimate tissue effects.

Malignancies of the auricle such as basal cell carcinoma, melanoma, and squamous cell carcinoma can be treated with the laser because of its thermal destructive properties and nonthermal biostimulation. Large lesions may be excised in cutting mode and sometimes require concomitant mastoidectomy and middle ear reconstruction. Argon, KTP-532, Nd:YAG, and pulsed heavy metal vapor lasers have been used successfully in photodynamic therapy (PDT). Both squamous cell carcinoma and melanoma can be pretreated with Rhodamine-123 (or other photosensitizing agents), increasing the sensitivity of the lesions. Some adjacent thermal destruction occurs, but the effect of the laser seems to be greatly augmented by the dye: Significant selective tumor destruction is seen.[14] Since most auricular cancers occur on the helix or the posterior auricular surface, the lesions can be easily observed and retreated as needed with very little distortion of the ear's structure or risk of complication.

A laser can be used to perform certain otoplasty techniques. Skin, soft tissues, and cartilage may be cut or bonded, depending on the laser power employed. Cartilage in the depths of the wound can be welded so that permanent sutures are not necessary in this area to create folds; this technique offers permanent stability and reduces foreign body reaction. Argon or KTP lasers with a hand-held fiber probe should be set at approximately 3 to 4 W, 100 msec, and a 1 mm spot size for best results in welding cartilage. The CO_2 laser hand-held probe is cumbersome and imprecise but can be used for this purpose, or the low-power CO_2 laser can be used with the operating microscope.

Meatoplasty can be done with the laser, but becomes a slow, tedious microscopic process. The surgery is more quickly handled with standard knife and cautery. Even in the canal recontour procedure of Perkins and Goode, the use of the laser has gradually disappeared as the technique has evolved and been modified.

The concept of biostimulation by laser is also of interest because of its potential for preventing periauricular keloids. Castro et al[15] have added Kodak Q-Switch II dye to treat cell cultures. The Nd:YAG laser with a wavelength of 1060 nm was used. The beam was delivered through an articulated arm or an optical fiber. At physiologic temperatures, cell inhibition was seen, and at 36°C cell destruction was seen. These effects were not seen with the laser used alone. Obviously further experimentation is needed, but there is promise for the treatment of all collagen deposition disorders if fibroblast formation can be altered in this manner.

Auditory Canal Procedures

Ear canal lesions treatable with the laser include chronic infection, tumors, atresia, scarring, and webs.

Chronic ear canal infections, whether bacterial or fungal, tend to recur. If medical treatment does not cure the problem, surgical intervention may be necessary. Hunsaker[16] describes the conchomeatoplasty as treatment for chronic otitis externa, with canal widening effective in resolving the disease in all 30 ears treated. Stripping of ear canal skin and replacing with skin grafts has been done. The laser offers an advantage because it is able at low power density to spot weld the edges or corners of skin grafts, holding them in position and minimizing the amount of packing that is necessary.

If full removal of skin is not thought necessary, weeping areas of canal skin can be cauterized with the laser in sweeping parallel strokes (Fig. 8.1). The argon or KTP laser at 1.5 to 2.0 W power with a 1-mm spot size provides cauterization of the area extending to both the surface epithelium and the subepithelial layers. If lower power is used, no blister effect is seen in the tissue interaction. Healing of chronic disease is usually seen after one or two courses of cautery. This procedure can be performed without difficulty in the office on an outpatient basis under local anesthesia.

Polyps that partially or totally fill the ear canal generally originate from middle ear inflammatory disease but may also come from inflamed tissue in the ear canal or the tympanic membrane. A polyp may also be the first indication of a canal or middle ear carcinoma, or the leading edge of a glomus tumor. Prudent judgment would advise against avulsing these polyps, and a biopsy, even though indicated, might cause severe bleeding. The laser proves extremely useful in such situations. Polyps can be biopsied with very little bleeding, or they can be removed a portion at a time under microscopic vision for good hemostatic control. Complications such as scarring, fistula formation, or ossicular disruption are avoided (Figs. 8.2 and 8.3). The red, granular appearance of inflamed polyps makes them especially treatable with a blue-green laser such as the argon or an emerald green laser such as the KTP

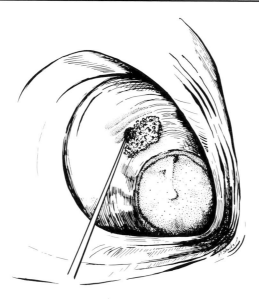

Figure 8.1. Chronic otitis externa with granulations cauterized at low power in parallel strokes.

because of their absorption characteristics (see Table 8.1). Surgery can be performed under local anesthesia.

Carcinoma of the ear canal may present as a nonhealing, painful ulcer, as a polypoid growth, or as granulation tissue. Biopsy specimens from these areas may be taken by using the laser to remove samples of skin and cartilage. Lasers are of no help in formal treatment of the carcinoma by resection of the ear canal en bloc, mastoidectomy, partial or total parotidectomy, or high cervical neck node dissection.

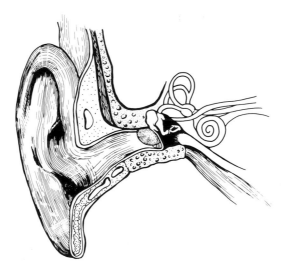

Figure 8.2.   Ear canal polyp.

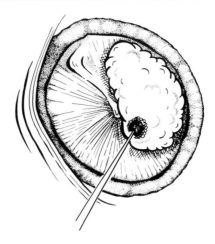

Figure 8.3. Canal polyp cauterized or biopsied.

Acquired ear canal atresia or stenosis, usually secondary to chronic infection or previous surgical procedures, can be treated successfully with the laser. Dissection of thickened fibrotic subcutaneous tissue superiorly can be performed by incising just lateral to the anulus so that quadrant strips of ear canal skin can be rolled laterally and the underlying fibrosis vaporized, leaving skin intact. Alternatively, a meatal incision can be made and the laser used to vaporize fibrotic tissues as they are rolled medially, as in Figure 8.4. With either technique, hemostasis is excellent, and quick healing with minimal postoperative edema is usually obtained. The same effect can be achieved with sharp scissors dissection. Dissection with most instruments tends to pull, tear, and macerate the tissues instead of resecting them cleanly.

TABLE 8.1. *Comparison of Argon/KTP and CO_2 Lasers*

Visible Wavelength *Argon/KTP*	*Invisible Wavelengths* *CO_2*
Advantages	
Optical precision	Tissue-related properties
Small spot size	Good power at tissues
Aiming and laser beams same	Moderate hemostasis
Fiberoptic transport	Surface active
Excellent calibration	
Excellent hemostasis	
Pigment absorption	
Disadvantages	
Low power	Separate aiming beam
Requires plumbing	Bulky
Pigment absorption	Hollow tube transport

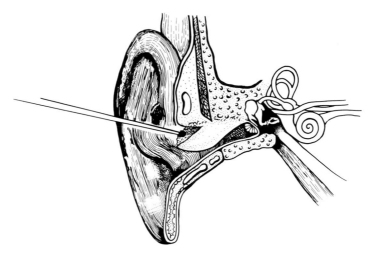

Figure 8.4. Fibrous subcutaneous tissue exposed and vaporized through a lateral meatal incision.

Tympanic Membrane Procedures

Myringotomy

The laser has been used for controlled perforation of the tympanic membrane in an effort to create a hole that would stay open for two to three months, allowing the middle ear to heal from episodes of otitis media or effusion without requiring insertion of a ventilation tube. Goode[5] consistently produced a 1.5- to 2.0-mm tympanic membrane perforation using a CO_2 laser at 12 W, applying a single 100-msec pulse through a 200-mm objective. Of 11 ears, 10 healed within six weeks and 5 remained free of middle ear fluid. Tube placement was avoided and cost reduced. Goode noted that when the laser was directed against the tympanic membrane and the middle ear was free of fluid, a "small burn spot" was produced on the medial wall of the middle ear. Outpatient laser myringotomy was thus advocated as a safe screening procedure in infected or fluid-filled ears to identify patients who would eventually need ventilation tube placement.

Lipman[17] had a 60% success rate in over 100 cases of CO_2 laser myringotomy for treatment of chronic otitis media with effusion. A 0.8-mm perforation was produced and stayed open two to four weeks.

Tympanoplasty/Myringoplasty

Sealing of temporalis fascia to tympanic membranes in the manner previously described seems to be successful but probably unnecessary in most tympanoplasties. Recurrent perforations with several failures, or very anterior perforations, would seem to lend themselves to this particular treatment. The temporalis fascia can be delicately welded to anterior canal skin, tympanic membrane, or anulus, maintaining the most anatomically correct position of the future tympanic membrane sulcus.

The exact mechanism by which spot welding or bonding of tissues occurs is unknown. Schober et al[18] feel that thermal coagulation and protein denaturation (particularly collagen) play a role. Vale[19] contends that laser thermal effects accentuate the spread of polymerized fibrogen across the anastomotic site. Apparently, a combination of processes promote bonding, and different lasers may enhance certain of these processes.

Marquet,[20] in describing his treatment of cholesteatoma, suggests that an atelectatic tympanic membrane can be cleansed from the ossicles and pulled laterally by fine suction. The everted edges of excessive tissue can then be removed with scissors, leaving a more firm, taut, healthy membrane. If this technique is employed, the edges may be sealed with the laser to produce firm bonding rather than simply allowing overlapping and adhesion of the edges as they heal with time.

Middle Ear Procedures

The middle ear space is where the laser was first used in otology. Here good technique and the appropriate laser can greatly facilitate microsurgery. The tight confines of this area, the tendency for scarring, the delicate nature of ossicular connections and movement, all have limited the rate of success in middle ear surgery. The goal of laser use would be to improve this success rate.

Middle ear adhesions can be vaporized with minimal manipulation of the ossicles. The amount of laser energy required to vaporize these scars will vary, however, according to the amount of pigment and the size and location of the lesion. As a general rule, the KTP or argon laser is used with a spot size of 200 μm and a power of 1.0 to 2.0 W delivered to the tissue. If the tissues to be removed are actually impinging on the stapes or promontory, the spot size should be reduced to 150 μm and, if necessary, the power dropped to 8 mW. Granulation tissue around the stapes footplate and superstructure and adhesions around other ossicles can be vaporized. Attachments to the tympanic membrane and promontory restricting ossicular movement can be removed in similar fashion. A peristapedial fibrous tent causing stapes fixation following otitis media should be easily treatable without stapedectomy by vaporization of the fibrous adhesions. Attention to the course of the facial nerve must be maintained during these maneuvers.

The CO_2 laser has sufficient power to cleanse middle ear disease. Most examiners consider it safe. Its biggest drawbacks are the cumbersome bulk of the microscope and its attached articulated arms, and the imprecision of this type of laser. The microspot micromanipulator has been developed to improve laser precision.[21] Spot diameters are about one-third those of conventional CO_2 lasers, thus allowing a tenfold increase in power density for any set power level. The helium-neon aiming beam that formerly caused reflected glare and focusing problems in the middle ear has been superseded by a beam carried through an adjustable fiberoptic cable with a movable focal plane. The aiming spot thus produced is visible to the surgeon through the microscope but does not actually show up on the tissues. There is also a power defocus that enlarges the spot size incrementally for coagulation. These changes make middle ear work more precise and make CO_2 laser middle ear surgery practical for the first time. Power settings of 0.2 to 1 W can be used for cutting, coagulation, and welding.

The bulk of the CO_2 laser system and its need for rigid tubes instead of fiberoptic cables limit its use in otology, but attempts at correcting these problems continue.

Polycrystalline infrared optical fibers and hollow fiber wave guides have been created for use with both the superpulse and the continuous wave CO_2 lasers. A 600 μm hollow fiber can be used through a 1.5 mm steel tube, but the rigidity of this system still is a limiting problem.

Lasers may also be used to remove middle ear keratoma persisting after conventional removal of diseased tissue. Minute deposits around the ossicles can be vaporized under direct vision or by use of a reflecting mirror. The anterior variant of congenital pediatric cholesteatomas can be quite easily handled with or without tympanic membrane grafting, since the mastoid in these patients is usually free of disease and well pneumatized.[22]

Choristoma is technically a hamartoma—a collection of normal tissue in an abnormal location. Middle ear choristoma is generally salivary gland tissue that secretes fluid to fill the middle ear cleft, but there are reported cases of neural tissue in the middle ear. Tumor removal has generally required ossicular sacrifice, which may be avoidable by laser vaporization.[23]

Rhabdomyosarcoma and other malignant tumors presenting in the middle ear space generally present as a granular or polypoid mass. Lasers may be used in obtaining biopsy specimens. These lesions require multiple modality therapy for definitive management.

In 1864 VonTröltsch described an entity that has come to be known as **tympanosclerosis**. This lesion appears to consist of a failure of the healing process after inflammatory disease of the middle ear. Degeneration of the lamina propria occurs on the mucosal surface of the tympanic membrane, and the basement membrane in the middle ear thickens. Fibrous adhesions form, followed by hyaline degeneration, calcification, and new bone deposition in the middle ear space. There appear to be two separate subtypes: sclerosing mucositis involving surface elements, and invasive mucoperiostitis that may actually erode into the cochlear promontory and the otic capsule. The argon, KTP, and milliwatt CO_2 lasers are effective in vaporizing deposits of tympanosclerosis. Pieces can be freed from the ossicle with the laser and then removed with forceps, avoiding thermal damage to surrounding structures from prolonged laser use. We have performed laser stapedotomy in tympanosclerotic, fixed footplates after removal of peristapedial disease. This procedure averts removal of the anterior footplate, which may have saccular adhesions from invasive tympanosclerosis.

Paraganglioma should be considered if the patient reports pulsation or ringing in the ear and examination reveals fullness or bulging of the tympanic membrane or discoloration of the middle ear space. Further audiometric and radiographic testing should be undertaken. If a vascular tumor confined to the middle ear space, such as glomus tympanicum, is found, surgical resection with the laser should be possible. Paragangliomas may occur anywhere that glomus tissue exists: apex of the jugular bulb, course of Jacobsen's and Arnold's nerves, hypotympanum, cochlear promontory, or medial tympanic membrane. Consequently, the presentation of these tumors varies.

Glomus tympanicum tumors confined to the promontory, middle ear space, and hypotympanum can be successfully removed through either a transmeatal or transmastoid approach. The tumor is cauterized with the laser in essentially the same fashion as an acoustic tumor, and the edges tend to simply roll toward the center, freeing the tumor from the promontory or the undersurface of the tympanic membrane (Fig. 8.5). Surprisingly little bleeding is seen with this procedure if the tumor

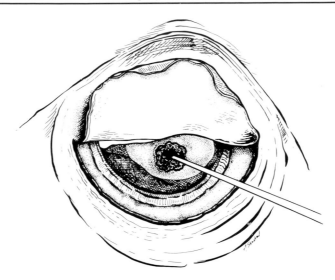

Figure 8.5. Glomus tympanicum vaporized and cauterized beginning centrally through a transmeatal approach.

has not deeply invaded bone. The KTP laser is preferred for glomus tympanicum tumors because of its absorption by the pigmented cells of the tumor (Fig. 8.6) and its slightly more effective power.

Before leaving the area of middle ear surgery, one must consider the debate regarding the use of microscopic laser manipulation versus hand-held probes. The fiber probes are attractive because of the ease in bringing them into the opera-

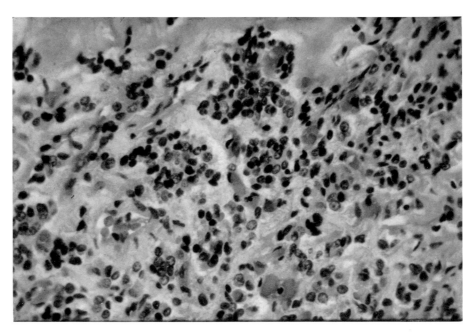

Figure 8.6. Glomus tympanicum paraganglioma with vascular spaces and typical cell pattern of "*zellballen*" clusters.

TABLE 8.2. *Characteristics of Laser Types*

	Argon	KTP/532	Nd:YAG	CO₂
Medium	Gas	Crystal	Crystal	Gas
Wavelength	488–514 nm	532 nm	1060 nm	10,600 nm
Color	Blue-green	Green	Invisible	Invisible
Smallest spot size	.150 mm (at 200 mm micro) .100 mm (at 100 mm probe)	.150 mm (at 200 mm micro) .100 mm (at 100 mm probe)	0.3 mm	.45 mm (200 mm micro) .09 mm (50 mm probe)
Power maximum	15 W (4–10 W at tissue)	15 W (4–10 W at tissue)	100 W	Usually 100 W (50 W at tissue)
Transport	Fiberoptic Microslad	Fiberoptic Microslad	Fiberoptic Microslad	Rigid hollow tubes Microslad
Absorption	Pigment	Pigment	Deep tissue	Water-surface

155

tive field without changing the microscope. Instrument manufacturers are increasingly advocating probes. Gillis[13] describes the difficulty in making precise lesions using hand-held fiberoptic laser transports. Silverstein[24] had significant problems with hand-held probes in two cases of stapedotomy: with 40% loss of discrimination in one case and massive granulation formation leading to total hearing loss in the second case. It seems unwise to abandon the search for precision and to adopt the use of fiberoptic tips and hand-held probes in some types of middle ear work when observers repeatedly have shown that misdirected laser beams can damage the inner ear.

Mastoid Procedures

Laser surgery of the mastoid serves an adjunctive role in chronic ear disease. With a microscope-coupled laser or through use of hand-held probes, granulation tissue can be removed from the mastoid bowl, bleeding points cauterized, and muscle and fascial grafts removed. Mucosa that extends along cellular tracts can also be cauterized. McGee[25] reported the use of the argon laser with spot sizes ranging from 150 μm to 2 mm in over 2000 tympanomastoid operations without any laser-related complications. He described the use of the laser to incise scar tissue when reexploring old mastoidectomy cavities using 4 to 6 W of power on continuous mode to cut through the tissue.

Table 8.2 summarizes the characteristics of three common laser systems. At present there is really no role for the Nd:YAG laser in general otology. Table 8.1 compares CO_2 and visible light lasers. The visible spectrum lasers (argon and KTP) are optically excellent, having the advantage of precision. The CO_2 lasers have excellent tissue interaction characteristics but lack the precise optical control of the visible wavelength lasers. Theoretically, with time, the desired optical qualities can be engineered for the CO_2 laser. Uses for both types can be found in current otologic practice, and these uses continue to expand.

CONCLUSIONS

The laser is simply a tool. As with any other tool, its safety and efficiency is dependent principally on the skill and understanding of the surgeon who controls it. There have always been, and always will be, certain surgeons who are gifted with exceptional dexterity, but for the majority of surgeons, any tool that might extend their skill and provide a buffer of safety for any mistake they might make is a tool of great value. During the 15 years the author has used lasers in surgery and the eight years since he assisted Dr. Perkins in expanding the initial series of stapedotomy patients, the equipment has been much refined, and the understanding of physiological responses to laser surgery has greatly matured. The underlying need for creativity in addressing disease remains the same.

8B
Lasers in Otology: Neurotology

Steven D. Rowley

Neurotologic work with lasers currently involves three main categories: benign and malignant tumor removal, work on nerves including nerve section and nerve anastomosis, and vascular anastomosis and cautery.

TUMOR REMOVAL

Both benign and malignant tumors can occur in the temporal bone, the posterior fossa, or the base of the skull. Tumors from the breast, kidney, lung, gastrointestinal tract, prostate, larynx, and thyroid may metastasize to the temporal bone hematologically. Parotid and nasopharyngeal tumors invade locally or by perineural spread. Melanoma can exhibit meningeal metastases around the internal auditory canal.[26] Lymphoma, lymphosarcoma, and Hodgkins disease may occur anywhere in the temporal bone including the middle ear and eustachian tube area, the internal auditory canal, and the facial nerve canal.[27] Squamous carcinoma from the auricle, auditory canal, or middle ear may also invade the temporal bone.

Acoustic neuroma accounts for 8% of intracranial tumors and 90% of posterior fossa tumors and is, along with other less common lesions such as cholesterol cysts and granulomas, meningiomas, neurofibromas, and facial nerve neuromas, amenable to treatment with the laser. Attempts have been made at laser cauterization of glomus jugulare paraganglioma, but to date these have not been particularly successful.

Better diagnostic tools such as magnetic resonance imaging (MRI) and evoked response audiometry help discover earlier and smaller tumors. Since the first description of acoustic neuroma removal in 1894 by Sir Charles Ballance,[28] lower morbidity and mortality in surgical removal have been attained through advances in technique including the use of the operating microscope, better anesthesia, and the understanding and treatment of complications. Acoustic neuromas originally were associated with a mortality of about 80%, but Cushing was able to lower that to 30% by 1917 and to 4% by 1932.[29] Clearly, mortality will always be lower for surgeons with exceptional skill, but the overall mortality and morbidity for removal of these types of tumors continue to improve. Future generations of investigators will decide whether the use of lasers in debulking these tumors has further reduced morbidity and mortality to a significant extent. Rand[30] recently described 31 cases of acoustic neuroma in which lasers were employed. Total removal of the tumor was achieved in 93% with a mortality of only 2%. Smith and Lager[31] described 15 cases of tumor; facial nerve function was preserved in 80% of the patients by means of a suboccipital approach and use of the CO_2 laser. Mortality was 6%, and total tumor removal was accomplished in 14 of the 15 patients.

Cerullo[32] compared 21 patients whose acoustic neuromas were removed conventionally (1974–1980) with 22 whose tumors were removed by CO_2 laser (1980–1984). Facial nerve preservation and function was better in the laser group, and these patients were able to return to work sooner.

Surgical Technique

A translabyrinthine, retrolabyrinthine, or suboccipital approach is performed in standard fashion, exposing the dura. The proposed opening of the dura is demarcated with the defocused laser used to cauterize vessels. Either sharp scissors or the laser in cutting mode may be used to open the dura. Care should be taken to maintain the arachnoid sheath when removing tumor contents and capsule. This is generally facilitated by placing moist cottonoids around the area of tumor. The tumor is debulked from center to periphery. Finally, the capsule is removed.

Neurofibromas and many neurolemmomas are rather dense, and laser vaporization or morselization of the tumor is faster than using the Urban dissector or the Cavitron Ultrasonic Surgical Aspirator (CUSA). The laser is much faster than using cup forceps and bipolar cautery. In Glasscock's 1981 series of acoustic tumor removal, the argon laser was used and tumor resection was somewhat slow.[33] Since then the increased power of the KTP-532 laser or CO_2 laser has allowed much faster tumor vaporization. Most tumors can be vaporized with power settings between 5 and 10 w using a 0.45- to 1.0-mm spot size. Single pulses should be used initially to verify the effect of the laser, but continuous mode can be employed in the center of the tumor for debulking (Fig. 8.7) because the use of irrigating fluids and the spinal fluid bathing the tumor will counteract any thermal effect. As char forms over the tumor it should be removed by scraping or suction. Such desiccated debris can reach temperatures well above 100°C. Indisputable thermal damage to tissues can occur if this debris is not removed. The laser is used in strokes, much like a paintbrush, over the central portion of the tumor to avoid deep holes in the tumor mass. As the central parts of the tumor are vaporized, the edges roll toward the center so that dissection can be readily continued.

If the KTP-532 laser is used, a 5-w power setting is generally employed and tumor vaporization may be accomplished by microscopic visualization or using hand-held fiberoptic probes. This author prefers the precision of microsurgery, but many neurosurgeons use the hand-held probes.

If a suboccipital or retrolabyrinthine approach is employed, the laser may also be used to remove periosteal dura from the posterior surface of the internal auditory canal prior to drilling and tumor removal in this area.

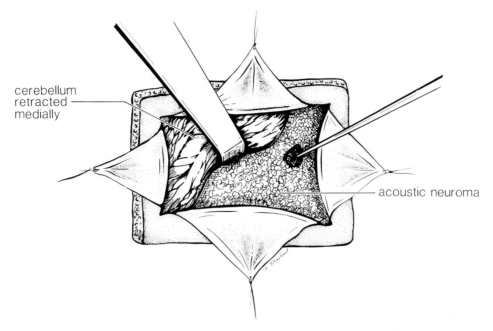

Figure 8.7. Acoustic neuroma filling cerebellar–pontine angle as seen through the subocciput, right side. Tumor vaporization begins centrally.

Electrical monitoring of eighth cranial nerve action potentials has been accomplished during acoustic neuroma surgery. Silverstein[34] describes placing a silver wire electrode against the eighth cranial nerve and holding it in place with cottonoids during tumor removal. The tumor was debulked with the Sharplan 733 CO_2 laser set between 10 and 20 w in continuous mode. Their findings suggested that the latency of the nerve's action potential improved as tumor size diminished. Extensive use of the laser on the area of the tumor above the cochlear nerve seemed to cause transient decreases in the amplitude of the action potential. However, it was later noted that contact of the electrode with the nerve had been poor, and the amplitude of the action potentials increased after the electrode was replaced. Following surgery, the patient had a temporary reduction in speech discrimination but improved during the subsequent week.

Saunders[35] and associates placed electrodes and monitored somatosensory-evoked potentials while vaporizing spinal cord lesions with the CO_2 laser in cats. They demonstrated that single and multiple exposures totaling 287 to 43,750 J did not cause any permanent impairment in these responses.

During tumor vaporization, one must constantly be aware of the contiguous and deep structures. Overheating of the tumor from excessive use of the laser must be avoided. Penetration through tumor into deeper structures should not occur.

For removal of the last remnants of tumor and capsule from the facial and cochlear nerves and the brain stem, some surgeons prefer to employ conventional techniques instead of the laser. It appears that as surgeons gain more skill and understanding of laser/tissue interactions, they will be able to dissect tumor from these areas, thus taking full advantage of the minimal trauma inherent in laser surgery (Fig. 8.8). Certainly, as surgeons vaporize the periphery of the neoplasm,

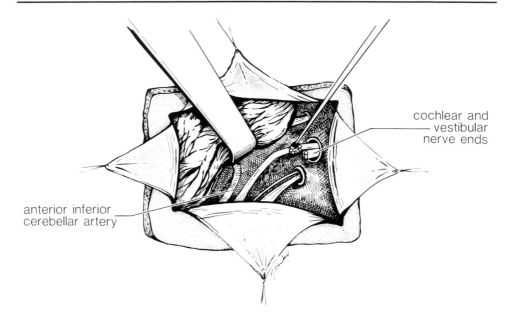

cochlear and
vestibular
nerve ends

anterior inferior
cerebellar artery

Figure 8.8. Cerebellopontine angle after tumor removal. Last remnants of tumor vaporized from facial nerve.

they should avoid any prolonged exposures in the continuous mode which would result in heat injury to adjacent normal tissues. These concerns are not as paramount when the surgeon is working on the central portion of the tumor and all adjacent tissue consists of neoplasm. Pulsed mode CO_2 lasers may form sharper edges at the treatment spot with reduced thermal spread, providing more precise dissection over these final delicate areas.

NEURAL SURGERY

Nerve Section

Vestibular nerve section through the posterior fossa can be easily and safely done. Moist cottonoids are placed to isolate the neural bundle from surrounding brain stem areas and from vascular structures coursing between the facial and vestibular nerves. Eighth nerve monitoring after the fashion suggested by Silverstein[34] can be performed. Precise cutting with the laser is employed. When changes in cochlear nerve action potential are seen, the dissection is stopped. In this fashion there is essentially no traction on the cochlear nerve and its microcirculation. Silverstein reports that if eighth nerve anteroposterior latency recovers to within 0.4 msec of preoperative level and there is less than a 40% decrease in amplitude, postoperative hearing will be within 20 dB, and discrimination within 20% of preoperative levels.

After the posterior fossa dura has been opened and the cistern decompressed, the cochleovestibular complex is examined. In patients in whom a clear cleavage plane between the vestibular and cochlear nerve components is seen (75% of cases),

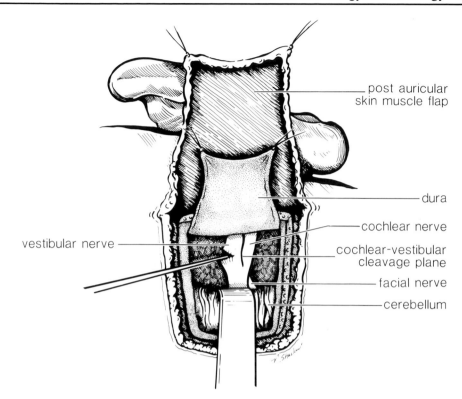

post auricular
skin muscle flap

dura

cochlear nerve

vestibular nerve

cochlear-vestibular
cleavage plane

facial nerve

cerebellum

Figure 8.9. Retrolabyrinth approach to vestibular nerve. Laser microsection technique allows fibers to retract after being cut. Moist cottonoids have been omitted for better visualization.

the KTP laser at 3 w or a milliwatt CO_2 laser at 300 to 500 mw is used to section the vestibular portion while protecting the deep facial nerve and blood vessels with moist cottonoids. As the fibers are vaporized beginning at the nerve edge, they pull away from each other, making dissection easier (Fig. 8.9). This technique avoids any traction on the cochlear nerve or circulation and should enhance hearing results.

If a cleavage plane is not visible (25% of cases), the dissection can proceed in the same fashion, but fibers near the cochlear portion are vaporized almost one at a time while the eighth nerve action potential is continually monitored. As soon as the first small nonreversible change is seen, dissection is stopped. This technique should enhance the surgical treatment of vertigo by giving a more precise resection, thereby maintaining hearing levels. If a retrosigmoid approach is used, the bone over the internal auditory canal (IAC) can be removed, and the superior vestibular nerve and singular nerve can be selectively vaporized.

Neuroma

Electron microscopy has demonstrated that high energy laser transsection of peripheral nerves permanently seals the endoneural tubules, thus preventing axon regeneration past the point of transsection. This concept can be used effectively in the

treatment of painful neuromas, but it could also be used to prevent neuroma formation in ear surgery. Studies have shown less neuroma formation using the low power
CO_2 laser in nerve cutting than with the scalpel technique. The Nd:YAG laser is
even better, with smaller, less reactive neuromas being formed.

Anastomosis

In 1932 Ballance and Duel[36] reported on facial nerve grafting using epineural repair
techniques. In 1982 Crumley[37] described the spatial orientation of individual fascicles. This finding led to the concept of interfascicular perineural nerve anastomosis.

Nishihira[38] reported results of nerve grafts performed by a two-stitch epineural
suture technique and by fibrin glue apposition. He concluded that compound action
potentials were significantly better in the sutured nerves.

Incomplete regeneration is believed to be caused by mechanical trauma, uneven
cutting of nerve ends, crushing during cutting, and edema or mushroom swelling
of sutured ends in such a way that axons are misdirected. These problems were
addressed by a reconnection technique in which the nerve endings are cooled and
bathed in a physiologic solution. Results using this technique on rat sciatic nerves
seem promising. A 300 to 400% improvement is seen in comparison with the
average amount of functional recovery that one can expect from standard epineural
repair.[39]

The laser may have a role in nerve anastomosis using a very small spot size and
a very low power for welding. Investigation of this concept is needed, but studies
to date show less neuroma formation and better functional results with low power
CO_2 laser–assisted anastomosis than with conventional suture techniques. (See
Chapter 13.)

VASCULAR SURGERY

A variety of vascular work has been done with CO_2, argon, and Nd:YAG lasers,
including coagulation of aneurysms, coagulation of blood vessels, laser-assisted microvascular anastomosis, and coring of intravascular deposits for improved perfusion. (See Chapter 13.)

Most anastomotic failure is thought to be related to inflammatory thrombosis,
often in response to the presence of suture material. A laser may be used to weld
vessels at an anastomotic site, reducing or entirely averting use of foreign body
suture material and thereby reducing the risk of thrombosis. This concept was
investigated by Ruiz-Razura and associates,[40] who performed laser-assisted end-to-
side microvascular anastomoses on the iliac arteries of 150 rats. The technique
consisted of placing four stay sutures and then using a CO_2 laser to spot weld
between the stay sutures.

High pressure anastomoses had patency rates of 96% with the laser and 92%
with conventional methods. An aneurysm rate of 44% was seen in the laser-assisted
cases. In anastomoses under lower pressure there was 98% patency with the laser
and 92% without. There was no evidence of aneurysm formation, leading the

investigators to postulate that aneurysm formation was related to the amount of tension on the anastomotic suture line.

Vale and associates[41] reported on the use of the laser in forming anastomoses in the carotid arteries of rats. The CO_2 laser was used at 100-mw power and 0.2-mm spot size. Twenty to 30 pulses were used for each vessel anastomosis. Pathologic examination showed some desiccation of the vessel media and intima and some collagen damage, which theoretically could lead to aneurysm formation.

Jain[42] performed extracranial–intracranial anastomoses in rats using the YAG laser and was able to achieve a rate of greater than 90% patency. His studies showed early endothelialization (2 to 3 days) and some collagen fibrosis. He theorized that thermal effects of the laser caused collagen denaturization and this helped seal the anastomotic site. This hypothesis may explain why all investigators report redoing a laser anastomosis is very difficult, because the collagen protein has already been affected.

Jain[41] performed superficial temporal artery to middle cerebral artery bypass in five patients. The YAG laser was used at 18 w power and 0.1-sec pulse. It was passed through a 600-μm quartz fiber to create a spot size between 300 and 400 μm. A prototype ophthalmologic handpiece was used to manipulate the laser. Jain performed an anastomotic closure, then allowed blood to accumulate over this site and performed a second closure on top of this. He concluded that the laser anastomosis was easier and faster than conventional suture techniques; no foreign-body reaction occurred. Nine months postsurgically he found excellent results with no evidence of aneurysm formation and patent vessels in all five cases.

Fried[43] used a milliwatt CO_2 laser at 0.23 w-power and 0.3-mm spot size with repeated 0.1-sec exposures to perform microvascular anastomosis. He considered that operations were easier to perform and saved time compared with conventional techniques. Revision surgery was difficult, however.

Studies of the tensile strength of anastomoses show equal early results in CO_2 laser versus conventional suture technique. Six weeks postoperatively, however, the laser-assisted anastomotic sites are generally stronger than sutured ones.

The Nd:YAG 1318 nm laser has also been used through a 200-μg catheter with excellent results (88% long-term success).[44]

Nd:YAG LASER

To date the argon, KTP-532, and CO_2 lasers are much more widely used than the YAG laser because of the difficulty in precisely controlling depth of tissue damage. Ophthalmologists have recently begun using the YAG laser to perform iridotomy as treatment for acute angle glaucoma and have noted that the YAG laser is much more efficient than the argon laser. Its higher power enables it to rupture the iris with a single exposure of energy.

Perhaps this same treatment concept can be applied to the treatment of petrous cholesterol cysts and arachnoid cysts. These lesions tend to be difficult to treat because they re-form and often require repeat surgery or long-term drainage. The Nd:YAG laser is capable of rupturing the cyst walls and maintaining a patent opening. The laser can be used at the depths of ventricles or cisterns and has been used to remove third-ventricle colloid cysts effectively.[45] It is also being used in computer-assisted stereotactic biopsy and removal of intracranial neoplasms. Malignant brain tumors seem to respond to the hyperthermic environment created by these lasers, offering some hope for unresectable tumors.

Other vascular applications of the Nd:YAG laser appear promising. This laser can close arterotomies in major vessels as well as clearing vessels of intraluminal deposits using intraluminal fiberoptic catheters or metal probes. Arteriovenous malformations can be treated with this laser because of its coagulative properties.

Collagen deposition can apparently be diminished by the use of the Nd:YAG laser when coupled with dye (photo dynamic therapy).[46]

FUTURE CONSIDERATIONS

Lasers are here to stay. They are dramatically changing the technology available for neurotologic surgery. There continue to be problems related to laser surgery and instrumentation. It is anticipated that future argon lasers will have greater power output, and that combining multiple lasers will be developed. For otologic and neurotologic purposes a combination of a milliwatt CO_2 laser coupled to a visible light laser such as the KTP would be ideal. We anticipate the creation of computer programs and remote control of laser systems, making it possible to control the aiming and movements of lasers more precisely. Numerous new laser wavelengths will be available because of improved ability to manufacture crystals. Heavy metal vapor lasers and variations of pulsing patterns will provide lasers more specifically suited to specific pathologic entities.

8C

Lasers in Otology: Otosclerosis

S. George Lesinski
Jay Paul Willging

The concept of using laser energy to perform stapedotomy and stapedectomy revision is an attractive one. Lasers could vaporize a precise, round stapedotomy in the stapes footplate regardless of its thickness or degree of fixation. Mechanical trauma to the inner ear would be eliminated, introducing an elegant simplicity to a sometimes difficult operation. In revision of a previously failed stapedectomy, lasers could enable the otologic surgeon to vaporize the obliterating oval window tissue atraumatically, thus precisely identifying margins and depth of the oval window and the relationship of the stapes prosthesis to these landmarks. The exact mechanism of the conductive failure could then be safely determined. The laser could create a stapedotomy in the oval window neomembrane, thereby stabilizing the new prosthesis and minimizing the risk of recurrent prosthesis migration—the most common cause for stapedectomy failure.

Lasers have been developed to permit precise, controlled delivery of energy to the microscopic operative field. A choice between visible lasers (argon, 514 nm and KTP-532, 532 nm) and invisible lasers (CO_2, 10,600 nm), however, needs to be made, based on their physical properties. The optical and tissue characteristics of these two groups of lasers are dramatically different. The visible lasers possess ideal optical properties but less than ideal tissue characteristics for otosclerosis surgery. Conversely, the CO_2 laser possesses ideal tissue characteristics, but less than ideal optical properties (Fig. 8.10).

This chapter reports the author's experience in attempting to answer the question of which is the best type of laser for use in otosclerosis.

HISTORICAL REVIEW

The advantages of stapedotomy over stapedectomy have been demonstrated by Fisch,[47] Marquet,[48] Smyth,[49] Causse,[50] and others. Conceptually, laser vaporization

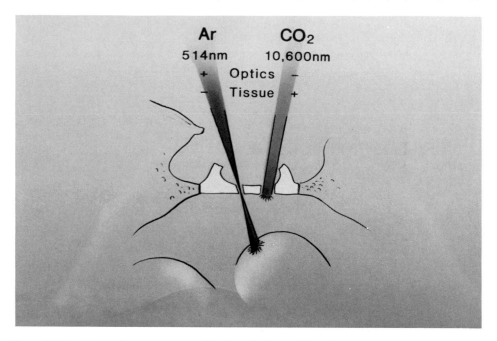

Figure 8.10. Argon laser possesses ideal optical precision for stapedotomy, but less than ideal tissue characteristics. Its energy is only partially absorbed by the whitish stapes footplate and readily penetrates clear perilymph to be selectively absorbed by pigmented cells and blood vessels in the utricle and saccule. The CO_2 laser has ideal tissue characteristics (completely absorbed by the stapes footplate and surface perilymph without significant penetration) but poses an optics dilemma that until recently rendered it too imprecise for otosclerosis surgery. (From Lesinski SG, Palmer A: Lasers for otosclerosis: CO_2 vs. argon and KTP-532. *Laryngoscope* 99 [suppl 46]:1–8, 1989. With permission.)

of the stapedotomy opening will eliminate mechanical trauma to the inner ear. In 1980 Perkins[51] reported the first successful series of human stapedotomies using the laser (argon, 514 nm), which was followed by other successful series from McGee,[52] DiBartolomeo,[53] Marquet, and others. No vertigo or sensorineural hearing loss was reported in these series. Gantz[54] published his histologic study of stapedotomies performed with the argon laser in the cat, showing the potential danger of the visible laser. Three saccule perforations were demonstrated in these eight stapedotomies. Silverstein's 1989 study[55] illustrated the potential consequences of such damage. He reported that 40% of the KTP-532 stapedotomy patients had significant postoperative vestibular symptoms, and two of the stapedectomy revisions performed with a hand-held HMG argon laser led to significant sensorineural hearing loss.

The surgical use of the CO_2 laser was delayed because of technical complexities inherent in aligning an invisible CO_2 laser beam with a second visible aiming laser beam. It was not until 1984 that Sharplan Laboratories introduced refined optics allowing the precision required for otosclerosis surgery. On the basis of the physical properties of the long wavelength of the CO_2 laser, Wilpizeski[56] proposed that this type of laser would theoretically minimize the risk to inner ear structures because the CO_2 laser energy is completely absorbed by tissue and fluid regardless of their color. DiBartolomeo[53] warned, however, that the CO_2 laser may "boil" perilymph, but this risk was not substantiated in the experimental stapedotomy studies reported by Gardner[57] and later by Coker.[58] Both of these surgeons actually recommended use of the CO_2 laser in humans. In 1987 Lesinski reported the first successful clinical series of CO_2 laser stapedotomies.[59]

GENERAL PRINCIPLES OF LASER USE

The safe, effective use of electromagnetic energy requires a thorough understanding of each wavelength's physical properties and its effect on tissue. Laser energy (*l*ight *a*mplification through *s*timulated *e*mission *r*adiation) is monochromatic (one wavelength), collimated (parallel), and in phase (positive and negative waves aligned). When applied to tissue, the laser energy can ionize molecules or have a thermal effect on tissue resulting in warming, photocoagulation, or vaporization. The specific tissue effects are dictated by three parameters: the wavelength of the laser beam, the power density (W/cm^2), and the duration of application.

Visible Lasers: Argon (512 nm) and KTKP-532 (532 nm)

Visible lasers possess ideal optical properties for microscopic otologic surgery. Because of their short wavelengths, these lasers can easily be transmitted through fiberoptic cables, delivered through a Microslad® adapter attached to the microscope, and focused to a small spot size (50 μ) at a 250-mm focal length. Because these lasers are visible, the same beam is used for both aiming and vaporizing. Therefore, with the argon and KTP lasers, the aiming beam and firing beam are focused to the same exact spot (parfocal, coaxial). These optical properties of the visible lasers provide the convenience and precision required for otosclerosis microsurgery.

On the other hand, tissue absorption characteristics of the visible laser energy are less than ideal for otosclerosis surgery. Two tissue properties imparted by the relatively short wavelengths of the visible lasers are undesirable: energy absorption and thermal scatter.

Tissue Absorption Coefficient

The absorption rate of laser energy in the visible light spectrum depends on tissue color. Opposite or complementary tissue colors will maximally absorb visible light laser energy. The blue-green argon or KTP-532 beam is absorbed best by dark red–pigmented colors. When applied to the stapes footplate, only a portion of the laser energy will be absorbed by the footplate bone, vaporizing it. The remaining energy passes readily through the clear fluid (perilymph) in the vestibule, to be absorbed by blood vessels and pigmented cells in the inner ear (Fig. 8.10).

Thermal Scatter

Because of their short wavelengths, the energy of visible lasers penetrates tissue deeper, with more thermal scatter than the long wavelength invisible CO_2 beam. These characteristics make the argon and KTP-532 lasers ideal for retinal surgery but somewhat risky for oval window surgery. If visible laser energy is applied directly to an open oval window it will readily pass through the perilymph to be absorbed by inner ear structures. Theoretically, then, the visible lasers should be used with care when performing stapedotomy. Direct application of the visible laser energy to the perilymph should be avoided. Since surgical techniques for revision stapedectomy often require vaporizing thin soft tissue in the oval window, the visible lasers probably should be used with extreme caution for stapedectomy revision.

Carbon Dioxide Laser (10,600 nm)

The CO_2 laser possesses ideal tissue absorption characteristics for otosclerosis surgery but poses an optics dilemma for the microscopic surgeon. Because of its long wavelength, the CO_2 laser is invisible. Therefore, a second visible aiming beam (HeNe—614 nm) is required. Both of these beams must be focused to a small spot size; they must be parfocal and coaxial. Figure 8.11 demonstrates the inherent optics dilemma—a principle of optical physics called chromatic aberration. When light passes through a lens, the amount of refraction (bending of that light beam) will be inversely proportional to its wavelength. Therefore, as these two different laser beams pass through the same lens, the shorter wavelength HeNe beam will be bent much more than the CO_2 beam. It is physically impossible to focus both beams on the same spot while passing them through the same lens. In 1984 Sharplan Laser Laboratories introduced significant engineering advances in the optics of the CO_2 laser, allowing consistent delivery of the CO_2 beam within 0.1 mm of the

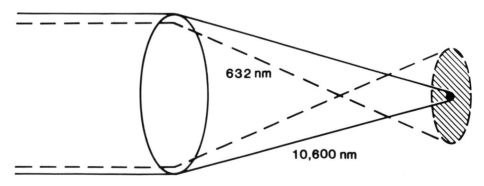

Figure 8.11. Chromatic aberration. Passing through the same lens, the HeNe beam (632 nm) is refracted much more than the CO_2 beam (10,600 nm). This phenomenon of optical physics made it nearly impossible to keep the aiming HeNe beam and the functioning CO_2 beam parfocal and coaxial. (From Lesinski SG, Palmer A: Lasers for otosclerosis: CO_2 vs. argon and KTP-532. *Laryngoscope* 99 [suppl 46]:1–8, 1989. With permission.)

center of the HeNe aiming laser beam. The CO_2 and HeNe laser beams are delivered to the microscope by a series of precisely aligned mirrors and lenses (often a dozen or more), compounding the inherent optics problem many times over. In contrast to the visible laser, the CO_2 laser cannot be efficiently passed through a fiberoptic cable.

The CO_2 beam, because of its long wavelength, possesses ideal tissue characteristics for otosclerosis surgery. Carbon dioxide laser energy is rapidly absorbed by tissue or fluid, regardless of color. The CO_2 type has the least tissue penetrance and energy scatter among the medical lasers. With proper energy parameters, the CO_2 laser should be completely absorbed by the stapes footplate when performing a stapedotomy. Carbon dioxide laser energy that might strike surface perilymph should be absorbed instantaneously by the fluid at the surface.

Laboratory experiments performed by the senior author verify these theoretical laser principles. Stapedotomies and stapedectomy revisions were performed with visible lasers and the CO_2 laser on human temporal bones while computerized pyroelectric detectors analyzed the energy "packets" delivered to the operative field and ultrasensitive thermocouples positioned in the vestibule measured energy transfer to the inner ear.

LABORATORY ANALYSIS: ARGON, KTP-532, AND CARBON DIOXIDE LASERS

Three specific tissue effects must be considered if the laser is to be used safely and effectively for otosclerosis surgery:

1. Vaporization of stapedotomy opening into the stapes footplate or in the soft tissue, obliterating the oval window (stapedectomy revision)
2. Thermal effect on vestibular perilymph and endolymph
3. Energy penetration of perilymph causing damage to blood vessels and neuroepithelium of the inner ear

Laser energy absorption by a particular tissue varies with the wavelength of the laser energy and the power density of the focused beam (W/cm^2), as well as the precise time (pulse duration) and the mode of delivery (continuous vs pulsed) by which the energy is applied to the tissue. To understand potential tissue effects one must consider more than the simple power settings and pulse duration (Example: 2 W in 0.1 sec) of the laser beam. The precise mode (continuous, quasicontinuous, chopped, pulsed) used to deliver this power to the tissue will determine its effect on that tissue (warming, coagulation, vaporization, and thermal spread). In these experiments, wave analyzers (pyroelectric detectors) were employed to measure precise energy parameters being delivered to the operative site. Then operating conditions were duplicated, and stapedotomies and stapedectomy revisions were performed in human temporal bones while heat transferred to the inner ear was measured with an ultrasensitive thermocouple strategically placed in the vestibule.

Wave Analysis

Each laser beam was directed into a pyroelectric detector (Molectron, Inc. J-2HR Detector) connected to an oscilloscope (Tektronix 2221) linked to a dot matrix printer. A qualitative and quantitative graphic analysis of each laser beam's "package" was performed. During a 0.05-sec pulse duration, the laser energy may be delivered to the operative field in a continuous (argon), quasicontinuous (KTP-532), or pulsed (CO_2 superpulse) model. Our analysis included the peak-to-peak wattage of each micropulse (its "on" time), its frequency and duty cycle (percentage of each cycle that laser is "on"), and a calculation of the amount of work (millijoules) delivered to the tissue in each miniburst and during the entire 0.05-sec pulse duration.

Argon Laser

Electronically stimulating argon gas produces a blue-green visible laser beam whose principal wavelength is 514 nm. With the argon laser (Coherent Model 920) set at 2 W of average power and a 0.05-sec pulse duration, a continuous nonpulsed beam with a peak-to-peak power of 2 W is delivered (Fig. 8.12). During the 50-msec pulse, 100 mj of work are delivered to the operative field in a continuous manner (100% duty cycle) with no off-time to limit thermal spread.

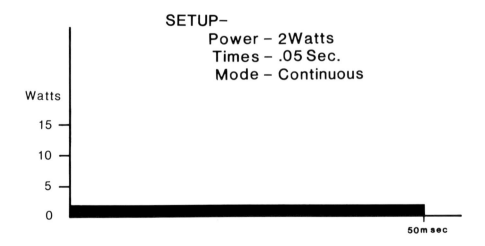

Figure 8.12. At 2 W power setting, the Coherent 920 argon laser delivers a continuous 2 W of power for 50 msec, which equals 100 mj of work. (From Lesinski SG, Palmer A: Lasers for otosclerosis: CO_2 vs. argon and KTP-532. *Laryngoscope* 99 [suppl 46]:1–8, 1989. With permission.)

KTP-532 Laser

In the KTP-532 laser (Laserscope Model 100501), a neodymium-YAG crystal is optically pumped to produce an invisible 1064 nm laser beam. This invisible beam is electronically Q-switched at 7600 Hz. The pulsed beam is then passed through a crystal that doubles its frequency and halves the laser wavelength to 532 nm, a visible green beam.

When the KTP-532 console is set to 2 W and 0.05-sec duration, 3800 tiny "pips" of energy are delivered in 50-msec (Fig. 8.13). Each tiny pulse has a peak-to-peak power of 6 W and an on-time of 4 μsec, producing 24 μJ of work per pip; together, these tiny pips deliver a total of 91 mJ of work to the operative field during a 0.05-sec pulse. The KTP-532 energy is on for 30% of each pulse and off for 70% (30% duty cycle). This high frequency Q-switching of the KTP-532 energy exerts quasicontinuous energy on the tissue, somewhat diminishing thermal spread compared with a continuous argon beam.

The recommended power settings for both the argon and KTP-532 lasers are 2 W, single pulse, pulse duration of 0.1 sec. During that 0.1-sec pulse duration the argon delivers 200 mJ of work in a continuous mode and the KTP-532 delivers 182 mJ of work in a quasicontinuous mode.

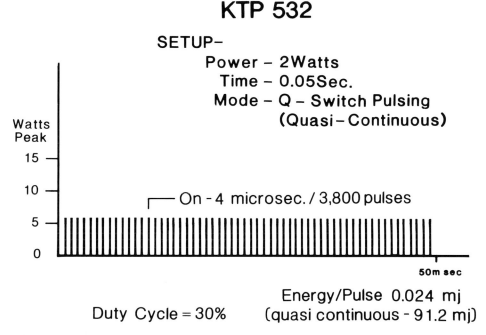

Figure 8.13. The KTP-532 (Laserscope) set at 2 W average power delivers 3800 micropulses during the 50-msec pulse duration. Each micropulse has a peak-to-peak power of 6 W and is on for 4μsec. During this 50-msec pulse duration with a duty cycle of 30%, 91.2 mj are delivered. (From Lesinski SG, Palmer A: Lasers for otosclerosis: CO_2 vs. argon and KTP-532. *Laryngoscope* 99 [suppl 46]:1–8, 1989. With permission.)

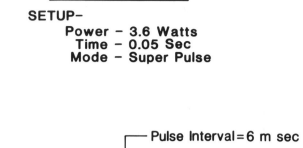

SHARPLAN 734

Figure 8.14. The CO_2 laser (Sharplan 734) set at 3.6 W superpulse mode delivers 8 micropulses during the 50-msec pulse time. Each micropulse has a peak-to-peak power of 36 W and an on-time of 0.6 msec, providing 21.6 mj of work. In the 50-msec pulse duration a total of 172 mj of energy is delivered in divided microbursts with a duty cycle of 10%. (From Lesinski SG, Palmer A: Lasers for otosclerosis: CO_2 vs. argon and KTP-532. *Laryngoscope* 99 [suppl 46]:1–8, 1989. With permission.)

Carbon Dioxide Laser

By electrically exciting CO_2 gas, a 10,600-nm invisible CO_2 laser beam is produced. A Sharplan 734 laser is equipped with an electronic switching mechanism (superpulse) that pulses this CO_2 laser in tiny microsecond bursts. When the power is set at 3.6 W, 0.05-sec pulse duration, superpulse mode, eight micropulses of energy are delivered (Fig. 8.14). Each individual micropulse has a peak-to-peak power of 36 W and an on-time of 0.6 msec; it delivers 21.6 mJ of work. During the entire 0.05-sec pulse duration, 172 mJ of work are delivered to the operative field, but the work is split up into eight tiny partitions (micropulses) with a long rest period (cooling time) between micropulses. During the first 0.6 msec, 21.6 mJ are delivered to the tissue. The CO_2 laser beam is then off for 6 msec, back on for 0.6 msec, and then off for 6 msec—a duty cycle of 10%. Therefore, during 90% of the 0.05-sec pulse duration the CO_2 laser beam is actually off. This pulsing of the CO_2 beam into tiny microbursts "sharpens" the vaporizing effect on the stapes footplate by limiting thermal spread in the bone and the underlying perilymph.

Thermocouple Experiments

Stapedotomy

Operating room conditions were duplicated, and 0.6-mm stapedotomy openings were vaporized into the center of human stapes footplates while temperature changes were measured with an ultrasensitive thermocouple placed in the peri-lymph-filled vestibule 2 mm below the footplate (Fig. 8.15).

Stapedotomy techniques for the visible lasers (argon and KTP-532) are similar. A beam size of 0.05 mm, a power setting of 2 W, and a pulse duration of 0.1 sec, are used to vaporize eight to ten tiny rosettes in a circumferential pattern to produce a 0.6-mm opening in the center of the stapes footplate. The delay between firings averaged 1 to 3 sec. As cautioned by Perkins,[51] meticulous care was taken not to apply the laser beam directly to the open oval window.

The CO_2 laser stapedotomies were performed with a 0.6-mm spot size, a power setting of 3.6 W, and a 0.1-sec pulse duration in superpulse mode (*Sharplan 734 model only*). Usually three to five bursts were required, firing at 2-sec intervals to vaporize a round 0.6-mm stapedotomy into a normal stapes footplate.

Figure 8.16A shows a typical temperature rise of 0.2 to 0.3°C measured in our vestibular thermocouple during CO_2 laser stapedotomy. Note also the configuration of the rise. It is smooth, with no initial spiking, and cooling is gradual. This pattern indicates that the CO_2 laser energy is completely absorbed at the footplate and that thermal spread from the surface perilymph down to the level of the saccule is almost negligible. Fifty percent of the energy from a carbon dioxide laser is absorbed in .0000/ cm. Therefore, carbon dioxide laser vaporization of the footplate can be performed by repeated firing of an equal-sized laser beam in the same place on the stapes footplate without fear that the laser energy will penetrate the surface perilymph.

When the visible laser energy (argon or KTP-532) was carefully applied to the stapes footplate so that the rosettes did not overlap, the thermocouple measurements were similar and quite satisfactory. Figure 8.16B is a typical temperature measured in the vestibule during a stapedotomy performed with the argon laser and shows a maximum rise of approximately 0.5°C when a stapedotomy is vaporized without overlapping the "rosettes." This should produce no significant thermal effect in the patient. Note, however, the character of the thermocouple temperature measurements observed during nearly all the stapedotomies performed with the visible lasers. The initial temperature spike represents the portion of energy that is not absorbed by the white stapes footplate but passes directly through the peri-lymph to be absorbed by the thermocouple. A second, slower rise in temperature represents the caloric effect in the surrounding perilymph.

Stapedotomies were also performed with the visible lasers while allowing the rosettes to overlap approximately 50%. Figure 8.17 is a typical temperature curve obtained with the KTP-532. A 200-μm spot size was used to permit a more accurate approximation of the overlap, but this reduces the power density (W/cm^2) of the beam to 1/16th that of the 50-μm spot size. These power settings produced an immediate temperature spike of 4.3°C. On the second direct application the temperature rose 6.3°C as the visible laser energy passed directly through a portion of the vaporized footplate, through the perilymph, and into the thermocouple.

Stapedectomy Revision

Revising a previously failed stapedectomy requires vaporization of the soft tissue obliterating the oval window and often direct application of the laser energy to the open vestibule. Theoretically, the short wavelength of the argon and KTP-532 visible lasers are potentially hazardous to the inner ear because visible laser energy

THERMOCOUPLE IN VESTIBULE

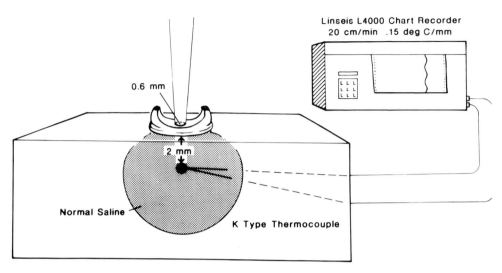

Figure 8.15. An ultrasensitive K-type thermocouple is inserted in the saline-filled vestibule 2 mm below the stapes. After appropriate standardization, temperature changes are recorded while laser stapedotomy and laser stapedectomy revision are performed with the argon, KTP-532, and CO_2 lasers. (From Lesinski SG, Palmer A: Lasers for otosclerosis: CO_2 vs. argon and KTP-532. *Laryngoscope* 99 [suppl 46]:1–8, 1989. With permission.)

readily passes through perilymph to be selectively absorbed by the blood vessels and pigmented cells in the inner ear. The CO_2 energy should be ideal for stapedectomy revisions because this long-wavelength energy should not penetrate perilymph at these low energy levels and any caloric effect could be minimized by pulsing the beam.

To evaluate the validity of this theory, the visible lasers and the CO_2 lasers were directly applied to the open saline-filled vestibule while a K-type thermocouple measured temperature change 2 mm below. Power settings used where those recommended as safe for stapedotomy. Figure 8.18 represents actual measurements obtained with the CO_2 and argon lasers while simulating stapedectomy revision.

Application of the CO_2 laser directly to the open vestibule produced temperature rises no greater than 0.5°C 2 mm below the surface. A single pulse of argon energy focused to a 0.6-mm spot size produced a 22.5°C temperature rise. The recommended 0.05 mm-spot size produced temperature rises as high as 175°C. Figure 8.19 is a microphotograph of a typical "pothole" melted into the submerged thermocouple by a single pulse of argon energy (2 W, 0.1-sec duration, 0.05-mm spot size). The melting temperature of the thermocouple metal is 175°C.

Application of the KTP-532 laser energy through the open vestibule produced temperature changes between 21° and 52°C in the thermocouple at spot sizes of 0.1 mm and 0.05 mm respectively. In contrast to the CO_2 laser, visible laser energy must travel approximately 227 feet through a medium before 50% of the energy is absorbed.

STAPEDOTOMY

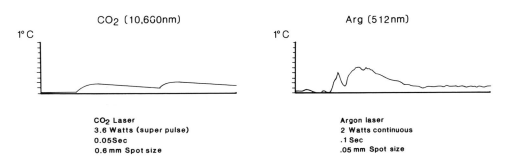

CO₂ (10,600nm)   Arg (512nm)

1°C   1°C

CO₂ Laser   Argon laser
3.6 Watts (super pulse)   2 Watts continuous
0.05 Sec   .1 Sec
0.6 mm Spot size   .05 mm Spot size

Figure 8.16. Thermocouple measurements during laser stapedotomy. Carbon dioxide laser increased thermocouple temperature 0.2 to 0.3°C during stapedotomy. The argon laser energy raised thermocouple measurements 0.5°C. Note immediate spike as argon energy passed through stapes footplate and perilymph to strike thermocouple directly, and then a delayed temperature rise secondary to caloric effect in the perilymph. (From Lesinski SG, Palmer A: Lasers for otosclerosis: CO_2 vs. argon and KTP-532. *Laryngoscope* 99 [suppl 46]:1–8, 1989. With permission.)

STAPEDOTOMY

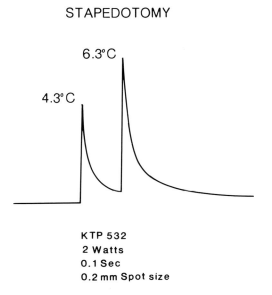

6.3°C

4.3°C

KTP 532
2 Watts
0.1 Sec
0.2 mm Spot size

Figure 8.17. Thermocouple measurements with KTP-532 during stapedotomy when rosettes are 50% superimposed. Some KTP-532 energy enters the open vestibule. (From Lesinski SG, Palmer A: Lasers for otosclerosis: CO_2 vs. argon and KTP-532. *Laryngoscope* 99 [suppl 46]:1–8, 1989. With permission.)

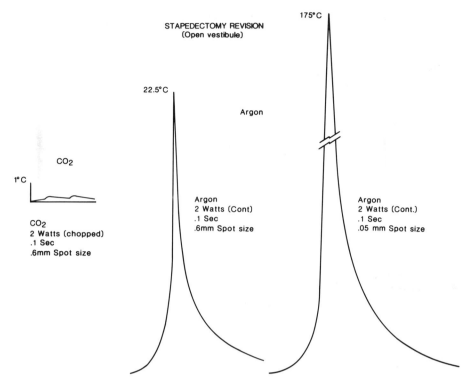

Figure 8.18. Thermocouple measurements with CO_2 and argon laser energy applied directly to open vestibule in simulated stapedectomy revision. (From Lesinski SG, Palmer A: Lasers for otosclerosis: CO_2 vs. argon and KTP-532. *Laryngoscope* 99 [suppl 46]:1–8, 1989. With permission.)

Use of Hand-Held Probes

Hand-held fiberoptic visible laser probes produce a noncollimated, non-coherent, defocused laser beam and thus require much higher energy levels for vaporizing the stapes footplate (stapedotomy) or the soft tissue obliterating the oval window (stapedectomy revision). Thermal scatter into the inner ear is therefore considerably greater and the risk to inner ear neuroepithelium and blood vessels theoretically higher.

Laboratory Data and Conclusions

Clinical Applications

In summary, visible lasers (argon and KTP-532) possess ideal optical properties for microsurgery and until 1984 were the only group of lasers optically precise enough for otosclerosis surgery. Unfortunately, the short wavelength of these visible lasers imparts tissue properties that are less than ideal for otosclerosis surgery. Visible laser energy is only partially absorbed by the white stapes footplate and readily

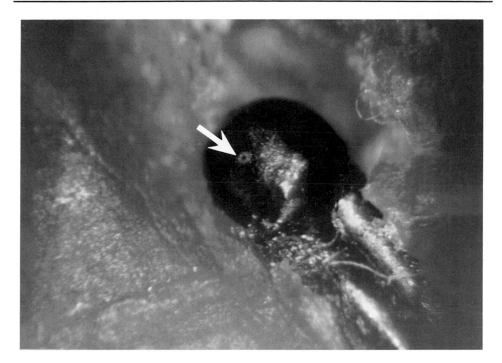

Figure 8.19.   Thermocouple following a single argon pulse at 2 W, 0.1 sec pulse duration, 50 micrometer spot size. A 60 micrometer "pothole" was melted into thermocouple 2 mm below surface of perilymph (melting temperature 175°C). (From Lesinski SG, Palmer A: Lasers for otosclerosis: CO_2 vs. argon and KTP-532. *Laryngoscope* 99 [suppl 46]:1–8, 1989. With permission.)

passes through the perilymph to be absorbed by pigmented cells of the inner ear (blood vessels, neuroepithelium, etc.). The argon and KTP-532 lasers should therefore be used with caution while performing stapedotomies. Care should be exercised not to overlap the "rosettes." Visible lasers should not be used for stapedectomy revisions because of the potential for direct application of the visible laser energy to the open vestibule, which the described experiments have shown to produce dramatic temperature rises (up to 175°C) in the vestibule at the level of the utricle and saccule.

The long wavelength of the invisible CO_2 laser imparts many optical problems that necessitated significant engineering advances to develop a precise Microslad® optical delivery system. The CO_2 laser beam and the HeNe laser aiming beam can now be delivered to the operative field satisfactorily parfocal and coaxial. The capacity to superpulse further refined the beam energy and minimized thermal spread. Tissue characteristics of this long-wavelength CO_2 energy are ideal for stapes surgery. Laboratory data confirm that with appropriate power settings, CO_2 laser stapedotomy can be performed without significant caloric effect in the vestibule. More important, the CO_2 laser can be applied to the perilymph in the open vestibule without significant penetration or caloric effect, this laser is therefore ideal for stapedectomy revision.

At present only the CO_2 laser should be used for stapedectomy revision. Both the visible lasers and the CO_2 laser can be safely used for stapedotomy, though the surgeon is cautioned to avoid applying the argon or KTP-532 lasers directly to the open vestibule. Future engineering advances in laser microsurgery will no doubt modify these recommendations.

Safe Energy Parameters

Safe energy parameters for each of Sharplan's CO_2 laser models (734, 1040, 1100A) were established in the laboratory before clinical use of the devices. Ultrasensitive pyroelectric detectors analyzed the precise energy "package" delivered to the operative field with these power settings. Figures 8.20, 8.21, and 8.22 illustrate the appropriate safe power settings for each model.

Energy parameters were considered safe if the power setting produced no more than a 0.3°C temperature rise in the vestibule during stapedotomy and no more than a 0.5°C rise during stapedectomy revision. Table 8.3 lists the safe energy parameters for each of the CO_2 models tested.

Following these guidelines, the CO_2 laser was then employed to perform stapedotomy[60] and stapedectomy revisions[61] in otosclerosis patients. The senior author has now performed over 250 consecutive operations with the CO_2 laser under local anesthesia. No patient has become dizzy while the CO_2 laser energy was being applied to the stapes footplate or to the oval window neomembrane. This clinical experience confirms the absence of significant caloric effect to the inner ear predicted by the laboratory's established safe energy parameters. More important, no patient has experienced significant postoperative sensorineural hearing loss in the speech range.

STAPEDOTOMY EMPLOYING THE CARBON DIOXIDE LASER

The advantages of stapedotomy over stapedectomy have been demonstrated by Fisch,[47] Marquet,[48] Causee,[50] and others. Better long-term hearing is obtained when a stapedotomy opening centered in the stapes footplate stabilizes the stapes prosthesis. Because the entire footplate is not removed, mechanical trauma to the inner ear is reduced, with a concurrent reduction in the risk of a postoperative perilymph fistula or serous labyrinthitis. Sensorineural loss and postoperative dizziness are also diminished. Unfortunately, the condition of the otosclerotic stapes footplate often prohibits mechanically drilling a symmetrically round stapedotomy opening into its center.

A partially fixed footplate often mobilizes during attempted mechanical drilling. A thin footplate often fractures. A thick, obliterative footplate requires extensive drilling with consequent vibratory trauma to the inner ear. With the CO_2 laser, a symmetrically round stapedotomy can be made at the center of the stapes footplate regardless of its thickness or degree of fixation, with no mechanical trauma being transmitted to the inner ear.

SHARPLAN 734

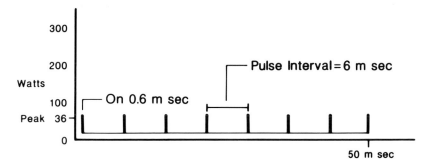

Duty Cycle-10%   Energy/Pulse 21.6 mj

Figure 8.20. Safe power settings for Sharplan Model 734 CO_2 laser. Average power of 3.4 W is delivered in superpulse mode by eight micropulses. Each micropulse has a peak-to-peak power of 36 W and on-time of 0.6 msec and delivers 21.6 mj of work. The pulse is then off for 6 msec (10% duty cycle), thus limiting thermal spread of the laser energy. (From Lesinski SG, Palmer A: CO_2 laser for otosclerosis: safe energy parameters. *Laryngoscope* 99 [suppl 46]:9–12, 1989. With permission.)

SHARPLAN 1040

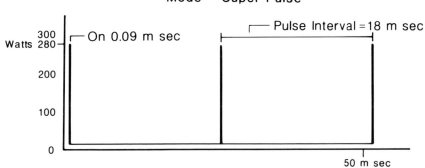

Duty Cycle-0.5%   Energy/Pulse 25.2 mj

Figure 8.21. Safe power settings for Sharplan CO_2 laser Model 1040. An average power of 2 W in the superpulse mode is delivered by 2 micropulses. Each micropulse has a peak-to-peak wattage of 280 W and on-time of 0.09 msec and delivers 25.2 mj of work. Pulse interval is 18 msec, giving a duty cycle of only 0.5%. This brief, high-powered burst of laser energy greatly minimizes thermal spread to the vestibule. The 280 W (25.2 mj) is the maximum energy per micropulse that will produce clean stapedotomy vaporization without a microscopic "flame." (From Lesinski SG, Palmer A: CO_2 laser for otosclerosis: safe energy parameters. *Laryngoscope* 99 [suppl 46]:9–12, 1989. With permission.)

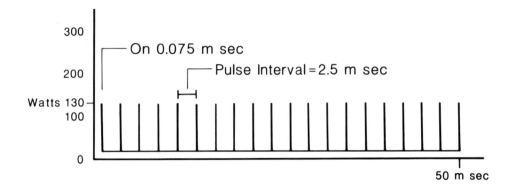

Figure 8.22. The Sharplan 1100A was adapted to deliver 1 to 5 W in a chopped mode. When set at 4 W power, this model delivers 20 micropulses, each with 130 W power, on-time of 0.075 msec, and an energy of 9.75 mj. Off-time is 2.5 msec (3% duty cycle). This energy package vaporized 0.6 mm stapedotomies with less than 0.1°C temperature rise in the vestibule. (From Lesinski SG, Palmer A: CO_2 laser for otosclerosis: safe energy parameters. *Laryngoscope* 99 [suppl 46]:9–12, 1989. With permission.)

TABLE 8.3. *Safe Energy Parameters*

Sharplan CO_2 Laser	Power	Pulse Duration	Mode
734	3.4 W	0.05 sec	Superpulse
1040	2 W	0.05 sec	Superpulse
1100A	4 W	0.05 sec	Chopped

Source: Lesinski SG, Palmer A: CO_2 laser for otosclerosis: safe energy parameters. *Laryngoscope* 99 (suppl 46):9–12, 1989. With permission.

Surgical Technique

The senior author has compiled a series of 153 consecutive laser stapedotomies over a five-year period using the following technique (Fig. 8.23). The CO_2 laser is adjusted to the appropriate power and mode (see Table 8.3). Under local anesthesia, a standard tympanotomy flap is raised. The stapedial tendon and posterior crus are vaporized. The incudostapedial joint is separated, and the anterior crus is fractured with a 1-mm right-angle pick. A 0.6-mm stapedotomy fenestration is vaporized into the center of the stapes footplate.

A thin footplate requires three to four "hits"; a thick footplate may require as many as fifty. The laser is fired at 2-sec intervals to avoid significant caloric effect in the vestibule. Throughout the procedure the patient is asked about subjective dizziness. The stapedotomy char is removed with a straight pick.

A 0.6-mm diameter stapedotomy prosthesis (teflon/platinum) of the appropriate length is then inserted in the stapedotomy. The platinum wire loop is passed over the neck of the incus and crimped. Clotted blood is placed in the oval window to seal the stapedotomy, as described by both Perkins[51] and Fisch.[52] The tympanotomy flap is then repositioned and the patient asked to repeat words that are softly whispered and to report any dizziness. Polysporin ointment is used as tympanotomy packing.

Results

Long-term (mean followup 32 mos.) postoperative hearing results are summarized in Figure 8.24, illustrating the efficacy of the technique. Comparison of postoperative and preoperative bone thresholds showed that no patient demonstrated a significant (10 dB or greater) sensorineural hearing loss in the speech range (500, 1K, 2K, 3K H2). No patient experienced vertigo while the CO_2 laser beam vaporized the stapedotomy opening or immediately afterward. Two weeks postoperatively, 8 of 153 (5%) reported some unsteadiness with rapid head movements. Three of these patients were found to have a perilymph fistula that was repaired. The other 5 patients were completely free of vestibular symptoms at one month postoperatively.

Complications

Over the 3- to 64-month followup period, the complication rate was exceptionally low. Eight of the 153 patients required revision surgery (4 for perilymph fistula (3 immediate, 1 delayed), 4 for hearing failure—3 of which were successfully revised). One other patient had had delayed facial weakness that cleared completely within 5 days. No postoperative tympanic membrane perforations occurred. There was no significant postoperative sensorineural hearing loss in the speech frequencies.

Conclusions

The CO_2 laser has provided this surgeon with a safe, precise instrument for performing stapedotomies in patients with otosclerosis. The absence of mechanical

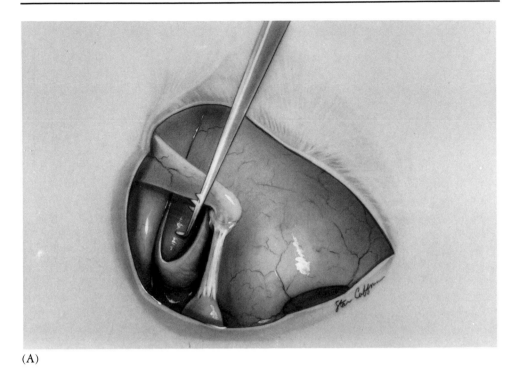

(A)

(B)

Figure 8.23.   Surgical techniques—*A*, Distance between stapes footplate and undersurface of incus is measured. *B*, Stapedius tendon and posterior crus are vaporized.

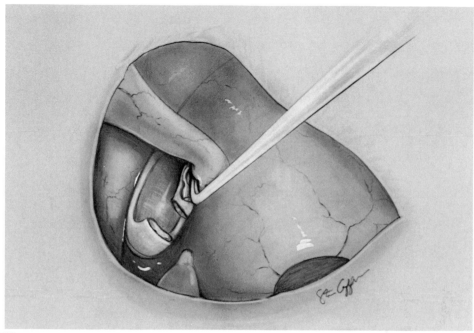

(C)

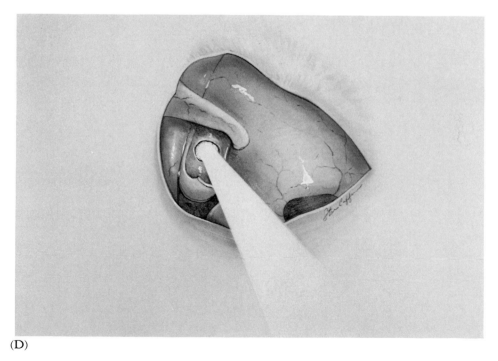

(D)

Figure 8.23. *C*, Incudostapedial joint is separated with a right-angle pick and anterior crus fractured. *D*, 0.6 mm stapedotomy is vaporized into center of the footplate.

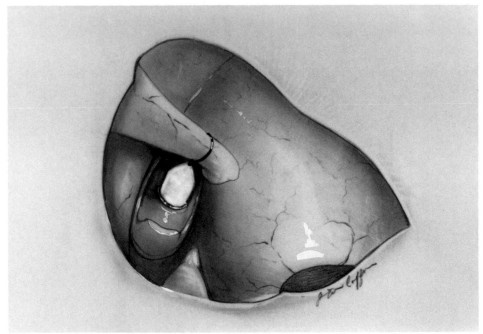

(E)

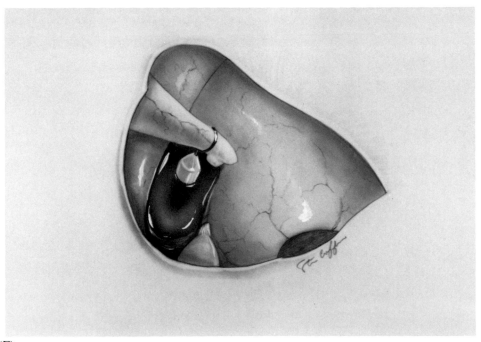

(F)

Figure 8.23. *E*, A Teflon platinum piston (0.6 mm diameter) of appropriate length is inserted into stapedotomy opening and crimped to neck of the incus. *F*, Drop of clotted blood is used to seal oval window. (From Lesinski SG, Stein JA: CO_2 laser stapedotomy. *Laryngoscope* 99 [suppl 46]:20–24, 1989. With permission.)

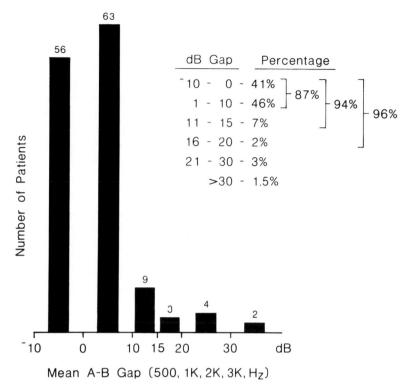

dB Gap	Percentage
$^-10$ - 0 -	41%
1 - 10 -	46%
11 - 15 -	7%
16 - 20 -	2%
21 - 30 -	3%
>30 -	1.5%

Figure 8.24. CO_2 laser stapedotomy (Hearing Results (S/P 6-64 mo.) 137 pts.) (From Lesinski SG, Stein JA: CO_2 laser stapedotomy. *Laryngoscope* 99[Suppl 46]:20–24, 1989. With permission.)

trauma to the inner ear has minimized postoperative complications. Of patients who have undergone CO_2 laser stapedotomy, 94% have maintained an air/bone gap closure to within 15 dB at a mean followup of almost 3 years. No patient incurred a significant sensorineural hearing loss. Vestibular symptoms following laser stapedotomy were dramatically reduced when compared with standard stapedectomy. A stable prosthesis, centered in a precise 0.6-mm stapedotomy, resists migration—the common underlying cause for most stapedectomy failures.

STAPEDECTOMY REVISION EMPLOYING THE CARBON DIOXIDE LASER

Present surgical techniques for revising failed stapedectomies achieve inconsistent hearing results and often damage the inner ear. Recent studies by many prominent otologists (Glasscock,[62] Sheehy,[63] Lippy,[64] Crabtree[65] have demonstrated that postoperative closure of the air/bone gap to within 10 dB is achieved in fewer than half the patients in whom revision is undertaken. After revision surgery, hearing worsened in 8 to 33 of the patients in these studies. The incidence of significant postoperative sensorineural hearing loss was 3 to 20%, and as many as 14% of patients had a profound loss of hearing. Every author cautioned against the hazards of trauma to the inner ear and recommended avoiding excessive manipulation of the prosthesis or the soft tissue obliterating the oval window.

Histopathologic studies of the temporal bone in post stapedectomy patients by Hohmann,[66] Linthicum,[67] and others demonstrate that adhesions may develop between the prosthesis or the neomembrane of the oval window and the utricle and saccule. Manipulation of the neomembrane could easily rupture these delicate inner ear structures, with resultant vertigo and sensorineural hearing loss.

Successful stapedectomy revision requires that the cause of initial failure be identified. Once the tympanotomy flap has been elevated, the surgeon is confronted with a dilemma (Fig. 8.25). To determine the reasons for the conductive failure, the surgeon must determine the mobility and integrity of the entire ossicular chain, the status of the oval window, and the precise relationship of the failed prosthesis to the vestibular entrance. Yet the surgeon can visualize neither the depth or lateral margins of the oval window nor what is underneath the obliterating membrane (especially if fat or fascia was used). The need for minimal manipulation of these structures to avoid trauma to the inner ear compromises the surgeon's ability to identify the pathophysiology underlying the hearing loss. The precise anatomic dimensions of the oval window, and the presence of a residual fixed stapes footplate must be estimated

On the basis of these estimates, the surgeon inserts a new prosthesis of approximate length into the estimated center of the soft tissue obliterating the oval window. If the oval window is free of residual pathology and the surgeon has guessed correctly, the patient's hearing will improve—initially. Postoperative prosthesis migration, the cause for two-thirds of all standard stapedectomy failures can still occur. Considering these unfavorable factors, the 30 to 50% reported success rate for revising failed stapedectomies is quite remarkable.

The CO_2 laser allows the surgeon to atraumatically remove tissue from the oval window area that obscures his view of the underlying anatomy. For this reason the CO_2 laser represents an elegant technical advance that offers patients undergoing revision stapedectomy a reduction in procedure-induced hearing loss and the best possible long-term hearing. The senior author performed CO_2 laser stapedectomy revisions on 59 consecutive patients during a five-year clinical study. The procedure and results are discussed below.

Surgical Technique

Transcanal exploratory tympanotomy is performed under local anesthesia augmented by intravenous sedation. Once a tympanotomy flap has been elevated, the cause of conductive hearing loss is assessed. The malleus and incus are inspected and palpated. The precise relationship of the stapedectomy prosthesis to the oval window is defined in the following manner:

At the appropriate power settings (see Table 8.3), one of the Sharplan CO_2 lasers is employed to gradually vaporize obliterating tissue, concentrically thinning the tissue surrounding the prosthesis to allow its atraumatic removal (Fig. 8.26). Soft tissue vaporization continues, thinning the area of the oval window until its exact

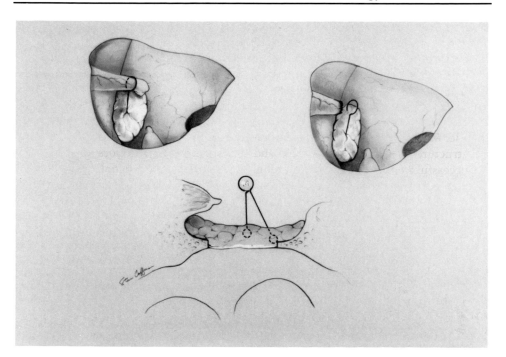

Figure 8.25. Stapedectomy revision: a diagnostic problem. Typical appearance of middle ear at time of stapedectomy revision (right ear). Soft tissue obliterates the precise margins and depth of the oval window and possible underlying residual fixed stapes footplate. Prosthesis may be too short or may have migrated out of the oval window to become fixed to the otic capsule. (From Lesinski SG, Stein JA: Stapedectomy revision with the CO_2 laser. *Laryngoscope* 99 [suppl 46]:13–19, 1989. With permission.)

lateral margins and depth are identified. A 0.6-mm stapedotomy is then vaporized in the center of the oval window neomembrane. Stapedotomy is not complete until the vestibule with its clear perilymph is visible. Next, a 0.6-mm diameter prosthesis (usually 4.5 to 4.75 mm long) is inserted into the stapedotomy and crimped to the neck of the incus (Fig. 8.27). The opening is then sealed with clotted blood.

If the incus is eroded, a homograft incus columella of appropriate size is created and the stapedotomy is enlarged to 0.8 mm. A 2×3 mm-perichondrial graft must be placed over the enlarged stapedotomy to support the weight of the columella. The homograft incus columella is then centered with its long process in the reinforced stapedotomy opening and its notched short process under the malleus.

To evaluate the CO_2 laser's thermal effect in the vestibule, each patient was asked about dizziness intraoperatively, both during and immediately after the application of the CO_2 laser. No patient experienced perioperative vertigo or dizziness.

Results

Table 8.4 lists the causes for stapedectomy failure found at the time of CO_2 laser revision in this series. In about 20% of the patients more than one abnormality

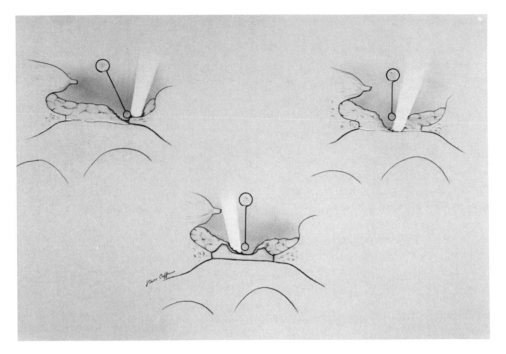

Figure 8.26. Reasons for failure of stapedectomy. Concentric vaporization of the obliterating soft tissue reveals (*A*) an eccentric prosthesis fixed against the otic capsule, (*B*) a too-short prosthesis, or (*C*) a residual fixed stapes footplate. (From Lesinski SG, Stein JA: Stapedectomy revision with the CO_2 laser. *Laryngoscope* 99 [suppl 46]:13–19, 1989. With permission.)

was identified as responsible for the conductive loss. The common underlying cause for stapedectomy failure seen in two-thirds of these patients was migration of an unstable prosthesis.

Use of the CO_2 laser allows visualization of the oval window sufficient for precise diagnosis without undue risk of trauma to the inner ear. The condition or conditions causing the conductive loss can then be corrected, leading to a high success rate in closing the air/bone gap.

Conductive Hearing Repair

Table 8.5 analyzes the mean postoperative air/bone gaps obtained from the most recent postoperative audiograms obtained from these patients (6 to 60 mos. postoperatively). Successful closure of the air/bone gaps to within 20 dB was maintained in 91% of the patients in whom the prosthesis was at fault, 81% of the patients in whom the incus required repair, and 72% of those in whom a fisula of the oval window had occurred.

Sensorineural Hearing Loss

To evaluate any damage to the inner ear related to CO_2 laser stapedectomy revision, the most recent postoperative pure tone bone thresholds were compared with

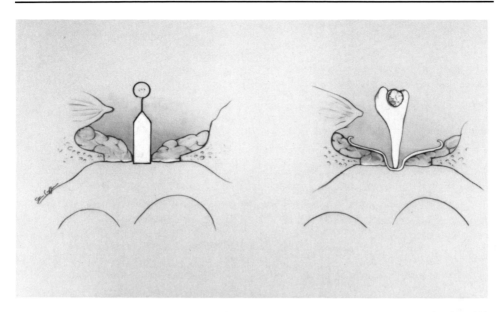

Figure 8.27. CO_2 laser stapedotomy in neomembrane stabilizes new prosthesis—(A), Incus intact. (B), Incus eroded. Note perichondrium supporting incus columella when incus is eroded. (From Lesinski SG, Stein JA: Stapedectomy revision with the CO_2 laser. *Laryngoscope* 99 [suppl 46]:13–19, 1989. With permission.)

TABLE 8.4. *Causes of Stapedectomy Failures in 59 Patients*

Prosthesis	
Displaced	37
Short	8
Loose	2
Stapes	
Fixed footplate	6
Oval window fistula	7
Incus	
Eroded	10*
Dislocated	4
Fixed	2
Malleus	
Fixed	3

*In 9 of 10 cases with an eroded incus, the prosthesis had migrated out of the oval window and was fixed against the otic capsule bone.
Source: Lesinski SG, Stein JA: Stapedectomy revision with the CO_2 laser. *Laryngoscope* 99 (suppl 46):13–19, 1989. With permission.

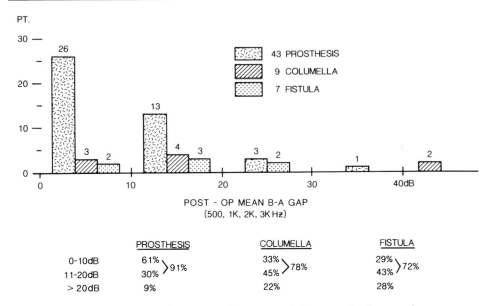

	PROSTHESIS		COLUMELLA		FISTULA	
0–10dB	61%		33%		29%	
11–20dB	30%	91%	45%	78%	43%	72%
> 20dB	9%		22%		28%	

Table 8.5. CO_2 laser stapedectomy revisions conductive repair.

preoperative levels. In the speech range (500, 1K, 2K, 3K Hz) no patient experienced significant sensorineural hearing loss (mean 10 dB or greater). Three percent (2/59) lost more than 15 dB at 4K Hz.

Carbon Dioxide Laser and Traditional Technique Compared

Conductive Repair

Table 8.6 compares long-term conductive hearing results attained in this series with four recent series of standard stapedectomy revisions.[47-50] Of the patients in whom the CO_2 laser revision was performed, an air/bone gap of 10 dB or less was maintained in 66%, whereas a similar sound-conduction efficiency was maintained in 39 to 49 percent of patients in whom standard techniques were employed. Glasscock[62] stated that only 40% of the stapedectomy revisions he performed for

TABLE 8.6. *Stapedectomy Revisions CO_2 Laser vs "Standard" Conductive Repair*

Mean B-A Gap (Pre op bone Post op air)	Lesinski (CO_2)	Standard			
		Glasscock (1987)	Sheehy (1981)	Lippy (1980)	Crabtree (1980)
0–10dB	66%	39%	44%	49%	46%
11–20dB	23% 89%	25% 64%	27% 71%	5% 54%	"Improved"

Source: Lesinski SG, Stein JA: Stapedectomy revision with the CO_2 laser. *Laryngoscope* 99 (suppl 46):13–19, 1989. With permission.

hearing failure actually improved hearing, and Crabtree reported 46%.[65] Of the 52 patients undergoing CO_2 laser stapedectomy revision for hearing loss in this series, 48 (92%) had an improvement in hearing demonstrated by both postoperative SRTs and air/bone gaps.

These improvements in postoperative conductive hearing results can be attributed to the CO_2 laser. It provides the revising surgeon with greater safety and precision, first in diagnosing the pathophysiology of the conductive loss and then in stabilizing the new prosthesis in the center of the oval window by means of a laser stapedotomy in the neomembrane.

Sensorineural Loss

To evaluate any damage to the inner ear related to CO_2 laser stapedectomy revision, the most recent postoperative pure tone bone thresholds were compared with preoperative bone thresholds. Table 8.7 compares these results with three conventional stapedectomy revision series. Though each used different criteria for significant damage to the inner ear, comparing postoperative pure tone one thresholds (mean dB at 500, 1K, 2K, 3K Hz), 20% of Crabtree's patients and 3% of Glasscock's patients showed >15 dB sensorineural hearing loss. Seven percent of Sheehy's patients developed a 30 dB or greater sensorineural loss or a 33% drop in spech discrimination postoperatively. Of particular note is the risk of profound deafness (no useful hearing) associated with standard stapedectomy revision—2 to 14% in these series.

In the 59 patients undergoing CO_2 laser stapedectomy revision, none developed a sensorineural loss of >10 dB in the speech range (mean dB 500, 1K, 2K, 3K Hz). In two of the patients (3%), speech discrimination was reduced by more than 16% (36 and 48%). In neither case was this due to a postoperative decrease in pure tone thresholds, but rather was due to converting a flat mixed hearing loss to a sloping high frequency sensorineural loss through successful closure of the air bone gap. The CO_2 laser, when used at appropriate power settings to vaporize soft

TABLE 8.7. *Stapedectomy Revisions: CO_2 Laser vs "Standard" S-N Loss*

Postoperative results	Lesinski (CO₂)	Glasscock (1987)	Sheehy (1981)	Crabtree (1980)
> 15 mean dB decrease (at 500, 1K, 2K, 3K H₂) in bone conduction. Post op bone	0	3%	(worse 30dB)	20%
> 16% decrease in speech discrimination	3%*	11%	7% (worse 35%)	?
Profound S-N Loss	0	2%	3%	14%

Source: Lesinski SG, Stein JA: Stapedectomy revision with the CO_2 laser. *Laryngoscope* 99 (suppl 46):13–19, 1989. With permission.

tissue in the oval window, clearly causes less trauma to the inner ear than mechanical dissection.

Conclusions

The CO_2 laser provides the otologic surgeon with three distinct advantages over standard techniques for revising previously failed stapedectomies:

1. *Improved diagnostic precision:* The ability to atraumatically vaporize the obliterating soft tissue in the oval window allows the surgeon to precisely identify the pathophysiology underlying the conductive hearing loss with no mechanical trauma to the inner ear.
2. *Increased stability of prosthesis:* By vaporizing a precise stapedotomy in the stapes footplate or in the neomembrane of a stapedectomy revision, the surgeon can stabilize the prosthesis in the center of the oval window, thereby decreasing postoperative migration of the prosthesis—the most common cause of stapedectomy failure.
3. *Reduction of inner ear trauma:* Standard techniques for stapedotomy and stapedectomy revision require mechanical manipulation of the stapes footplate, the prosthesis or the obliterating tissue of the oval window, often leading to significant inner ear trauma. At recommended power settings, the CO_2 laser can be used for atraumatic dissection of strictures in the oval window without significant caloric effect or vestibular damage.

Visible lasers (argon and KTP-532) should be used only with great caution for stapedectomy revision. Direct application of these visible lasers to the open vestibule has the potential to produce dramatic temperature changes and consequent damage to inner ear structures.

Modern lasers offer considerable potential for solving many of the problems confronting the otologic surgeon. The safe, effective clinical application of laser energy for otologic microscopic surgery is predicated upon an accurate understanding of laser physics confirmed by laboratory experimentation.

REFERENCES

General Otology

1. Maiman TH: Stimulated optical radiation in the ruby. *Nature* 187:493–494, 1960.
2. Wilpizeski CR: Otological applications of laser. In Wolbarsht MK (ed): *Laser Applications in Medicine and Biology,* New York, Plenum, 1977, vol 3, pp 289–328.
3. Escudero LH, Castro AO, Drummond, et al: Argon laser in human tympanoplasty. *Arch Otolaryngol* 105:252–253, 1979.
4. Perkins RC: Laser stapedotomy for otosclerosis. *Laryngoscope* 90:228–241, 1980.
5. Goode RL: Carbon dioxide laser myringotomy. *Laryngoscope* 92:420–423, 1982.
6. Palva T: Argon laser in otosclerosis surgery. *Acta Otolaryngol* 104:153–157, 1979.
7. DiBartolomeo JR, Ellis M: The argon laser in otology. *Laryngoscope* 90:1786–1796, 1980.
8. McGee TM: Argon laser in chronic ear and otosclerosis. *Laryngoscope* 93:1177–1182, 1983.

9. Vollrath M, Schreiner C: Influence of argon laser stapedotomy on cochlear potentials. *Acta Otolaryngol* 385 (suppl):1–31, 1982.

10. Gantz BJ, Kischimoto S, Jenkins HA, et al: Argon laser stapedotomy. *Ann Otol Rhinol Laryngol* 91:25–26, 1982.

11. Norris CW, Mullarky MB: Experimental skin incision made with the carbon dioxide laser. *Laryngoscope* 92:416–419, 1982.

12. Hall RR: The healing of tissues incised by a carbon dioxide laser. *Br J Surg* 58:222, 1971.

13. Gillis TM, Strong MS, Shapshay SM, et al: Argon laser and soft tissue interaction. *Otolaryngol Head Neck Surg* 92:7–12, 1984.

14. Castro DJ, Saxton RE, Fetterman HR, et al: Phototherapy with argon lasers and rhodamine-123 for tumor eradication. *Otolaryngol Head Neck Surg* 98:581–588, 1988.

15. Castro DJ, Saxton RE, Fetterman HR, et al: Bioinhibition of human fibroblast cultures sensitized to Q-Switch II dye and treated with the Nd:YAG laser: a new technique of photodynamic therapy with lasers. *Laryngoscope* 99:421–428, 1989.

16. Hunsaker DH: Conchomeatoplasty for chronic otitis externa. *Arch Otolaryngol* 114: 395–398, 1988.

17. Lipman S, Guelcher RT, Anon JB, et al: Carbon dioxide laser myringotomy: a retrospective analysis of 91 patients. *Lasers Surg Med,* in press

18. Schober R, Ulrich F, Sander T, et al: Laser-induced alteration of collagen substructure allow microsurgical tissue welding. *Science* 232:1421–1422, 1986.

19. Vale BH, Frenkel A, Trenka-Benthin S, et al: Microsurgical anastomosis of rat carotid arteries with CO_2 laser. *Plast Reconstr Surg* 77:759–766, 1986.

20. Marquet J: My current cholesteatoma techniques. *Am J Otol* 10:124–130, 1989.

21. Shapshay SM, Wallace RR, Kventon JF, et al: New microspot micromanipulator for CO_2 laser application in otolaryngology-head and neck surgery. *Otolaryngol Head Neck Surg* 98:179–181, 1988.

22. Parisier SC, et al: Management of congenital pediatric cholesteotomas. *Am J Otol* 10: 121–123, 1989.

23. Gulya AJ, Glasscock ME, Pensak ML: Neural choristoma of the middle ear. *Otolaryngol Head Neck Surg* 97:52–56, 1988.

24. Silverstein H, Rosenberg S, Jones R: Small fenestra stapedotomy with and without KTP laser: a comparison. *Laryngosocope* 99:485–488, 1989.

25. McGee TM: Lasers in otology. *Otolaryngol Clin North Am* 22:233–238, 1989.

Neurotology

26. Morton AL, Butler SA, Kuhn A, et al: Temporal bone metastases—pathophysiology and imaging. *Otolaryngol Head Neck Surg* 97:583–587, 1987.

27. Paparella M, El Fiky FM: Ear involvement in malignant lymphoma. *Ann Otol Rhinol Laryngol* 81:352–363, 1972.

28. Ballance C: *Some Points in the Surgery of the Brain and its Membranes.* London, Macmillan, 1907.

29. Cushing H: *Intracranial Tumor.* Springfield, IL, Charles C Thomas, 1932.

30. Rand RW: Suboccipital transmeatal microneurosurgical resection of acoustic tumors. *Ann Surg* 174:663–671, 1971.

31. Smith MFW, Lagger RL: Hearing conservation in acoustic neurilemmoma surgery via the retrosigmoid approach. *Otolaryngol Head Neck Surg* 92:168–175, 1984.

32. Cerullo LJ, Mkrdichian EH: CO_2 laser in acoustic tumor removal. *Lasers Med Surg* 7:224–228, 1987.

33. Glasscock ME, Jackson CG, Whitaker SR: The argon laser in acoustic tumor surgery. *Laryngoscope* 91:1405–1416, 1981.

34. Silverstein H, Norrell H, Hyman SM: Simultaneous use of CO_2 laser with continuous monitoring of eight cranial nerve action potential during acoustic neuroma surgery. *Otolaryngol Head Neck Surg* 92:80–84, 1984.

35. Saunders ML, Young HF, Becker DP, et al: The Use of the Laser in Neurological Surgery. *Surg Neurol* 14:9, 1980.

36. Ballance C, Duel AB: The operative treatment of facial palsy by introduction of nerve grafts into the fallopian canal and by other intratemporal methods. *Arch Otol* 15:1–70, 1932.

37. Crumley RL: Spacial anatomy of facial nerve fibers. In Graham MD and House WF (eds): *Disorders of Facial Nerve*. New York, Raven Press, 1982, p 33.

38. Nishihira S, McCaffrey TV: Repair of motor nerve defects: comparison of suture and fibrin adhesive techniques. *Otolaryngol Head Neck Surg* 100:17–21, 1989.

39. Wikholm RP, Swett JE, Torique Y, et al: Repair of severed peripheral nerve: a superior anatomic and functional recovery with a new "reconnection" technique. *Otolaryngol Head Neck Surg* 99:353–361, 1988.

40. Ruiz-Razura A, Lan M, Cohen BE: The laser-assisted end-to-side microvascular anastomosis. *Plast Reconstr Surg* 83:511–517, 1989.

41. Vale BH, Frenkel A, Trenka-Benthin S, et al: Microsurgical anastomosis of rat carotid arteries with CO_2 laser. *Plast Reconstr Surg* 77:759–766, 1986.

42. Jain KF: Sutureless extra-intracranial anastomosis by laser. *Lancet* 2:816, 1984.

43. Fried MP, Moll ERS: Microvascular anastomoses. *Arch Otolaryngol* 113:968–973, 1987.

44. Ulrich F, Dürsek R, Schober R: Long term investigation of laser-assisted microvascular Nd:YAG laser. *Lasers Surg Med* 8:104, 1988.

45. Abernathy CD, Davis DH, Kelly RJ: Colloid cysts. *J Neurosurg* 70:525–529, 1989.

46. Castro DJ, Saxton RE, Fetterman HR, et al: Bioinhibition of human fibroblast cultures sensitized to Q-switch II dye and treated with the Nd:YAG laser: a new technique of photodynamic therapy with lasers. *Laryngoscope* 99:421–428, 1989.

Otosclerosis

47. Fisch U: Stapedotomy vs. stapedectomy. *Am J Otol* 4:112–117, 1982.

48. Marquet J: Stapedotomy technique and results. *Am J Otol* 6:63–67, 1985.

49. Smyth GDL, Hassard TH: Eighteen year's experience in stapedectomy. The case for the small fenestra operation. *Ann Otol Rhinol Laryngol* 87(49):3–36, 1978.

50. Causse J: Stapedotomy techniques and results. *Am J Otol* 6:68–71, 1985.

51. Perkins R: Laser stapedotomy for otosclerosis. *Laryngoscope* 90:228–241, 1980.

52. McGee T: The argon laser in surgery for chronic ear disease and otosclerosis. *Laryngoscope* 93:1177–1182, 1983.

53. DiBartolomeo J: A versatile argon microsurgical laser. *Otolaryngol Head Neck Surg* 90:139–141, 1982.

54. Gantz B: Argon laser stapedotomy. *Ann Otolaryngol* 91:25–26, 1982.

55. Silverstein H: Comparison of small fenestra stapedotomies with and without KTP-532 laser. Presented at Southern Section Triological Society Meeting, Naples, FL, January 14, 1989.

56. Wilpizeski C: Letters to the editor. *Laryngoscope* 91:834–835, 1981.

57. Gardner G: CO_2 laser stapedotomy. Is it practical? *Am J Otolaryngol* 5:109–117, 1984.

58. Coker NJ: Carbon dioxide laser stapedotomy: a histopathologic study. *Am J Otolaryngol* 4:253–257, 1986.

59. Lesinski SG: CO_2 laser for otosclerosis. Presented at Midsection Triological Society Meeting, Chicago, January 1986.

60. Lesinski SG, Stein JA: CO_2 laser stapedotomy. *Laryngoscope* 99(46):20–24, 1989.

61. Lesinski S: Stapedectomy revision with the CO_2 laser. *Laryngoscope* 99(46):13–19, 1989.

62. Glasscock M: Revision stapedectomy surgery. *Otolaryngol Head Neck Surg* 96:141–148, 1987.

63. Sheehy J: Revision stapedectomy: a review of 258 cases. *Laryngoscope* 91:43–51, 1981.

64. Lippy W: Stapedectomy revision. *Am J Otol* 2:15–21, 1980.

65. Crabtree J: An evaluation of revision stapes surgery. *Laryngoscope* 90:224–227, 1980.

66. Hohmann A: Inner ear reactions to stapes surgery (animal experiments). In Schuknect HF (ed): *Otosclerosis,* Boston, Little, Brown, 1982, pp 305–317.

67. Linthicum F: Histologic evidence of the cause of failure in stapes surgery. *Ann Otol Rhinol Laryngol* 80:67–68, 1971.

SUGGESTED READING

General Otology

Clark TE: Electrolysis of exostoses of the ear. *Br Med* 2:656–657, 1873.

Javan A, Bennet WR, Herriott DR: Population inversion and continuous optical maser oscillation in a gas discharge containing a He-Ne mixture. *Phys Rev Lett* 6:106–110, 1961.

McKenzie D: *Diathermy of Otolaryngology.* New York, MacMillan, 1930.

Mulwert H, Voss O: Eine neue physicalische Behandlungsmethode chronischer Schwerhörigheit und deren Ergebnisse. *Acta Oto Laryngol* 12:63, 1928.

Sataloff H: Experimental use of laser in otosclerotic stapes. *Arch Otolaryngol* 88:58–60, 1967.

Snitzer E: Optical laser action of Nd in Ba crown glass. *Phys Rev Lett* 7:444, 1961.

Stahle J, Hobert L: Laser and the labyrinth. Some preliminary experiments in pigeons. *Acta Otolaryngol* 60:367–374, 1965.

Stahle J, Hobert L, Engstrom B: The laser as a tool in inner ear surgery. *Acta Otolaryngol* 73:27–37, 1972.

Neurotology

Brown TE, True C, McLaurin RL, et al: Laser radiation: I. Acute effects on cerebral cortex. *Neurology* 16:730, 1966.

Fox JL, Hayes JR, Stein MN: The effects of laser radiation on intracranial structures. First

Annual Biomedical Laser Conference of the Laser Medical Research Foundation, Boston, 1965.

Garden JM, O'Banion K, Shelnitz LS, et al: Papillomavirus in the vapor of carbon dioxide laser-treated verracoa. *JAMA* 259:1199–1202, 1988.

Ieppner F: The laser scalpel on the nervous system. In Kaplan I (ed): *Laser Surgery II.* Jerusalem, Jerusalem Academic Press, 1978, pp 79–80.

Liss L, Roppel R: Histopathology of laser-produced lesions in cat brains. *Neurology* 16:783, 1977.

Maira G, Mohr G, Panisset A, et al: Laser photocoagulation for treatment of experimental aneurysms. *J Microsurg* 1:137, 1979.

Ossoff R, Keller G, Rowley S: Laser Safety Guidelines, to be published by AAO Laser Surgery Committee.

Stellar S: A study of the effects of laser light on nervous tissue, in *Proceedings of Third International Congress of Neurological Surgery,* series No 110, Copehagen, 1965.

Stellar S, Polanyi TG, Bredemeier HC: Experimental studies with the carbon dioxide laser as a neurosurgical instrument. *Med Biol Eng* 8:549, 1970.

Takiyawa T: Laser surgery of brain tumors. *No Shinkei Geka* 9:743, 1978.

9
Laryngology

Edward C. Weisberger

When Jako and Polanyi used laser-delivered energy to ablate portions of human cadaver vocal cords in 1965,[1] they placed the cornerstone in the edifice of laser laryngology. Today that structure is rising and expanding at an exponentially increasing rate. Initially, a neodymium laser was used, but in 1967 the carbon dioxide laser was introduced for treatment of laryngeal disease and has subsequently been the "workhorse." Jako's Triological thesis presented in 1972[2] described the initial clinical applications of the carbon dioxide laser for treatment of laryngeal disease. The laser was delivered to the tissues using a Zeiss operating microscope and binocular vision.

The carbon dioxide (CO_2) laser offers several unique advantages for the treatment of laryngeal disease.[1-9] The ability to ablate or dissect tissue of the larynx using the optics and magnification of the operating microscope, without having to use an interposed microforceps or scissors, certainly enhances visibility. The almost bloodless field provided by the hemostatic properties of the laser improves accuracy and precision. The CO_2 laser will seal vessels up to 0.5 mm in diameter,[5] which provides adequate hemostasis for most laryngeal surgery—especially regarding surgery of the laryngeal glottis and subglottis. For more extensive resections in the supraglottic area, or for the resection of malignant disease, standard electrocautery using a shielded conductor is occasionally required to seal larger bleeding vessels.

Currently available lasers allow a new level of precision in laryngeal surgery. The initial spot size used by Jako was approximately 3 mm in diameter.[1] Currently available CO_2 lasers provide a spot diameter one third to one tenth of that size (1 to 0.3 mm diameter at a focal length of 400 mm).[10] This corresponds to a surface area up to 100 times smaller than the earliest lasers. The surgeon now has the ability to excise tissue precisely from the larynx and not merely to vaporize tissue.

The nature of the interaction between the CO_2 laser and biologic tissue affords certain advantages over conventional surgery. Several investigators have demonstrated a diminished rate of formation of collagen and scar tissue in CO_2 laser wounds.[11-13] However, other aspects of laser–tissue interaction may be detrimental, such as the delayed coverage of laser wounds by epithelial cells, documented by some investigators.[13,14] The CO_2 laser seems to seal lymphatics,[15] potentially modifying postoperative edema involving the airway. The properties of the CO_2 laser, as described above, allow successful endoscopic treatment of some laryngeal lesions that would previously have required an open surgical procedure. In many such cases tracheotomy is no longer needed.

BENIGN NODULES AND POLYPOID DEGENERATION OF THE VOCAL CORD

Singers' nodules of the true vocal cord involve the middle one third and are almost always bilateral, although one side usually predominates. Conservative measures to modify identifiable vocal abuse should be tried before surgery is recommended. A very conservative approach is employed in children.

Mature nodules are removed with the CO_2 laser, using a shaving technique. A moist cottonoid or a protective metal platform is placed in the subglottis to protect the subglottis and trachea from inadvertent laser impacts. The laser beam is aimed so as to strike the medial extent of the nodule tangentially. The beam is then slowly moved laterally with each subsequent impact so that the lesion is "shaved" off the true vocal cord, leaving a slight depression.[16] The patient is encouraged to use a soft, relaxed voice for 1 to 2 weeks postoperatively.

Granulomas that involve the vocal cord over the vocal process can present with hoarseness and discomfort. Pain is often referred to the ear on the ipsilateral side. These lesions can be removed with the laser, but the cure rate has been disappointing.[17] Often there is a smoldering perichondritis if the lesion has followed endotracheal intubation. Also, certain patterns of voice abuse such as habitual throat-clearing and glottal attack can cause the lesion to recur. Gastroesophageal reflux can also cause recurrence of the lesion after laser excision unless the reflux is addressed and corrected.

Polypoid degeneration usually involves both true vocal cords symmetrically from the anterior commissure to just in front of the vocal process. The vocal cords have a gelatinous appearance. The patients are usually middle-aged and are cigarette smokers. Histologically, Reinke's space (the superficial layer of the lamina propria) is involved.[18-20] Attempts to simply ablate the edematous tissue and overlying mucosa often cause prolonged hoarseness lasting several months.[21] If both true vocal cords are treated simultaneously and all the mucosa at the anterior commissure is ablated, an anterior web and stenosis can result.

The poor voice quality that occurs after simple ablation of polypoid tissues and the overlying mucosa is associated with findings on laryngeal stroboscopy of an absence of the mucosal wave.[18] It has been shown on histologic examination that true vocal cord mucosa that regenerates after CO_2 laser excision has abnormal neural elements.[22] This may also relate to the poor voice quality noted. If charred and desiccated debris that accumulates during the procedure is not conscientiously removed, a foreign body reaction may impart a granular texture to the regenerated mucosa, with a corresponding deterioration of voice quality.

In a technique described by Hirano,[23] the CO_2 laser is used to incise the superior aspect of the true vocal cord, and the mucosa is retracted medially with a microsuction or microcup forceps (Fig. 9.1A). The subepithelial edematous tissue stroma is ablated (Fig. 9.1B,C). A medially based mucosal flap is carefully preserved and re-placed over the area of resection (Fig. 9.1D). A CO_2 laser having a spot size of less than 1 mm at a focal length of 400 mm affords the necessary precision to perform this procedure. An improved, satisfactory voice is usually evident by 2 weeks postoperatively.

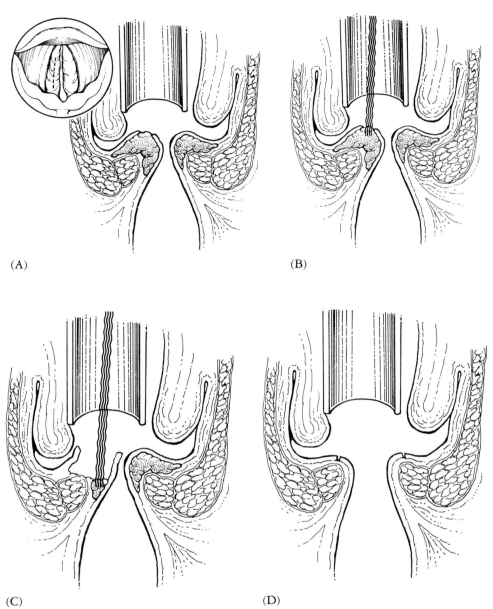

(A)

(B)

(C)

(D)

Figure 9.1 (*Inset*) Proposed line of laser incision on superior surface of true vocal cord involved by polypoid degeneration. (*A*) Sagittal view after laser incision on superior surface of true vocal cord. (*B*) Beginning of CO_2 ablation of gelatinous submucosal polypoid tissue. (*C*) Completion of laser ablation of submucosal polypoid tissue. (*D*) Completion of procedure where bilateral ablation of submucosal polypoid tissue has been accomplished and the true vocal cord resurfaced with a medially based mucosal flap.

NEUROGENIC DISEASES OF THE LARYNX

Bilateral vocal cord paralysis can significantly obstruct the upper airway. Several corrective techniques have been proposed. Surgical alternatives include an extra-laryngeal approach for removal of the arytenoid, such as employed by Woodman,[24] laryngofissure with excision of the arytenoid,[25] reinnervation of the posterior crico-arytenoid muscle,[26] and endoscopic excision of the arytenoid.[27] The anterior portion of the glottis, consisting of the membranous true vocal cords, is most important in voice production. The posterior glottis provides the space necessary for respiration. Successfully performed arytenoidectomy has the potential to leave the anterior phonatory portion of the glottis relatively undisturbed while improving respiration by enlarging the space in the posterior larynx.

Arytenoidectomy can be performed endoscopically, using the CO_2 laser,[28-33] for neurogenic laryngeal paralyses or when trauma or scarring has led to fixation of the cricoarytenoid joint. In the latter situation there is often an associated laryngeal stenosis, and the prognosis for establishment of an adequate airway is somewhat diminished. The surgeon should carefully check for a "tethering" band between the vocal processes. Such a band can impede cricoarytenoid joint motion and masquerade as a true vocal cord paralysis. When this band is identified, its division usually suffices to reestablish an adequate airway, and arytenoidectomy is not required.

The technique employed for endoscopic arytenoidectomy with the laser is as follows. The larynx is exposed with a Dedo laryngoscope, using the Lewy suspension device. The barrel of the laryngoscope is pointed at the posterior larynx. The mucosa and the corniculate cartilage are ablated with the CO_2 laser, using a power density of approximately 1500 W/cm^2 (Fig. 9.2A). Since the water content of the arytenoid cartilage is 62% versus 85% for the mucosa, the power density required for resecting the former is approximately twice that required for mucosal ablation, or 3000 W/cm^2. As the vocal process and muscular process of the arytenoid are approached, the power is decreased to 1500 W/cm^2 (Fig. 9.2B–D). This is done to avoid excessive heat trauma to the interarytenoid tissues, which are very prone to the formation of cicatrix. Some of the adjacent posterior aspect of the vocalis muscle is removed (Fig. 9.2E). Prophylactic antibiotics are employed for 1 week. The wound usually heals in approximately 1 month (Fig. 9.2F). Decannulation can usually be performed in 6 to 12 weeks.

In addition to performing the arytenoidectomy, an endoscopic laser approach can be used to excise additional soft tissues from the vocal cord in a patient in whom an arytenoidectomy has not achieved an adequate airway. There are some disadvantages and potential complications to this technique. The increased power density required to ablate cartilage and the propensity for scarring exhibited by the interarytenoid tissues has been discussed. In the relatively smaller larynx of a child, the probability of posterior commissure stenosis occurring after this technique is increased. We prefer laryngofissure and non-laser microsurgical excision of the arytenoid when treating bilateral vocal cord paralysis in children. Other potential problems occurring after laser excision of the arytenoid are perichondritis with associated granulation tissue and foreign body inflammatory reactions to residual char and desiccated debris.

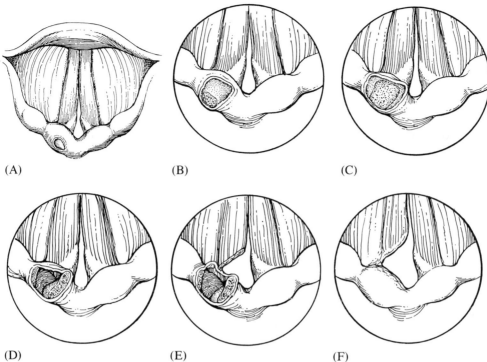

(A)   (B)   (C)

(D)   (E)   (F)

Figure 9.2 (*A*) Initial removal of mucosa with the laser over the corniculate cartilage. (*B*) More extensive removal of mucosa and beginning of removal of the arytenoid cartilage. (*C*) Most of the arytenoid cartilage has been removed. (*D*) Arytenoid cartilage has been removed down to the cricoarytenoid joint. Some cartilage is preserved medially to avoid thermal damage to the interarytenoid area and resultant scarring. (*E*) Some of the soft tissues in the region of the vocal process and posterior aspect of the true vocal cord are excised. (*F*) The areas ablated by the laser have resurfaced with mucosa, leaving a wider opening in the posterior or respiratory portion of the glottis.

The CO_2 laser can play a role in the treatment of spastic dysphonia[34]; 90% of these patients are cured by resection of the recurrent laryngeal nerve on one side. If spasticity and significant voice aberrations recur, a revision procedure as described by Dedo can be performed.[34]

A "trough" is created on the superior surface of the true vocal cord on the side of recurrent laryngeal nerve section. The trough extends from the anterior commissure to just lateral to the vocal process and measures approximately 2 mm in width and 8 mm in depth. The resultant vocal cord thinning will benefit approximately two thirds of these patients.

LARYNGEAL PAPILLOMATOSIS

Laryngeal papillomas are wartlike growths that have a predilection for the larynx when they involve the head and neck area. Although this disease usually begins during early childhood, the first evidence of involvement may not present until adulthood.[35] These patients report airway obstruction and a change in voice. Histological examination reveals increased keratinization, maturational immaturity, and a predominant basal layer hyperplasia.[36] Usually a papillary morphology is present. Human papilloma virus (HPV) particles have been identified in these lesions on electron microscopy and immunoperoxidase staining.[36] HPV subtypes 11 and 6 are most commonly implicated in laryngeal disease.

Other head and neck sites, including the soft palate, tonsillar pillars, nasopharynx, oropharyngeal walls, nasal cavity, pulmonary parenchyma, and trachea, are involved in 25 to 30% of cases. A positive history of genital warts in the mother at the time of delivery has been reported in about 50% of children with laryngeal papillomatosis. Since latent genital infection by HPV in pregnant women might approach 30%, the actual incidence of maternal infection may be significantly higher.[36] Microsurgical removal of the papillomas has been the mainstay of treatment. Many patients have required more than 10 microlaryngoscopies for papilloma removal and still have persistent disease. Latent HPV DNA has been detected in adjacent tissues that appeared clinically uninvolved under the operating microscope.[36,37] This partially explains the phenomenon of recurrence, even after apparent total excision of abnormal tissue.

The CO_2 laser has proved to be an excellent instrument for microsurgical excision of laryngeal papillomas. The papillomas are friable, and the decreased bleeding noted with laser excision facilities precise removal. A power density of 1200 to 1500 W/cm^2 is employed, with a spot size of approximately 0.8 to 1 mm and a continuous wave. If significant airway obstruction exists, the anesthesiologist allows the patient to ventilate through a mask and to slowly achieve a plane of surgical anesthesia. We prefer a technique of maintaining anesthesia that avoids having an endotracheal tube in the airway. A markedly improved visualization facilitates removal, especially in the posterior portion of the larynx. The risk of airway fire is also reduced. With this in mind, apneic anesthesia with intermittent ventilation, spontaneous ventilation or jet ventilation techniques can be employed; these are described in Chapter 4B of this volume.

If a patient's disease is very aggressive they must be treated every 2 to 4 weeks to avoid tracheotomy. All papillomas are removed completely at each microlaryngoscopy, including those at both sides of the anterior commissure. Anterior webbing or blunting can be a problem in such cases. However, because the denuded areas quickly resurface with rapidly proliferating papillomatous tissue, webbing probably occurs less often than expected even after total removal of papillomas. In patients whose disease progresses more slowly, the surgeon tries to preserve 2 mm of mucosa at the anterior commissure to avoid anterior web formation.

It is important to avoid damaging adjacent normal mucosa,[38,39] since raw surfaces and mucosal breaks encourage the seeding of papillomatous tissue.

Papillomatous involvement of the trachea has been correlated with the performance of tracheotomy, with seeding of the tracheotomy wound being implicated.[35,38] However, patients who require tracheotomy obviously have more biologically aggressive disease. Also, tracheotomy has been shown to induce mucosal changes and metaplasia in patients without papillomas. Therefore, seeding of a raw wound may not be the mechanism of pathogenesis. Instead, posttracheotomy tracheal involvement may be related to activation of latent virus in adjacent normal-appearing tissue.[36,40] In one series, only 50% of patients who had pulmonary parenchymal involvement had a prior tracheotomy.[38] This finding supports reactivation as the mechanism of dissemination. If viral seeding were the sole means of spread, one would expect more patients to have parenchymal involvement; patients frequently report "coughing up" particles of papillomatous tissue. This means that such tissue is commonly aspirated into the lower tracheal bronchial tree. The actual incidence of pulmonary parenchymal involvement is less than 5%.

Methylprednisolone is administered parenterally during surgery to reduce swelling after laser excision. Cool mist for humidification of the airway, and sometimes racemic epinephrine, is given in the recovery room. These precautions diminish the need for postoperative reintubation and the associated trauma that might play a role in activation of additional disease.

Most surgeries are performed on an outpatient basis. Patients are observed in the recovery room and day surgery area for approximately 5 hours.

The CO_2 laser is a very precise instrument, but its repeated use for removal of papillomas from the larynx is not without associated trauma to this organ. Patients who require frequently repeated treatment of aggressive disease can develop complications of anterior blunting and laryngeal scarring with associated stenosis.[35,39,41] The posterior commissure is especially vulnerable to injury and scarring. Because the papillomas are quite friable, char tends to build up on the surfaces where the laser strikes the lesions. This desiccated debris heats up above 100°C after repeated laser impacts and provides a mechanism for excessive heat transfer to adjacent tissues. It should therefore be frequently suctioned away.

Significant voice changes have been noted after frequent surgical excision. The voice is often lower pitched and diplophonic in quality. Some children habitually whisper. Stroboscopically, a decreased amplitude of vibration, an absence of mucosal waves, and incomplete glottic closure have been identified.[39] These findings are consistent with increased stiffness and mass of the true vocal cords.

Because laryngeal papillomas tend to recur, even after total surgical excision, numerous adjunctive therapies have been tried and include the following: vaccination, transfer factor,[42] interferon,[43,44] immunostimulant therapy with isoprinosine,[45] accutane (13-*cis*-retinoic acid),[46] topical podophyllin,[38] and topical 5-flurouracil.[47] The best results in terms of remission (defined as no evidence of disease on microlaryngoscopy for more than 1 year) have been reported by Dedo and coworkers.[38] They achieved a remission rate of 41.3% using laser excision in conjunction with topical application of podophyllin to the involved areas.

Remission is significantly lower in children who develop disease prior to age 5.[38] Strong and associates[35] note that patients who have required more than 10 microlaryngoscopies rarely achieve remission. Although puberty has been identified as a potential cause of remission by some authors, others have noted no significant improvement associated with this endocrine event.[35] It should be recalled that remission is not equivalent to cure, as papillomata can recur after a 20-year disease-free interval.

Of the adjunctive therapies mentioned, topical 5-fluorouracil,[47] topical podophyllin,[38] and parenteral interferon seem most effective. However, 5-fluorouracil has been associated with the histologic appearance of dysplasia in papillomas.[47] Interferon can induce remission in 25 to 30% of cases and partial remission in another 30%. The mechanism of action seems to be its antiviral and antiproliferative properties.[43] Interferon seems to induce morphologic changes in the gross appearance of the papillomata. The lesions are flatter and less exophytic, so that they obstruct the airway less.[39] Interferon would appear especially useful for patients who require surgical removal every 2 to 3 weeks, both because of the inconvenience associated with these frequently performed surgical procedures and because of the higher risk of inducing laryngeal stenosis. The side effects of interferon therapy include neutropenia, fever, malaise, and nausea.[43,46] All of these respond to a decrease in the dose.

Accutane is a vitamin A derivative that has antiproliferative properties. It is frequently used by dermatologists to treat cystic acne. A response rate of 60% has been reported in a small series of patients.[46] If, as previously suggested, the pathogenic mechanism causing papilloma growth is a defect in maturation rather than an increased rate of proliferation, the failure of accutane in some cases is explained.[36] Teratogenic effects have been noted and therefore accutane should not be used in adult females who might be pregnant.[46]

The frequency of performing microlaryngoscopy for treating laryngeal papillomatosis with the laser varies from institution to institution. Some recommend removing disease as infrequently as possible and only when obstruction of the airway mandates surgical therapy.[41] Others recommend that papillomas be removed often after the disease initially presents in an attempt to attain early remission.[39] If this fails, the interval between treatment is expanded. We prefer removal on a regularly scheduled basis every 2 to 3 months unless forced to operate more frequently because of airway obstruction.

SUBGLOTTIC HEMANGIOMAS

Subglottic hemangiomas are hamartomatous lesions that develop in the first 6 months of life and masquerade as recurrent and prolonged episodes of "croup."[48,49] About 50% of children with laryngeal subglottic hemangiomas have concomitant cutaneous hemangiomas.[49] Most of the time the lesion can be strongly suspected on the basis of anterior, posterior, and lateral soft tissue x-rays of the neck that show an asymmetry in the subglottic region.[50,51] The diagnosis is confirmed at the time of endoscopy, however. A smooth compressible swelling involving the posterior larynx and extending to one side is noted. It need not be purplish or bright red as cutaneous lesions are. In studies employing biopsy, the lesion has almost always been a capillary hemangioma and is not cavernous.[48,49] In most cases the clinical picture is so pathognomonic that biopsy is not required unless the appearance or presentation is atypical.

These lesions are generally very amenable to definitive resection with the CO_2 laser. An exception would be extensive external involvement of the neck and mediastinum with a large hemangiomatous mass; here the main mechanism of airway obstruction is external compression. Other modes of treatment have been tried: a tracheotomy may be employed while awaiting spontaneous involution. Corticosteroid therapy may afford temporary relief, but in most cases, airway obstruction recurs when it is discontinued.[49,51] These lesions do tend to spontaneously involute[52] but in some children this may not occur until well after age 2, prolonging the time a tracheotomy must be in place.

Some authors recommend the use of the Nd:YAG[53] or argon laser[54] for resecting these lesions because these wavelengths are more specifically absorbed by pigmented tissues. It is postulated that less bleeding would occur. However, because of the capillary histology of these lesions, significant bleeding rarely occurs when they are resected with the CO_2 laser. The Nd:YAG and argon lasers have the disadvantage of interacting with a relatively larger volume of tissue. The associated greater heating of adjacent tissues increases the risk of laryngeal scarring and stenosis.

With smaller lesions where no tracheotomy is to be employed, apneic anesthesia or jet ventilation is used. We usually prefer to use a temporary tracheotomy if a moderate or more extensive lesion exists. Extensive lesions may require serial resection to avoid scarring.[55] When moderate or larger lesions are resected without tracheotomy, repeat endoscopies are often required in the postoperative period to remove eschar and maintain the airway.[48] Prolonged intensive care unit support with oxygen and humidification may be necessary. In most patients the tracheotomy tube can be removed in 3 to 5 weeks after an adequate airway has been documented on repeat endoscopy.

In most cases a single treatment with the CO_2 laser is adequate for reestablishing the airway. An important technical consideration in using the CO_2 laser for resecting subglottic hemangiomas is to avoid injury to the perichondrium and exposure of cartilage, which would cause excessive granulation tissue and scarring. Also, injury to the arytenoid and cricoarytenoid joints should be judiciously avoided. In friable lesions, eschar should be removed frequently during the procedure to avoid excessive heat injury to adjacent tissues.

LARYNGEAL STENOSIS

In stenotic lesions of the upper airway, using the laser and an endoscopic technique has the attraction of avoiding a more extensive open procedure. Experimental work in animals has shown that the CO_2 laser wound displays a decreased rate of collagen formation but also seems to be associated with a decreased rate of epithelialization.[56,57] The potential for decreased scar formation makes it attractive for treating stenotic lesions of the larynx. The neodymium:YAG laser has been employed by some surgeons,[58,59] but it is a less precise laser modality, associated with greater heat injury to adjacent tissues. It may be of some use in subglottic lesions because it can be delivered through a fiberoptic cable. Shapshay and coworkers[59] have described a technique for increasing the precision of the neodymium:YAG laser by tattooing the tissue to be excised with India ink, increasing absorption of Nd:YAG laser energy.

Factors Affecting Prognosis

Evaluation of the lesion is critical. The anatomic location of the lesion, its extent, and the type of tissue causing the stenosis directly affect the prognosis. Lateral soft tissue x-rays of the neck and CT scans have proved useful adjuncts to endoscopy.[60] Nevertheless, a contrast laryngogram using a liquid or powdered contrast agent remains an elegant way to display the entire extent of a stenotic lesion of the airway on one film.[61]

In regard to laser management, the following factors generally apply:

Supraglottic lesions are almost always composed solely of soft tissue and therefore respond readily to laser reduction.

Lesions of the glottis that cause significant webbing or blunting of the anterior commissure usually do not respond to simple excision but require a stent or flap technique.[61-63]

Posteriorly located glottic lesions are most problematic if there is marked scarring of the interarytenoid area or cricoarytenoid joint fixation.[60,61,64,65]

Subglottic lesions have a poorer prognosis for successful laser treatment if greater than 80% of the lumen is involved[56] or a hard stenosis composed mainly of cartilage is present.[66]

Soft tissue stenoses involving the subglottis are usually composed of more mature granulation tissue, submucosal mucous gland hypertrophy, and submucosal fibrosis and are therefore more amenable to laser excision.[66]

Factors indicating a poor prognosis for laser management of airway stenosis are circumferential lesions, lesions having a vertical height greater than 1 cm, concomitant loss of cartilaginous support, and lesions associated with tracheal stenosis.[56,60,61,64-69] Some prognostic factors are interrelated. For instance, lesions that involve cricoarytenoid joint fixation and interarytenoid scarring have a poor prognosis in part because they usually extend vertically for more than 1 cm.

Adjunctive Measures and Techniques

Adjunctive measures and techniques have been combined with laser excision of stenoses. Steroids may reduce the amount of acute and subacute granulation tissue seen in the immediate period after trauma or after removal of an endolaryngeal stent.[56,70,71] They may also reduce acute edema postoperatively providing a margin of safety in patients without a tracheotomy. The prolonged use of steroids after laser excision of scar tissue in the airway is not recommended, however, because a delay in epithelialization is associated with their use.[60,71] Although a concomitant decrease in the deposition of collagenous tissue and scar tissue can be beneficial, steroids may also impair the cartilaginous support of the airway.[61] Certain lathyrogenic agents such as pencillamine or N-acetylcysteine may be used in the future to decrease crosslinkages between polypeptide chains of collagen and in this manner reduce scarring.[72]

Stenting does provide a spacer while epithelialization occurs,[56,60,64,65] but stents can also reduce epithelial migration and can cause a foreign body reaction with granulation tissue and scarring.[57] Stents that fit poorly in the posterior commissure of the glottis can cause pressure necrosis in the region of the arytenoid and vocal process, with resultant posterior commissure scarring that is very difficult to manage. Many authors recommend a stent as an adjunct to endoscopic laser resection with more severe stenosis,[60,65] but these are the same lesions that often require open laryngotracheoplasty.

Certain principles apply to most of the techniques for treating stenoses of the airway with the CO_2 laser. Circumferential wounds should be avoided as they almost always lead to a circumferential scar. In addition, they interrupt the mucociliary flow of a segment of the airway.[58] Injury to perichondrium and exposure of cartilage should be avoided because these poorly vascularized tissues often support the formation of granulation tissue and subsequent rescarring. The procedure should be designed to provide mucosal coverage, which hastens wound healing and minimizes granulation tissue formation. Excessive thermal injury to adjacent tissues should be averted by frequent removal of char and by keeping laser radiation times short to allow tissue cooling between impacts.

Anatomic Sites

Supraglottic stenoses may require multiple excisions if the lesion is circumferential, as is often seen after caustic ingestion, severe gastroesophageal reflux, or trauma. Approximately one third of such a circumferential supraglottic stenosis should be removed at each laser treatment. When only redundant tissue is present, as is often the case after partial laryngectomy for cancer, one simple laser reduction often suffices for successful treatment. In posttraumatic lesions in which the petiole of the epiglottis has been displaced far posteriorly, an open procedure is usually required to reestablish patency of the airway.

Glottic stenoses usually involve the anterior or posterior part of the glottis. Small anterior glottic webs can be treated with simple laser excision.[61] Moderate-sized or larger areas of anterior blunting require division and insertion of a keel,[62] which is placed and anchored endoscopically, or division and creation of a mucosal flap. The flap technique has been described in detail by McGuirt and colleagues.[63] The CO_2 laser was used to create a mucosal flap on one side of the superior surface of the anterior web. This flap was then spot-welded to the surface of the underlying vocal cord. Additional laryngoscopies were required to smooth irregularities with the laser. This technique yields excellent postoperative voice production.

If the *posterior commissure of the glottis* is the primary site of stenosis, treatment can be more problematic. It should be remembered that patients who have been intubated for some time and then receive a tracheotomy can develop a scar band between the vocal process areas of the vocal cords. An endotracheal tube may lead to pressure necrosis over the vocal process, to perichondritis, and to the formation of granulation tissue. Subsequent tracheotomy has been shown to reduce vocal cord excursion and mobility,[73,74] setting the stage for opposing granulations and formation of a scar tether. If this condition is recognized at endoscopy, simple division with the laser is often successful.

In more advanced scarring of the posterior commissure, the interarytenoid tissues seem on endoscopy to be at the same level as the anterior surface of the arytenoids.[61] A mucosal-lined sinus tract may be seen behind the anterior aspect of the scar. Occasionally this tract extends from the interarytenoid area to the subglottis and represents a complete fistula. If a sinus or fistula is present, the anterior scar tissue can be divided with the laser and the mucosa of the sinus or fistula preserved by protecting it with a suction tip or moist packing.[61] This provides more rapid healing of the wound and tends to prevent the posterior commissure stenosis from re-forming.

If the posterior commissure presents dense scarring without a sinus tract and extending for over 1 cm vertically, laser excision alone is unlikely to cure the situation. In less advanced posterior commissure scars with no sinus tract, the microtrapdoor technique described by Dedo can be used successfully (Fig. 9.3A–D). Beginning at the superior aspect of the posterior commissure scar, the submucosal cicatrix is excavated with the CO_2 laser, leaving overlying mucosa intact. Lateral incisions are extended inferiorly using microscissors, creating an inferiorly based mucosal flap that provides partial coverage of the wound, facilitating healing without granulation tissue.

Subglottic stenoses that cause less than 80% narrowing of the lumen often respond to serial laser excision. Approximately one third of the circumference of a circular scar is excised at each operation. This can be combined with the microtrapdoor technique described above. A subglottiscope is useful for operating in this area.[60] An alternative technique is radial excision of the subglottic scar with gentle dilatation.[59] Using an endoscopic laser excision technique, Holinger[66] found that tracheotomy could be avoided in approximately one half of the patients who would have otherwise required one.

All these techniques for removing subglottic scar require several procedures. Prophylactic antibiotics are recommended, as Sasaki and coworkers[75] have clearly shown that infection of wounds in the upper airway is associated with increased scar formation. In circumferential stenoses that occupy more than 80% of the airway, a stent is usually required after laser excision. In fact, many of these lesions require an open laryngotracheoplasty for correction. If the stenosis is primarily cartilaginous or if there is significant loss of cartilaginous support, endoscopic management is unlikely to be successful.

PREMALIGNANT AND MALIGNANT LESIONS OF THE LARYNX

The concept of endoscopic excision for cure of premalignant and early malignant lesions of the larynx is not new. A comparable cure rate to radiation therapy was achieved. It is only natural that this concept of endoscopic excision be extended to laser surgery of the larynx for early malignant lesions. In 1975, Strong[76] presented a series of 11 patients with early laryngeal cancer who were treated endoscopically with laser excision. Three of these patients, interestingly, had prior radiation therapy. There were no instances of recurrent disease in this initial series.

Figure 9.3 (*A*) Hypothetical drawing of stenosis involving the posterior commissure, subglottis, and upper trachea. The stippled areas represent submucosal scar tissue. (*B*) Sagittal view after initial CO_2 laser ablation of the mucosa over the submucosal scar, in preparation for the performance of the microtrapdoor technique. (*Inset*) View from above, showing initial mucosal ablation over submucosal scar tissue. (*C*) Coronal view showing initial CO_2 ablation of mucosa over submucosal scar tissue. (*D*) Completion of microtrapdoor technique in which submucosal scar has been ablated with the CO_2 laser and remaining overlying mucosa preserved as a flap that helps cover raw areas.

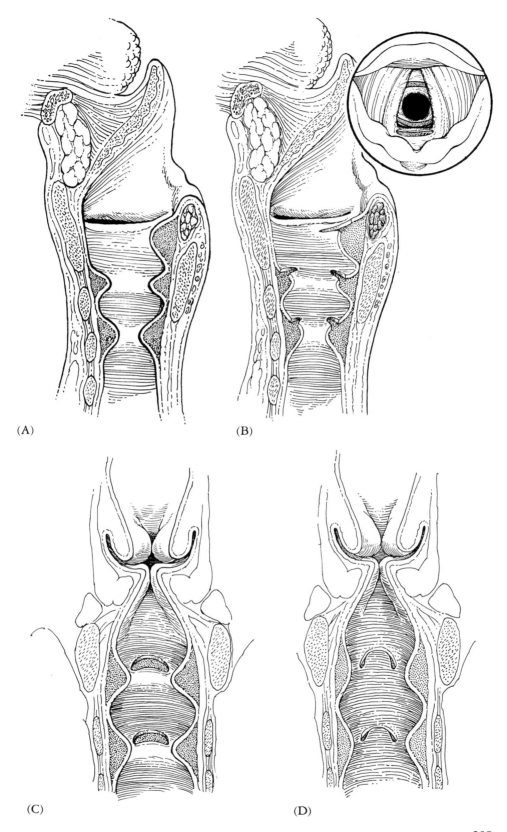

(A)

(B)

(C)

(D)

209

Further investigation and clinical trials at several centers have refined the principles of laser excision of malignant laryngeal disease and have extended its use. This technique has been used to debulk obstructing laryngeal cancers, thereby avoiding tracheotomy.[77-79] It has been used as a staging tool to provide information to select proper treatment.[79] In Europe, the concept of laser cytoreduction of more extensive laryngeal cancer, followed by radiation therapy, has been advocated in place of open surgical procedures.[80]

Carcinoma of the Glottic Larynx

The anatomic parameters and limitations of endoscopic laser resection have been outlined by Davis and associates.[81] Achieving adequate excision with a margin of normal tissue is most difficult at the anterior commissure, since, in this location, there is only 2 mm to traverse until the thyroid cartilage is encountered. At the midcord level the distance to the thyroid cartilage is 5 to 6 mm, while at the vocal process the distance is 9 mm. As the resection proceeds subglottically at the anterior commissure, the cricothyroid membrane is approached, providing a limit to the resection. So long as the inferior extent of excision at the anterior commissure is 5 mm or less, the cricothyroid membrane is not violated.

It is difficult to excise tissue posterior to the vocal process through an endoscopic approach. If the tumor extends laterally into the laryngeal ventricle, it becomes difficult to achieve excision out to the thyroid cartilage unless some of the false vocal cord is resected for exposure. For these anatomic reasons, many surgeons have limited their initial attempts to treat malignant disease of the larynx with the laser to T1 lesions involving the midportion of one vocal cord and without extension to the anterior commissure, vocal process, or lateralmost extents of the laryngeal ventricle.[82,83] Our indications for curative resection of early laryngeal cancer, using an endoscopic approach and the carbon dioxide laser, are as follows:

1. The lesion is a T1 glottic lesion, implying normal mobility of both vocal cords.
2. The full extent of the lesion and the anterior commissure are readily exposed endoscopically.
3. The vocal process and arytenoid are free of disease.
4. The lateralmost extent of the laryngeal ventricle is not involved.
5. No invasion of the thyroid cartilage is identified through the operating microscope.
6. Mucosal margins and deep margins are free of tumor. (This requires that biopsy specimens of adequate size be taken at the time of surgery so that the margins are evaluated for evidence of neoplasia.)
7. No evidence of recurrent tumor or suspicious lesions are noted at follow-up microlaryngoscopy.

The surgical technique is done as follows: Apneic anesthesia may be used for smaller lesions that require a relatively short time for resection. For longer procedures, jet ventilation is employed, using a Dedo laryngoscope with a 12- to 14-gauge spinal needle clamped to its proximal portion. It is also helpful if a suction device is clamped to the proximal portion of the scope or a No. 12 Frazier suction tip is inserted into one of the fiberoptic light channels of a scope that is supplied by two fiberoptic light cables. If significant anterior commissure involvement exists and "miniresection" of the anterior thyroid cartilage is to be performed (see below), a tracheotomy is usually employed to give anesthesia and maintain the airway post-operatively.

The CO_2 laser is employed. It should have a spot size of ≤ 1 mm at a 400-mm working distance. A power density of 1500 W/cm^2 is used.

The lesion is grasped firmly with cup forceps and retracted medially. The counter traction is very important in facilitating dissection and also brings more laterally located mucosa into view. The tissue should be regrasped as seldom as possible, and when this is necessary, only tissue that is to be excised is grasped to avoid contamination or seeding of normal tissues. The excision is conducted in a posterior-lateral to a medial-anterior direction.

When the lesion has been excised, it is placed on filter paper or on a tongue blade in the presence of the pathologist. In addition, representative biopsies of the deep and mucosal margins are obtained from the remaining laryngeal tissue. One of the problems with laser endoscopic excision of malignant neoplasms is that even with a 0.8-mm spot size, the kerf or trough created along the line of excision can impair interpretation of the margins because some normal tissue is vaporized by the laser. Also, the tissues being excised tend to tear as they are retracted medially with the cup forceps. The most difficult place to obtain an evaluable soft-tissue margin is at the anterior commissure.

If there is significant involvement of the anterior commissure (Fig. 9.4A), the endoscopic laser excision is combined with a limited open procedure in which a small portion of the anterior thyroid cartilage is included with the resection. In these cases, a 2-cm horizontal incision is made over the midportion of the thyroid cartilage and taken down to perichondrium. The perichondrium is incised and elevated laterally. An 8- to 10-mm diameter disk of thyroid cartilage is outlined and cut, centered over a point along the midline of the thyroid cartilage and one-half the distance between the thyroid notch and inferior border of the thyroid cartilage (Fig. 9.4B). A precise cut is made with a dental burr 0.6 mm in diameter and designed to cut in a lateral direction. These dental burrs are commonly used in orthognathic surgery.

The cut is made 80% through the thickness of the thyroid cartilage and then completed with a sharp cottle elevator. This avoids entry into the soft tissues at the anterior commissure, which might be involved with neoplasm. The inner perichondrium is elevated for a short distance around the edges of the cartilage disk so that it is completely mobilized. The disk is now depressed toward the endolarynx. A small piece of Gelfilm® is used to wedge the cartilage disk inwardly (Fig. 9.4C). The wound is irrigated and closed.

Suspension microlaryngoscopy is used to complete the endoscopic laser excision as described, and the specimen is pedicled at the anterior commissure. The resection is completed at the anterior commissure to include the disk of anterior thyroid cartilage with its inner perichondrium (Fig. 9.4D).

Follow-up laryngoscopy is performed in 2 weeks if the anterior commissure technique has been employed. This is to break up adhesions at the anterior commissure and, in some cases, to place a keel to prevent webbing at the anterior commissure. The keel is placed and anchored endoscopically, using a silicone button located at the anterior midline of the neck. The keel is placed only if the margins of

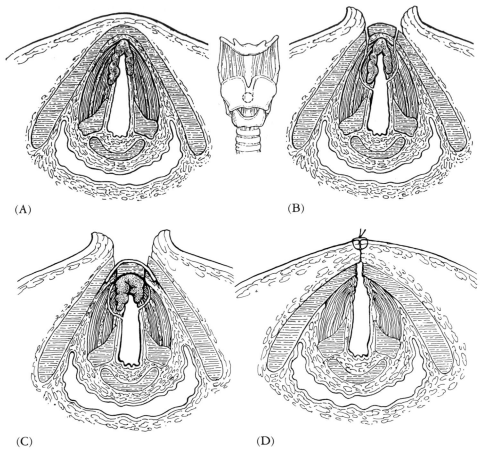

Figure 9.4 (*A*) T1 squamous cell carcinoma involving both true cords and the anterior commissure. (*B*) Incision of an anterior disk of cartilage overlying the anterior commissure and CO_2 laser excision of the lesion with adjacent tissue of the true vocal cords. (*Inset*) Anterior view of proposed disk of thyroid cartilage to be incised. (*C*) The anterior disk of cartilage is pushed into the larynx and held there by a small piece of Gelfilm®. (*D*) Cartilage disk, along with the lesion and adjacent soft tissues, has been removed. The surgical defect has been closed.

resection were shown to be clear of tumor to preclude any seeding of tumor that could occur when the anchoring sutures are passed.

All patients in whom endoscopic laser excision has been performed are given prophylactic antibiotics for 5 days. Humidified air is provided, using a mist shield for 24 to 48 hours. Depending on the extent of resection, the patient is discharged at 24 to 48 hours. If a tracheotomy has been performed, the patient is discharged in 72 hours.

If a deep margin is found to be positive for neoplasia on permanent section, the patient is referred for curative radiation therapy.

If the thyroid cartilage is found to be invaded, either at the time of microlaryngoscopy or on examination of the permanent histopathologic sections, a more extensive surgical resection is required.

If limited involvement of the mucosal margins is noted, the patient can receive repeat endoscopic laser excision of the involved mucosa.

If the mucosal margins are more diffusely involved, then the patient should be referred for definitive radiation therapy.

In T1 lesions limited to the glottis, it is not necessary to treat the neck prophylactically with radiation or surgery, because the incidence of metastasis to cervical nodes is 1% or less.

Endoscopic excision of early laryngeal cancers provides equivalent control of disease to curative radiation therapy.[76,78,83-85] Voice quality after laser excision is good to excellent if the lesion was located in the midportion of the vocal cord, only a small amount of vocalis muscle was removed, and the anterior commissure was not involved.[85-87] A neocord forms that has been shown stroboscopically to have the capacity to vibrate in phase with the other cord.[88] A decreased amplitude of vibration associated with a decrease in voice range almost always occurs.[89] Fundamental voice frequency often rises.[86] It should be remembered that similar changes have been documented after radiation therapy of early glottic cancer.[86]

If the anterior commissure is involved, voice quality relates closely to the degree of anterior blunting that occurs postoperatively.[78] This can be minimized by breaking up any forming adhesions and granulation tissue at a subsequent laryngoscopy 2 weeks after initial treatment. In some cases, endoscopic placement of a laryngeal keel may be required. When greater amounts of vocalis muscle are resected with the laser, an acceptable phonatory voice results, but voice quality is impaired.[85]

In summary, endoscopic excision of early glottic laryngeal squamous cell carcinomas with the laser provides a precise excision under magnification in a bloodless field. An equivalent control of disease is provided when comparing this modality to radiation therapy. Voice quality is excellent in early midcord lesions. In some cases, more accurate staging of disease occurs as early invasion of the thyroid cartilage is detected that was not evident on CT scanning.[81] This upgrades the lesion to a T4 stage, requiring more aggressive treatment. Endoscopic laser excision is a more expedient means of treating the neoplasm than $6\frac{1}{2}$ to 7 weeks of radiation therapy.

Supraglottic Laryngeal Squamous Cell Carcinoma

It is attractive to consider treating early squamous cell cancers of the supraglottic larynx with endoscopic laser excision.[90,91] However, these lesions have a significantly higher incidence of cervical lymph node metastases than cancers limited to the glottic larynx. If the lesion is limited to the suprahyoid epiglottis the incidence of lymph node metastases is approximately 16%.[92] If the infrahyoid epiglottis is involved, the incidence of lymph node metastases is approximately 33%.[92] Therefore, even small T1 lesions limited to the tip of the epiglottis require treatment of the neck with radiation therapy or modified neck dissection concomitant with treatment of the primary lesion.

We reserve endoscopic excision of small supraglottic carcinoma for limited lesions confined to the suprahyoid epiglottis and where both sides of the neck have already been treated by neck dissection or radiation therapy for an earlier primary tumor of the head and neck. An example of such a case follows.

A 49-year-old male presented with an 8-mm lesion involving the tip of the epiglottis. It had rolled edges and an area of central ulceration. There were no palpable masses in the neck. The patient had received prior treatment $1\frac{1}{2}$ years previously for a squamous cell carcinoma of the right retromolar trigone. He received a surgical resection and bilateral modified neck dissections with postoperative radiation therapy. In this instance it was felt appropriate to attempt endoscopic laser excision of the epiglottic lesion. This was performed and the margins were confirmed to be clear of tumor.

The CO_2 laser can be used to debulk obstructing squamous cell carcinomas of the supraglottis and glottis to establish an airway without having to resort to tracheotomy.[77-79,90] Sometimes emergency tracheotomy must be performed to establish an airway in a patient with a large laryngeal cancer prior to definitive surgical resection. These cases are associated with an increased rate of wound infection and sepsis and possibly an increased rate of peristomal recurrence of tumor.[79,93] An alternative is emergency laryngectomy performed immediately after intubation or tracheotomy. This has several disadvantages: The decision to perform a major ablative procedure must be made on the basis of a frozen section. The patient's medical condition cannot be adequately evaluated. The procedure may have to be performed at night with a surgical team who may not be very experienced with head and neck procedures.

If laser debulking of a malignant lesion to establish an airway is elected, the surgeon should be prepared to perform an emergency tracheotomy or to intubate the larynx with a rigid bronchoscope. Most patients can be intubated with an endotracheal tube, using topical anesthesia. A metal foil–wrapped endotracheal tube is inserted and initial debulking is performed with the CO_2 laser. The endotracheal tube is removed and an operating laryngoscope equipped with a needle attachment for jet ventilation is inserted. The patient is ventilated by this means for the duration of the surgery, while further tumor is excised.

There have been some limited trials of using the CO_2 laser for endoscopic excision of larger squamous cell carcinomas and then employing radiation therapy postoperatively.[80] It is hoped that this approach, consisting of endoscopic laser cytoreduction followed by radiation therapy, will make open laryngectomy unnecessary in a number of cases. Experience is too limited at present to determine to what extent the larynx can be resected with the laser endoscopically and still maintain a functioning organ that can protect the lower tracheobronchial tree. Also, adequate reproducible data regarding control of tumor is not yet available.

Endoscopic laser excision can be applied to resection of other varieties of malignant laryngeal lesions. This has been done to a very limited extent. Pedunculated laryngeal pseudosarcomas can be treated by subtotal laryngectomy and, because the pedicle of attachment often involves a very limited portion of the anterior larynx, these lesions are often amenable to endoscopic laser excision.[94] Metastatic lesions such as melanoma that involve the larynx and obstruct the airway can be debulked for palliation, using an endoscopic laser technique.[95]

MISCELLANEOUS LARYNGEAL PATHOLOGY

Certain conditions that are encountered less frequently can be successfully treated with the CO_2 laser. Unusual conditions that can obstruct the airway and cause hoarseness include sarcoidosis, amyloidosis, congenital saccular cysts, lymphangiomas, and granular cell tumors.

Patients with *sarcoidosis* can present with a turban-shaped epiglottis and involvement of the aryepiglottic fold with airway obstruction.[96] The bulk of the aryepiglottic fold can be reduced with the CO_2 laser, often relieving the obstruction without tracheotomy being required.[96]

There are two types of *congenital saccular cysts*. The anterior saccular cyst is usually smaller and presents toward the anterior portion of the laryngeal ventricle. The lateral cyst is larger and more likely to obstruct the airway. It causes a bulging of the aryepiglottic fold and sometimes of the pharyngoepiglottic fold on the side of the lesion. The lesion originates from dilatation of the laryngeal saccule. Congenital saccular cysts have been treated by aspiration, or simply opening the cyst with the laser. When this technique is employed, repeat drainage procedures are often required because the fluid contents rapidly reaccumulate in the cyst.[97] A more complete opening of the cyst, eversion of the lining, and vaporization of the lining with the laser are more likely to cure the condition.

Saccular cysts present in the newborn but *laryngoceles* can be noted for the first time in any age group.[97] Some internal laryngoceles can be marsupialized definitively, using the CO_2 laser.[98]

Amyloidosis can present as a systemic disease with multiple sites of involvement or can be limited to a single organ such as the larynx.[99] The larynx is usually involved bilaterally. The disease presents as hoarseness but rarely as marked airway obstruction.[99] Total excision of the amyloid deposits may cure the disease, but in a number of cases repeat excisions are required before the lesion is totally eliminated.[100]

Patients with *neurofibromatosis* can have involvement of the head and neck with laryngeal infiltration. Often the scope of infiltration of the larynx and perilaryngeal structures is so extensive that total removal would require laryngectomy. However, partial excision of an obstructing lesion can be accomplished with the CO_2 laser, with long-term improvement in airway function. If a tracheotomy was performed for airway obstruction, it can be removed after adequate reduction in the bulk of laryngeal neurofibroma.

Unusual neoplasms such as a *granular cell myoblastoma* can be successfully excised with CO_2 laser.[101] These are usually located in the posterior one third of the larynx and are white or gray.

Laryngomalacia is a disease entity encountered in the first year of life. There is an inspiratory stridor, made worse by crying, feeding, and agitation. Stridor is often more prominent when the patient is in the supine position. In severe cases, retractions and cyanosis can occur. The epiglottis is often omega-shaped, and the aryepiglottic folds are very short. The mucosa over the arytenoid cartilages is redundant and prolapses into the glottis on inspiration. This redundant tissue over the arytenoids and involving the aryepiglottic folds can be removed with the CO_2 laser.

Also, dividing the aryepiglottic folds allows the arytenoid to retract posteriorly and the epiglottis to retract anteriorly, lengthening the entrance into the glottis and thereby relieving airway obstruction.[102]

Some patients with *dysphonia plicae ventricularis* have been shown to have irreversible hypertrophy of the false vocal folds. Histologic changes consist of a reduction in submucosal glandular elements, a dense submucosal connective tissue, and a prominent infiltration with lymphocytes.[103] Laser reduction of the false vocal cord can, in some cases, dramatically improve airway obstruction.[103]

Patients with *congenital cleft larynx* have a major problem with recurrent aspiration and pneumonia. However, another component of the problem can be partial airway obstruction due to a prolapse of postcricoid soft tissues through the cleft in the cricoid cartilage. These obstructing soft tissues can be reduced with the CO_2 laser.[104]

Lymphangiomas of the head and neck can involve the larynx. In many cases there is also involvement of other areas of the head and neck and of soft tissues adjacent to the larynx. Lesions that extrinsically compress the larynx can be treated by conventional surgical excision and, where appropriate, by tracheotomy. When the endolarynx is involved, excision with the CO_2 laser is often very helpful in relieving airway obstruction and averting a tracheotomy.[105]

REFERENCES

1. Jako GJ, Strong MS, Polanyi TG, et al: Experimental carbon dioxide laser surgery of the vocal cords. *Eye Ear Nose Throat Mon* 52:171–172, 1973.

2. Jako GJ: Laser surgery of the vocal cords. An experimental study with carbon dioxide lasers on dogs. *Laryngoscope* 82:2204–2216, 1972.

3. Hobeika CP, Rockwell RJ Jr: Laser microsurgery in experimental otolaryngology. *Trans Am Acad Ophthalmol Otolaryngol* 76:325–333, 1972.

4. Andrews AH Jr, Polanyi TG, Grybauskas VT: General techniques and clinical considerations in laryngologic laser surgery. *Otolaryngol Clin North Am* 16:793–800, 1983.

5. Vaughan CW: Transoral laryngeal surgery using the CO_2 laser: laboratory experiments and clinical experience. *Laryngoscope* 88:1399—1421, 1978.

6. Kirschner RA, Unger M: Introduction to laser surgery. *Surg Clin North Am* 64: 839–841, 1984.

7. Vaughan CW: Use of the carbon dioxide laser in the endoscopic management of organic laryngeal disease. *Otolaryngol Clin North Am* 16:849–864, 1983.

8. Andrews AH, Moss HW: Experiences with the carbon dioxide laser in the larynx. *Ann Otol Rhinol Laryngol* 83:462–470, 1974.

9. Healy GB: Current management of lesions of the pediatric larynx. *Ann Otol Rhinol Laryngol* 96:122–123, 1987.

10. Shapshay SM, Wallace RA, Kveton JF: New microspot micromanipulator for carbon dioxide laser surgery in otolaryngology: early clinical results. *Arch Otolaryngol Head Neck Surg* 114:1012–1015, 1988.

11. Toohill RJ, Duncavage JA, Grossman TW: Wound healing in the larynx. *Otolaryngol Clin North Am* 17:429–436, 1984.

12. Mihashi S, Jako GJ, Incze J, et al: Laser surgery in otolaryngology: interaction of CO_2 laser and soft tissue. *Ann NY Acad Sci* 267:263–294, 1976.

13. Durkin GE, Duncavage JA, Toohill RJ, et al: Wound healing of true vocal cord squamous epithelium after CO_2 laser ablation and cup forceps stripping. *Otolaryngol Head Neck Surg* 95:273–277, 1986.

14. Hall RR: Healing of tissues incised by a carbon dioxide laser. *Br J Surg* 58:222–225, 1971.

15. Schenk F: Effect of CO_2 laser on skin lymphatics, an ultrastructural study. *Langenbecks Arch Chir* 350:145–150, 1980.

16. Carruth JA: The role of lasers in otolaryngology. *World J Surg* 7:719–724, 1983.

17. Benjamin B, Croxson G: Vocal cord granulomas. *Ann Otol Rhinol Laryngol* 94:538–541, 1985.

18. Hirano M: Structure of the vocal fold in normal and disease states: anatomical and physical studies. In Ludlow CL, Hart MO'C (eds): *Proceedings of Conference on Assessment of Vocal Pathology*. ASHA Report, No 11, pp 11–30, 1981.

19. Lumpkin SM, Bishop SG, Bennett S: Comparison of surgical techniques in the treatment of laryngeal polypoid degeneration. *Ann Otol Rhinol Laryngol* 96:254–257, 1987.

20. Yates A, Dedo HH: Carbon dioxide laser enucleation of polypoid vocal cords. *Laryngoscope* 94:731–736, 1984.

21. Lyons GD, Lousteau RJ, Mouney DF: CO_2 laser laryngoscopy in a variety of lesions. *Laryngoscope* 86:1658–1662, 1976.

22. Leonard RJ, Gallia LJ, Charpied G, et al: Effects of stripping and laser excision on vocal cord mucosa in cats. *Ann Otol Rhinol Laryngol* 97:159–163, 1988.

23. Hirano M: *Microsurgery of the larynx*. (Videotape.) New York, The Voice Foundation Film, 1982.

24. Woodman DG: Bilateral abductor paralysis. *Arch Otolaryngol* 58:150, 1953.

25. Lore JM: *Atlas of Head and Neck Surgery*. Philadelphia, Saunders, 1988, pp 878–881.

26. Tucker HM: Human laryngeal reinnervation. *Laryngoscope* 88:598, 1978.

27. Thornell W: Transoral intralaryngeal approach for arytenoidectomy in bilateral vocal cord paralysis with inadequate airway. *Ann Otol Rhinol Laryngol* 66:364, 1957.

28. Ossoff RH, Sisson GA, Duncavage JA, et al: Endoscopic laser arytenoidectomy for the treatment of bilateral vocal cord paralysis. *Laryngoscope* 94:1293–1297, 1984.

29. Remsen K, Lawson W, Patel N, et al: Laser lateralization for bilateral vocal cord abductor paralysis. *Otolaryngol Head Neck Surg* 93:645–649, 1985.

30. Prasad U: CO_2 surgical laser in the management of bilateral vocal cord paralysis. *J Laryngol Otol* 99:891–894, 1985.

31. Lim RY: Laser arytenoidectomy. *Arch Otolaryngol* 111:262–263, 1985.

32. Eskew JR, Bailey BJ: Laser arytenoidectomy for bilateral vocal cord paralysis. *Otolaryngol Head Neck Surg* 91:294–298, 1983.

33. Abramson AL: Endolaryngeal carbon dioxide laser arytenoidectomy: evaluation using a flow-volume loop. *Bull NY Acad Med* 60:825–845, 1984.

34. Dedo HH, Izdebski K: Evaluation and treatment of recurrent spasticity after recurrent laryngeal nerve section. A preliminary report. *Ann Otol Rhinol Laryngol* 93:343–345, 1984.

35. Strong MS, Vaughan CW, Healy GB, et al: Recurrent respiratory papillomatosis: management with the CO_2 laser. *Ann Otol Rhinol Laryngol* 85:508–516, 1976.

36. Abramson AL, Steinberg BM, Winkler B: Laryngeal papillomatosis: clinical, histopathologic and molecular studies. *Laryngoscope* 97:678–685, 1987.

37. Steinberg BM, Toop WC, Schneider PSS, et al: Laryngeal papillomavirus infection during clinical remission. *N Engl J Med* 308:1261–1264, 1983.

38. Dedo HH, Jackler RK: Laryngeal papilloma: results of treatment with the CO_2 laser and podophyllum. *Ann Otol Rhinol Laryngol* 91:425–430, 1982.

39. Crockett DM, McCabe BF, Shive CJ: Complications of laser surgery for recurrent respiratory papillomatosis. *Ann Otol Rhinol Laryngol* 96:639–644, 1987.

40. Shikowitz MJ, Steinberg BM, Winkler B: Squamous metaplasia in the trachea: the tracheotomized rabbit as an experimental model and implications in recurrent papillomatosis. *Otolaryngol Head Neck Surg* 95:31–36, 1986.

41. Wetmore SJ, Key JM, Suen JY: Complications of laser surgery for laryngeal papillomatosis. *Laryngoscope* 95:798–801, 1985.

42. Lyons GD, Schlosser JV, Lousteau R, et al: Laser surgery and immunotherapy in the management of laryngeal papilloma. *Laryngoscope* 88:1586–1588, 1978.

43. Benjamin BN, Gatenby PA, Kitchen R, et al: Alpha-interferon (Wellferon) as an adjunct to standard surgical therapy in the management of recurrent respiratory papillomatosis. *Ann Otol Rhinol Laryngol* 97:376–380, 1988.

44. McCabe BF, Clark CF: Interferon and laryngeal papillomatosis: the Iowa experience. *Ann Otol Rhinol Laryngol* 92:2–7, 1983.

45. Élö J, Máté A: Combined therapy with isoprinosine and CO_2 laser microsurgery for the treatment of laryngeal papillomatosis. *Arch Otorhinolaryngol* 244:342–345, 1988.

46. Alberts DS, Coulthard SW, Meyskens FL Jr: Regression of aggressive laryngeal papillomatosis with 13-cis-retinoic acid (accutane). *J Biol Response Mod* 5:124–128, 1986.

47. Smith HG, Healy GB, Vaughan CW, et al: Topical chemotherapy of recurrent respiratory papillomatosis. A preliminary report. *Ann Otol Rhinol Laryngol* 89:472–478, 1980.

48. Healy G, McGill T, Friedman EM: Carbon dioxide laser in subglottic hemangioma. An update. *Ann Otol Rhinol Laryngol* 93:370–373, 1984.

49. Mizono G, Dedo HH: Subglottic hemangiomas in infants: treatment with CO_2 laser. *Laryngoscope* 94:638–641, 1984.

50. Wenig BL, Abramson AL: Congenital subglottic hemangiomas: a treatment update. *Laryngoscope* 98:190–192, 1988.

51. Narcy P, Contencin P, Bobin S, et al: Treatment of infantile subglottic hemangioma: a report of 49 cases. *Int J Pediatr Otorhinolaryngol* 9:157–164, 1985.

52. Cleland WJD, Riding K: Subglottic hemangiomas in infants. *J Otolaryngol* 15:119–123, 1986.

53. McCaffrey TV, Cortese DA: Neodymium:YAG laser treatment of subglottic hemangioma. *Otolaryngol Head Neck Surg* 94:382–384, 1986.

54. Parkin JL, Dixon JA: Argon laser treatment of head and neck vascular lesions. *Otolaryngol Head Neck Surg* 93:211–216, 1985.

55. Choa DI, Smith MCF, Evans JNG, et al: Subglottic haemangioma in children. *J Laryngol Otol* 100:447–454, 1986.

56. Duncavage JA, Ossoff RH, Toohill RJ: Carbon dioxide laser management of laryngeal stenosis. *Ann Otol Rhinol Laryngol* 94:565–569, 1985.

57. McGee KC, Nagle JW, Toohill RJ: CO_2 laser repair of subglottic and upper tracheal stenosis. *Otolaryngol Head Neck Surg* 89:92–95, 1981.

58. Mayer T, Matlak ME, Dixon J, et al: Experimental subglottic stenosis: histopathologic and bronchoscopic comparison of electrosurgical, cryosurgical, and laser resection. *J Pediatr Surg* 15:944–952, 1980.

59. Shapshay SM, Beamis JF Jr, Hybels RL: Endoscopic treatment of subglottic and tracheal stenosis by radial laser excision and dilation. *Ann Otol Rhinol Laryngol* 96:661–664, 1987.

60. Friedman EM, Healy GB, McGill TJI: Carbon dioxide laser management of subglottic and tracheal stenosis. *Otolaryngol Clin North Am* 16:871–877, 1983.

61. Dedo HH, Sooy CD: Endoscopic laser repair of posterior glottic, subglottic and tracheal stenosis by division or micro-trapdoor flap. *Laryngoscope* 94:445–450, 1984.

62. Parker, DA, Das Gupta AR: An endoscopic Silastic keel for anterior glottic webs. *J Laryngol Otol* 101:1055–1061, 1987.

63. McGuirt WF, Salmon J, Blalock D: Normal speech for patients with laryngeal webs: an achievable goal. *Laryngoscope* 94:1176–1179, 1984.

64. Strong MS, Healy GB, Vaughan CW, et al: Endoscopic management of laryngeal stenosis. *Otolaryngol Clin North Am* 12:797–805, 1979.

65. Simpson GT, Strong MS, Healy GB, et al: Predictive factors of success or failure in the endoscopic management of laryngeal and tracheal stenosis. *Ann Otol Rhinol Laryngol* 91:384–388, 1982.

66. Holinger LD: Treatment of severe subglottic stenosis without tracheotomy: a preliminary report. *Ann Otol Rhinol Laryngol* 91:407–412, 1982.

67. Duncavage JA, Piazza LS, Ossoff RH: The microtrapdoor technique for the management of laryngeal stenosis. *Laryngoscope* 97:825–828, 1987.

68. Schmidt FW, Piazza LS, Chipman TJ, et al: CO_2 laser management of laryngeal stenosis. *Otolaryngol Head Neck Surg* 95:485–490, 1986.

69. Shugar JM, Som PM, Biller HF: An evaluation of the carbon dioxide laser in the treatment of traumatic laryngeal stenosis. *Laryngoscope* 92:23–26, 1982.

70. Strome M: Subglottic stenosis: therapeutic considerations. *Otolaryngol Clin North Am* 17:63–68, 1984.

71. Koufman JA, Thompson JN, Kohut RI: Endoscopic management of subglottic stenosis with the CO_2 surgical laser. *Otolaryngol Head Neck Surg* 89:215–220, 1981.

72. Livingston GL, Schild JA: Lathyrogenic agents as therapy for subglottic stenosis—a pilot study. *Otolaryngol Head Neck Surg* 97:446–451, 1987.

73. Kirchner JA, Sasaki CT: Fusion of the vocal cords following intubation and tracheostomy. *Trans Acad Ophthalmol Otolaryngol* 77:88, 1973.

74. Sasaki CT, Suzuki M, Horiuchi M, et al: The effect of tracheostomy on the laryngeal closure reflex. *Laryngoscope* 87:1428–1433, 1977.

75. Sasaki CT, Horiuchi M, Koss N: Tracheostomy-related subglottic stenosis: bacteriologic pathogenesis. *Laryngoscope* 89:857–865, 1979.

76. Strong MS: Laser excision of carcinoma of the larynx. *Laryngoscope* 85:1286–1289, 1975.

77. Shapshay SM, Ruah CB, Bohigian RK, et al: Obstructing tumors of the subglottic larynx and cervical trachea: airway management and treatment. *Ann Otol Rhinol Laryngol* 97:487–492, 1988.

78. McGuirt WF, Koufman JA: Endoscopic laser surgery: an alternative in laryngeal cancer treatment. *Arch Otolaryngol Head Neck Surg* 113:501–505, 1987.

79. Davis RK, Shapshay SM, Vaughan CW, et al: Pretreatment airway management in obstructing carcinoma of the larynx. *Otolaryngol Head Neck Surg* 89:209–214, 1981.

80. Steiner W: Experience in endoscopic laser surgery of malignant tumours of the upper aero-digestive tract. *Adv Oto Rhino Laryngol* 39:135–144, 1988.

81. Davis RK, Jako GJ, Hyams VJ, et al: The anatomic limitations of CO_2 laser cordectomy. *Laryngoscope* 92:980–984, 1982.

82. Elner Å, Fex S: Carbon dioxide laser as primary treatment of T1S and T1A tumours. *Acta Oto Laryngol Suppl* 449:135–139, 1988.

83. Ossoff RH, Sisson GA, Shapshay SM: Endoscopic management of selected early vocal cord carcinoma. *Ann Otol Rhinol Laryngol* 94:560–564, 1985.

84. Wetmore SJ, Key JM, Suen JY: Laser therapy for T1 glottic carcinoma of the larynx. *Arch Otolaryngol Head Neck Surg* 112:853–855, 1986.

85. Koufman JA: The endoscopic management of early squamous carcinoma of the vocal cord with the carbon dioxide surgical laser: clinical experience and a proposed subclassification. *Otolaryngol Head Neck Surg* 95:531–537, 1986.

86. Hirano M, Hirade Y, Kawasaki H: Vocal function following carbon dioxide laser surgery for glottic carcinoma. *Ann Otol Rhinol Laryngol* 94:232–235, 1985.

87. McGuirt WF: Laryngeal carcinoma in situ: a therapeutic dilemma. *South Med J* 80: 447–449, 1987.

88. Večerina S, Krajina Z: Phonatory function following unilateral laser cordectomy. *J Laryngol Otol* 97:1139–1144, 1983.

89. Young JR: Laser surgery for T1 glottic carcinoma—the argument against. *J Laryngol Otol* 97:243–246, 1983.

90. Davis RK, Shapshay SM, Strong MS, et al: Transoral partial supraglottic resection using the CO_2 laser. *Laryngoscope* 93:429–432, 1983.

91. Annyas AA, VanOverbeek JJM, Escajadillo JR, et al: CO_2 laser in malignant lesions of the larynx. *Laryngoscope* 94:836–838, 1984.

92. Nadol JB Jr: Treatment of carcinoma of the epiglottis. *Ann Otol Rhinol Laryngol* 90:442–448, 1981.

93. Keim WF, Shapiro MJ, Rosin HD: Study of post-laryngectomy stomal recurrence. *Arch Otolargyngol* 81:183–186, 1965.

94. Leuszler RW, Shapshay SM, Strong MS: Conservation surgery for laryngeal pseudosarcoma. *Otolaryngol Head Neck Surg* 92:480–484, 1984.

95. Andrews AH Jr, Caldarelli DD: Carbon dioxide laser treatment of metastatic melanoma of the trachea and bronchi. *Ann Otol Rhinol Laryngol* 90:310–311, 1981.

96. Ruff T, Bellens EE: Sarcoidosis of the larynx treated with CO_2 laser. *J Otolaryngol* 14:245–247, 1985.

97. Abramson AL, Zielinski B: Congenital laryngeal saccular cyst of the newborn. *Laryngoscope* 94:1580–1582, 1984.

98. Komisar A: Laser laryngoscopic management of internal laryngocele. *Laryngoscope* 97:368–369, 1987.

99. McIlwain JC, Shepperd HWH: Laser treatment of primary amyloidosis of the larynx. *J Laryngol Otol* 100:1079–1080, 1986.

100. Motta G, Villari G, Motta G, Jr, et al: The CO_2 laser in the laryngeal microsurgery. *Acta Oto Laryngol Suppl* 433:1–30, 1986.

101. Goldofsky E, Hirschfield LS, Abramson AL: An unusual laryngeal lesion in children: granular cell tumor. *Int J Pediatr Otorhinolaryngol* 15:263–267, 1988.

102. Seid AB, Park SM, Kearns MJ, et al: Laser division of the aryepiglottic folds for severe laryngomalacia. *Int J Pediatr Otorhinolaryngol* 10:153–158, 1985.

103. Feinstein I, Szachowicz E, Hilger P, et al: Laser therapy of dysphonia plica ventricularis. *Ann Otol Rhinol Laryngol* 96:56–57, 1987.

104. Holinger LD, Tansek KM, Tucker GF Jr: Cleft larynx with airway obstruction. *Ann Otol Rhinol Laryngol* 94:622–626, 1985.

105. Cohen SR, Thompson JW: Lymphangiomas of the larynx in infants and children. A survey of pediatric lymphangioma. *Ann Otol Rhinol Laryngol Suppl* 127:1–20, 1986.

10A
Lasers in Tracheobronchology: Malignant Disease

Praveen Mathur

According to the American Cancer Society, an estimated 150,000 cases of lung cancer were newly diagnosed in 1987, and 135,000 persons died of this disease in that same year.[1] The female death rate for bronchogenic carcinoma, which had been low, increased significantly[2,3] and continues to increase, so that lung cancer is now a leading cause of cancer deaths in women.

Many patients with lung cancer succumb to respiratory failure and infection, largely because of neoplastic obstruction of the tracheobronchial tree. Laser technology has expanded possibilities for therapeutic bronchoscopy in such patients. The therapeutic use of bronchoscopy in bronchogenic carcinoma is not a new concept. Rigid bronchoscopy has long been used in cauterizing points of hemorrhage, obtaining material for biopsy, and mechanically removing fragments of neoplasm. The flexible bronchoscope has heretofore been used mainly in diagnosis. The development of laser technology has expanded the therapeutic role of rigid bronchoscopy and has provided a therapeutic role for the flexible bronchoscope because some types of lasers can be applied through a fiberoptic cable.

The laser has two major applications in the management of patients with neoplastic lesions in the tracheobronchial tree: (1) the photoresection of benign and malignant lesions that obstruct the tracheobronchial tree, and (2) detection and photoradiation of bronchogenic carcinoma in conjunction with the use of photosensitizers.

HISTORICAL REVIEW

Strong and Jako[4] first reported the use of the CO_2 laser in head and neck surgery in 1972. It was found to be extremely useful in removing benign tumors. The first application of the laser in the tracheobronchial tree occurred in 1974,[5] after development of a coupling system for use with a rigid bronchoscope. Ossoff and Karlan[6,7] developed modifications that allowed quick coupling. The rigid bronchoscope was also modified to provide ventilation and suction evacuation of smoke.

221

Persistent shortcomings of the CO_2 laser are difficult beam alignment and clumsiness of the articulated arm. Despite these problems, the CO_2 laser has been widely applied therapeutically in lesions of the tracheobronchial tree. Its lack of a suitable means of flexible fiberoptic delivery, however, has stimulated the use of other lasers. The argon laser, a blue-green laser with a wavelength in the 488 to 515 nm range, can be transmitted through fiberoptic delivery systems. It is well absorbed by hemoglobin pigment, making it suitable for hemostasis. The argon laser has not been popular as an adjunct to therapeutic bronchoscopy, however, because tissue necrosis is less predictable than with other types and wound healing is delayed.[8]

Toty[9] and Dumon[10] reported the successful application of the neodymium yttrium aluminum–garnet (Nd:YAG) laser in the tracheobronchial tree. Like the argon laser, the Nd:YAG laser is suitable for transmission with a fiberoptic fiber and thus can be used in both flexible and rigid bronchoscopy. Its wavelength of 1060 nm is in the invisible infrared spectrum. Soft tissue penetration occurs at this wavelength. In addition, the Nd:YAG laser wavelength is highly absorbed by pigmented tissue such as hemoglobin, which makes this laser ideal for hemostasis. The Nd:YAG laser has recently gained popularity among therapeutic bronchoscopists for the palliation of obstructing tumors in the tracheobronchial tree.[11-14]

Dougherty[15] reported that hematoporphyrin derivative (HPD), a photosensitive agent, is safe, effective treatment in selected cases of early and advanced tumors of the tracheobronchial tree. Hematoporphyrin derivative is eliminated more slowly from the tumor than from normal tissues. Seventy-two hours after administration, red light produced from an argon-powered dye laser (630 nm wavelength) induces a photochemical reaction within the tumor, generating oxygen radicals and thereby causing cytotoxic injury to the neoplastic vascular stroma as well as the tumor cells themselves.

Nd:YAG LASER

Resection of Endobronchial Tumor

Bronchial malignancy involving the tracheobronchial tree tends to occlude the major airways, causing obstructive pneumonitis and hypoxia. Treatment with ionizing radiation, chemotherapy, or a combination often leads to a temporary resolution of the obstructive lesions. One alternative treatment for these patients is to use the Nd:YAG laser to photoresect the endobronchial portion of the tumor, thereby relieving obstruction of the trachea or mainstem bronchi.[16-19]

The appropriateness of the Nd:YAG laser for this application is related to its physical characteristics and the nature of its interaction with tissue. With a wavelength of 1060, it can be transmitted through a flexible fiberoptic fiber. It also scatters widely in living tissue, so that energy penetrates deeply. In laser resection, most of the tissue is destroyed by heating with resultant coagulation of cellular proteins. A smaller amount of tissue is vaporized when its water content is heated to 100°C. The extent to which the tissue is penetrated depends on its pigmentation and color as well as the amount of blood flowing to it. The higher the blood flow in proportion to volume, the greater the tissue's ability to dissipate heat. Other factors that determine the nature of the tissue interaction are the duration of exposure, the power delivered by the laser, and the spot size, which is determined mainly by the diameter of the quartz fiber that delivers laser energy.

Tissue sloughing after Nd:YAG laser treatment exceeds the amount of tissue that is visibly affected during photoresection. The tissue necrosis and coagulation effects extend deeper than the visible changes noted, and the final effect is delayed by a few days.[12] Some necrotic debris may need to be removed mechanically several days after surgery.

Preoperative Evaluation

Patients considered for laser resection of an obstructing bronchial tumor should undergo a careful prior evaluation. Chest x-ray, CT scan of the thorax, and pulmonary function studies including a flow volume loop are routinely employed. Many patients may not be suitable candidates for any of the following reasons:

The patient's demise is imminent because of a massive tumor load.

The lung beyond the tumor obstruction is nonfunctional.

Tumor has invaded the cartilage and is located near the right or left pulmonary artery.

Airway obstruction is caused by extrinsic compression from a mediastinal mass rather than an endobronchial tumor.

Owing to the nature of its tissue interaction, the Nd:YAG laser is well suited to coagulating and necrotizing obstructive tumors and thereby to assisting in their removal. This maneuver can be life-saving in obstructing lesions of the trachea. Once improvement of ventilation is achieved in well-perfused areas of the lung, symptomatic and physiological improvements are expected.

Several investigators[10-14] have proposed the following indications for use of the Nd:YAG laser:

Existing or threatening atelectasis of one or more pulmonary segments.

Hemorrhage from endobronchial tumor.

Respiratory insufficiency or marked impairment secondary to neoplastic obstruction of the trachea or mainstream bronchi.

Pronounced retention of mucus and secretions due to obstruction of the airway, resulting in pneumonia.

Severe coughing caused by an oscillating exophytic tumor.

It is important to remember that in the foregoing situations the Nd:YAG laser is used only as palliative therapy.

Postoperative Evaluation

Neither subjective evaluation nor the observation of a widening of the bronchial lumen is sufficient to establish the effectiveness of therapy. Any "last resort" therapy has a major placebo effect. Objective parameters such as radiographic improvement and improvement in ventilation, oxygenation, and pulmonary function should be measured to evaluate the success of therapy. One investigator proposes the following system of rating immediate results:[12]

Excellent: Complete removal of the bronchial obstruction, obvious improvement in objective parameters, and significant symptomatic improvement

Fair: Only partial removal of obstruction and corresponding partial objective and symptomatic improvement

Poor: Resection was not possible and little or no objective improvement is noted.

Some patients in whom objective findings do not improve nevertheless are made more comfortable when hemoptysis from bleeding neoplastic tissue is controlled by coagulation.

Using these criteria, Unger[12] found excellent results in 49% of his patients, fair results in 30%, and had poor results in 21%. Similarly, Dumon[10] showed excellent results in 47%, fair results in 40%, and poor results in 13%. Palliative effects sometimes are quite remarkable, but improvement in quality of life has always been difficult to quantify.

Partial Resection for Relief of Obstruction

Another application of Nd:YAG laser therapy in tracheobronchial neoplasia is in partial resection of a malignant lesion to relieve obstruction before definitive resection by conventional means. An example would be a patient with a pedunculated adenoid cystic carcinoma of the cervical trachea. Existing near-total airway obstruction requires urgent therapy, which can be performed bronchoscopically with the Nd:YAG laser. After immediate relief of the obstruction, definitive therapy can be carefully planned. Segmental resection of the trachea with end-to-end anastomosis can then be promptly performed at a planned time.

When benign tumors of the tracheobronchial tree are treated with the laser, the therapeutic goal is curative resection and not just palliation of obstruction. With these lesions, the Nd:YAG laser can be used to achieve coagulation and the CO_2 laser can be used as a cutting tool for excision. Tumors such as bronchial carcinoids that are entirely endobronchial can be approached bronchoscopically with the laser in an attempt at curative resection.

Equipment and Technique

Several manufacturers produce medically approved Nd:YAG lasers whose output is adjustable up to 100 W. Similarly, the length of laser pulses can be varied from 0.1 to 9.9 sec, in 0.1-sec increments. The fiberoptic guide is surrounded by a Teflon sheath in which a coaxial flow of gases cools the tip of the fiber. The Nd:YAG laser's wavelength of 1064 nm is in the invisible spectrum. An aiming beam is provided by a Xenon lamp (white light) or an HeNe laser in the range of 630 (red light).

Either a flexible or a rigid bronchoscope can be employed to deliver the laser energy. A rigid bronchoscope is preferred because larger cup forceps can be employed to facilitate debulking of a previously coagulated endobronchial tumor. Also, with the rigid bronchoscope one does need not worry about igniting the flammable coating that is present on a fiberoptic bronchoscope. Most important, should a sudden increase in airway obstruction or bleeding occur, this can be more readily bypassed and tamponaded with a rigid bronchoscope. On the other hand, the procedure can be performed more easily under local anesthesia with a flexible bronchoscope. A compromise technique is to pass a rigid bronchoscope and then to perform some of the laser application and/or excision with cup forceps through a flexible bronchoscope that is passed through the rigid scope.

The quartz fiber can be passed through the working channel of a fiberoptic bronchoscope or of the rigid bronchoscope. The laser is aimed by moving the tip of the bronchoscope and therefore simultaneously directing the flexible quartz fiber. Once the laser is aimed, the operator can activate it by means of a foot pedal. The obstructing endobronchial lesion is visualized and its location and extent noted. The aiming beam should always remain in the bronchoscopic field of vision.

The laser tip should be positioned 5 to 10 mm from the target. Because of the penetrating effects of the Nd:YAG laser, its beam should be directed parallel or tangentially to the long axis of the bronchial or tracheal lumen, not perpendicularly to the bronchial wall. Any anatomic distortion due to loss of volume or mediastinal shift should be carefully noted. Anatomic changes should be anticipated if the patient has had previous surgery and radiation therapy.

The laser should be used in a continuous mode, with pulses of 1 to 2 sec, at a power of 30 to 40 W. On large tumors, the laser should not be directed for long intervals at a single point. Laser motion over the tumor should be kept parallel to the tracheobronchial walls to avoid the "popcorn effect" that occurs with sudden vaporization and explosion of submucosal tissue. With adequate hemostasis, mechanical ablation can be safely performed with a large forceps.

Complications

Major potential complications are bronchial perforation with pneumothorax, hypoventilation during anesthesia, hypoxia, and penetration of a large blood vessel such as the pulmonary artery, with life-threatening hemorrhage. The extensive experience of Dumon,[10] Unger,[12] and McDougal,[13] has led to a reduction in the rate of complications. The danger of serious bleeding and endobronchial fire can be minimized by using a less powerful beam (30 to 40 W), a shorter pulse time (30 to 60 sec), or both. There are reports of postoperative infections with fulminant pneumonia resulting from opening an area of abscess formation into the tracheobronchial tree. Hypoxemia, hypercarbia, and arrhythmia are generally related to the anesthetic technique or dislodgment of tumor fragments.

Contraindications to Nd:YAG laser therapy include a bleeding diathesis, vascular involvement by tumor, tracheoesphageal fistula, extrinsic compression, and total bronchial obstruction that has been present for more than four to six weeks.

CARBON DIOXIDE LASER

The CO_2 laser wavelength of 10,600 nm in the invisible infrared spectrum is almost completely absorbed by most tissue. Instantaneous elevation of the intracellular temperature to 100°C vaporizes cellular water.

There are a number of advantages and disadvantages to CO_2 laser use. The depth of penetration is shallow, thus inadvertent penetration of the tracheobronchial tree is less likely. Similarly, the discrete nature of the tissue interaction with little scatter reduces the edema formed in surrounding tissue. Hemostatic effect is minimal, although small lymphatic and vascular channels are sealed. The most limiting property of the CO_2 laser is that its beam travels in a straight line and cannot be transmitted by a quartz fiber. A rigid bronchoscope with coupler must therefore be used. The CO_2 laser is absorbed by water, and the field has to be clear of secretions. In addition, its shallow penetration lengthens the time needed to eradicate a lesion, which can be cumbersome with larger tumors.

As noted by Healy, the CO_2 laser may be best used in the tracheobronchial tree for benign lesions such as tracheal stenosis or papillomatosis[20-22] (see the discussion of benign lesions).

Criteria for Use

McDougall and Cortese[13] suggest the following criteria for employing the CO_2 laser in the treatment of malignant neoplasms of the tracheobronchial tree:

The lesion should be easily visualized by the endoscopy.
The lesion should be primarily endobronchial, without major extension through cartilage into surrounding tissues.
The length of the endobronchial component is 4 cm or less.
Functional lung tissue should exist beyond the obstruction.

Equipment and Technique

A number of manufacturers provide medically approved CO_2 laser instruments that can be operated in a continuous or intermittent mode. Power settings of 15 to 30 W are employed. The articulating arm connects to a coupler that is attached to a rigid bronchoscope. After calibration of the equipment and induction of general anesthesia, the rigid ventilating bronchoscope is passed into the trachea. Ventilation is maintained via the side arm of the bronchoscope.

The rigid bronchoscope is used for examination of the lesion being treated. Some authors[23] prefer using the fiberoptic bronchoscope intermittently during the procedure to remove secretions as well as to provide a more detailed examination of the lesion.

Outcome and Conclusions

In 1976 Laforet[24] reported the first case of palliation of an obstructive pulmonary lesion. Since then, several authors[23,25-27] have reported good palliation of symptoms such as dyspnea and hemoptysis as well as relief of obstructive pneumonitis. Because of the limited hemostatic effect of the CO_2 laser, difficulty with hemorrhage from friable tumor has been noted, and electrocautery has occasionally been required to stop bleeding.

In 44 palliative procedures employing the CO_2 laser reported by Ossoff in 1984,[28] seven episodes of minor bleeding occurred and two patients died. The Nd:YAG laser was therefore recommended for management of tumors with a potential for hemorrhage, since it has a greater hemostatic effect. McElvein[27] reported the use of the CO_2 laser in 135 patients with tracheobronchial tumors. Of these patients, 100 had malignant disease. At the time of the report, 45 patients had died after an average survival of 4.3 months; 55 had survived for an average of 15.2 months.

The CO_2 laser has several disadvantages in the treatment of tracheobronchial tumors. A limited hemostatic effect is associated with the wavelength. In addition, difficulty in transmitting this wavelength through a fiberoptic fiber limits its use in the distal tracheobronchial tree. Although the CO_2 laser is more precise in its soft tissue interaction, the ease of transmission of the Nd:YAG laser through flexible fiberoptics makes it the better modality for treating more distal lesions.

The ideal situation would be to use both types concurrently: the CO_2 laser for precise removal of tissue and the Nd:YAG laser for photocoagulation. Until combined systems are readily available, each laser will play its own role in the treatment of tracheobronchial disorders. Laser therapy does not cure cancer, but it provides a patent airway.

PHOTODYNAMIC THERAPY

In photodynamic therapy, excitation of a photosensitizer by light leads to excitation of oxygen radicals and thereby to chemical destruction of cellular components. Tumor cell kill depends on the degree to which the malignant tissue selectively retains the photosensitizer and the ability to deliver light to the tissue.

Hematoporphyrin derivative (HPD) is the most commonly employed photosensitizer. Dihematoporphyrin (DME) is an alternative photosensitizer that has enhanced photodynamic cytotoxicity with fewer side effects.[29-34]

DHE fluorescence in tissue that retains the photosensitizer is also a potentially useful aspect of photodynamic therapy. Fluorescence is light emitted by an excited molecule as it returns to ground state. Detection of occult lung tumors and carcinoma in situ by fluorescence of HPD was accomplished by Profio et al[35] and Doiron.[36] The time interval administration of the photosensitizers and the use of photodynamic diagnosis and treatment varies in clinical studies. Most investigators allow 48 to 72 hours to elapse after HPD or DME administration, to allow clearance from nonneoplastic tissue.

Equipment and Technique

When using red light, sufficient energy to achieve photodynamic activity can be delivered over an extended time by a low-wattage light bulb and filter.[37] The laser delivers light more effectively by emitting an intense, collimated monochromatic light energy. An argon-pumped dye laser is often used in photodynamic therapy. The laser excites rhodamine B or Kiton red in an appropriate optical cavity to produce red laser light. This light can be tuned to specific wavelengths.

A pulsed gold vapor laser that emits at 628 nm has been used for photodynamic therapy with equal cytoxic efficacy.[38] The laser can deliver sufficient light energy to tissues previously considered inaccessible for practical application of the photodynamic technique. The optimal light energy for maximal effect is still being evaluated experimentally. A level of 50 to 300 J/cm^2 appears sufficient for tumor destruction. Lower energies (10 to 50 J/cm^2) appear acceptable for carcinoma in situ.[39,40]

Outcome and Conclusions

Debulking of large tumors within the endobronchial tree subsequent to photodynamic therapy has been unsatisfactory. Interstitial treatment of solid tumor has been accomplished, but with limited success. In general, superficial and earliest stage primary cancers are treated. Balcham[33] has treated over 100 patients with bulky obstructive lung cancer. Most of these patients presented with obstruction, and removal of tumor provided palliation but did not affect survival. The cell type and location were variable and included nonsmall cell carcinoma of the bronchus and metastatic disease. Similarly, submucosal lesions and large mucosal tumors have been treated for palliation, with varying results. All patients, after photodynamic therapy, require a "cleanup" bronchoscopy to remove necrotic debris. If residual tumor is found, endobronchial resection is preferred.

Kato[41] reported a five-year disease-free survival in a patient with early stage squamous cell lung carcinoma treated by photodynamic therapy. This same investigator has also used photodynamic techniques to convert inoperable lung cancer to operable disease.[42] Seven of the ten patients needed less extensive surgical resection. Hayata[43] reported some complete responses for squamous cell carcinoma of the lung treated with this technique. These patients remained disease free by endoscopic, cytologic, and histologic evaluation for 11 to 36 months. In high-risk patients, fluorescent detection has been helpful for location of radiologically occult lung cancer.[34]

Complications have included death by hemoptysis[32] four to five weeks after treatment. Other complications include pneumothorax, pneumonia, fever, and excessive bronchial mucosal secretions. The major toxic complication is skin photosensitivity resembling that of patients with porphyria. Patients are asked to avoid both direct and indirect sun exposure for 8 to 12 weeks after intravenous injection. Other side effects of the photosensitizers have been liver toxicity, eye photosensitivity, nausea, and vomiting. No additional toxicity appears to be caused by photodynamic therapy in patients treated with radiation therapy or chemotherapy.

It is imperative that all personnel and the patient wear protective glasses with appropriate filters to prevent retinal damage from either direct or indirect laser light.

The success of clinical trials using photodynamic therapy offers encouragement for its future use. Before accounts of patient success can be considered fully accurate, however, many aspects of the technique must be refined. New photosensitizing agents are being evaluated.[44-46] Photosensitivity in the form of severe sunburn is by far the most commonly reported complication. The logical avenues of research are toward the development of photosensitizers that allow lower dosages and more rapid clearance and elimination with less skin reaction.

The differential partitioning of cytotoxic photosensitizers between tumor cells and normal tissue is great enough in certain malignancies to render this form of therapy efficacious. No adequately controlled trials have so far assessed survival duration or duration of complete remission. Permanent incorporation of photodynamic therapy in the clinical armamentarium to be used against bronchogenic carcinoma will depend on the development of better photosensitizing agents and improved fiberoptic and laser technology for delivery of an appropriate type of light.

10B
Lasers in Tracheobronchology: Benign Disease

Edward C. Weisberger
Ellen M. Friedman

The laser can be employed to treat benign disease involving the tracheobronchial tree. As in the treatment of malignant lesions of the tracheobronchial tree, the carbon dioxide and Nd:YAG lasers have been the types of laser most commonly employed.

TRACHEAL STENOSIS

Perhaps the most common benign condition of the tracheobronchial tree that is treated using the laser is tracheal stenosis.[47-54] Tracheal stenosis may be related to an acute or subacute process that involves active granulation tissue, or it may represent a mature scar and cicatrix.

When the airway obstruction consists predominantly of granulation tissue, treatment with the laser is almost always effective so long as the inciting cause of the granulation tissue (such as a tracheotomy or endotracheal tube) can be removed.[47,55] Not uncommonly, the granulation tissue mass will be large enough to obstruct the airway but will be attached to the tracheal wall by a rather narrow pedicle. In this situation, excision with the laser is especially easy. Granulation tissue can be quite friable and may bleed on manipulation. Bleeding induced by attempts at removal may contribute to an immediate increase in airway obstruction. This is especially a hazard in the pediatric patient with a small tracheal lumen. Because of this danger, the hemostatic properties of the laser are therapeutically important.

Sometimes the only factor precluding removal of a tracheotomy tube and decannulation of the patient is a mass of granulation tissue immediately above the tracheostomy stoma. Again, this is especially the case with pediatric patients. If the patient is otherwise ready for an attempted decannulation, the granulation tissue can be removed endoscopically with the laser. After the patient has recovered from the effects of general anesthesia, decannulation can be carried out.

In patients who have had a laryngotracheoplasty associated with a four-week or longer period of airway stenting, granulation tissue is often found partially obstructing the airway at the time of stent removal. Some of these granulations will diminish spontaneously upon removal of the foreign body. Especially exuberant granulation tissue can be reduced with the laser.

In patients who have tracheal stenoses requiring sleeve resection and reanastomosis, granulation tissue can be present in association with sutures used to accomplish the reanastomosis. If these contribute to airway obstruction, they can be excised endoscopically with a laser.[56]

The treatment of established and mature stenoses of the upper airway is a more challenging clinical problem.

The likelihood of success in treating a mature tracheal stenosis is directly related to the extent of the lesion. Several authors have noted that the following circumstances portend an unfavorable outcome for the use of endoscopic laser therapy in tracheal stenosis:[52-54,57]

A circumferential lesion.

A lesion that has a vertical extent exceeding 1 cm.

A transmural lesion that involves loss of tracheal cartilaginous support, with airway collapse.

Lesions meeting these criteria often require an open surgical procedure, with segmental resection of the involved trachea and reanastomosis.

Even when an open procedure is required, however, the laser has been used in an ancillary way. The ability of the laser used endoscopically to remove granulations associated with sutures along the line of reanastomosis has already been mentioned. In addition, early investigations in which the laser's tissue-welding abilities have been used to accomplish the anastomosis suggest that a foreign body inflammatory response is less likely to occur with this technique than with conventional reanastomosis.[58]

The lasers most commonly employed in treating tracheal stenosis are the CO_2 and Nd:YAG varieties. When the stenotic lesion involves the upper portion of the trachea, a subglottiscope may be used to expose the pathologic condition. In this modified laryngoscope the proximal end is wide enough to provide binocular vision through the operating microscope. The elongated distal end, which is shaped like a bronchoscope, permits the laryngoscope to be inserted below the vocal cords into the subglottis and upper trachea. Lesions of the trachea as far inferiorly as a tracheostomy stoma can often be approached in this manner. Since the operating microscope can be employed, the CO_2 laser, with its greater precision, can be used. The availability of a microspot micromanipulator for the CO_2 laser provides a spot size of 200 to 300 μm,[59] affording an unprecedented degree of precision for endoscopic surgery on the upper airway. The microspot also allows for a greater power density; a lower wattage can be used, reducing the over-all thermal effect on surrounding normal tissues and minimizing tissue injury and scarring. For stenotic lesions of the upper trachea, the microflap trapdoor technique mentioned in Chapter 9 can often be employed. The microspot micromanipulator used with the CO_2 laser is especially well adapted for this technique. The microspot micromanipulator also has a green aiming beam that is easier to see on red-colored tissues than the helium-neon red aiming dot used with other micromanipulators.

For more distally located lesions, a rigid bronchoscope is usually employed. When the CO_2 laser is used with a bronchoscope, the availability of a laser coupler with a joystick greatly facilitates aiming this laser.[60] However, when the CO_2 laser is employed, the magnifying optics are located proximally. The ability to deliver the ND:YAG laser through a flexible fiberoptic fiber allows it to be used in conjunction with specially designed laser bronchoscopes that employ magnifying telescopic rigid fiberoptics.[61,62] This system provides greatly superior visualization of the pathologic condition. Work is proceeding to design wave guides that would allow distal delivery of the CO_2 laser so that it could be used with a ventilating bronchoscope that incorporates telescopic fiberoptics.

The rigid bronchoscope is preferred. It is metal and therefore nonflammable. The flexible fiberoptic scope has a flammable sheath,[63,64] and ignition of such a sheath has been reported.[65] The rigid scope also can dilate a stenotic segment to enlarge the airway and immediately provide improved ventilation during endoscopic treatment.[66]

Excision of stenoses of the upper airway should *not* include circumferential vaporization of the stenosis. A contracting circular scar would form reproducing the obstructing lesion as healing occurs.

In the proximal trachea, as mentioned, a micro trapdoor method of excision can be employed. Distally, radial incisions can be made in the area of stenosis followed by gentle dilatation with the rigid scope.[48] If the Nd:YAG laser is to be used, the lines along which radial incision will be accomplished may be tattooed with India ink. The tattooing increases absorption of the laser beam and improves technical precision. A plastic suction catheter serves as the "pen." With the Nd:YAG laser, the amount of laser energy employed must also be considered. This type of laser is used in the continuous mode at a beam power of 50 W. If the radiation time exceeds 1 sec (>50 J), there is a definite risk of transmural penetration of the trachea with consequent excessive tracheal injury and scarring, eventually re-creating a stenotic lesion.[67]

Endoscopic laser excision of benign obstructions of the airway is most successful when acute or subacute soft tissue granulations are involved. It is least successful when a mature circumferential scar involves the full thickness of the tracheal wall. Investigators dealing with mature stenotic lesions, have reported success rates ranging from 33 to 50%.[49] When reporting success rates it is important to follow the patient for at least six months, as gradual recurrence of the airway stenosis can occur.

OTHER BENIGN LESIONS

Tracheal involvement by papillomatosis may obstruct the upper airway. Lesions located in the subglottis and proximal trachea can be managed with the CO_2 laser, using a subglottiscope and the operating microscope. If tracheal papillomatosis recurs rapidly and is obstructive, the clinician should consider the adjunctive use of interferon therapy.[68]

Amyloidosis can involve the tracheobronchial tree in multiple sites. Sometimes these lesions are quite friable, making the use of endoscopic laser management attractive.[47,57,69] Miscellaneous lesions that have been managed endoscopically, using lasers, include broncholiths,[47] embedded foreign bodies,[55] and rhinoscleroma.[70] The coagulative properties of the Nd:YAG laser are useful in the management of hemoptysis from tracheobronchial hemorrhage associated with any of a variety of inflammatory and neoplastic lesions.[55]

BENIGN NEOPLASIA

Benign neoplasms have also been managed with the laser. Granular cell myoblastomas can obstruct the airway and occasionally involve more than one site simultaneously in the tracheobronchial tree.[71,72]

REFERENCES

Malignant Disease

1. Silverberg E: Cancer statistics. *CA* 37:2–19, 1987.
2. Doll R, Peto R: The causes of cancer: quantitative estimate of available risks of cancer in the United States today. *J Natl Cancer Inst* 66:1191–1308, 1981.
3. Beard CM, Annegers JF, Woolner LB, et al: Bronchogenic carcinomas in Olmsted County, 1935–1979. *Cancer* 55:2026–2030, 1985.
4. Strong MS, Jako GJ: Laser surgery in the larynx: early clinical experience with continuous CO_2 laser. *Ann Otol Rhinol Laryngol* 81:791–798, 1972.
5. Strong MS, Vaughan CW, Polanyi T, et al: Bronchoscopic carbon dioxide laser surgery. *Ann Otol Rhinol Laryngol* 83:769–776, 1974.
6. Ossoff RH, Karlan MS: Universal endoscopic coupler for carbon dioxide laser surgery. *Ann Otol Rhinol Laryngol* 91:608–609, 1982.
7. Ossoff RH, Karlan MS: A set of bronchoscopes for carbon dioxide laser surgery. *Otolarngol Head Neck Surg* 91:336–337, 1983.
8. Gillis TM, Strong MS, Shapshay SM, et al: Argon laser and soft tissue interaction. *Otolaryngol Head Neck Surg* 92:7–12, 1984.
9. Toty L, Personne CL, Hertzog P, et al: Utilisation d'un faisceau laser (YAG) a conducteur souple, pour le traitement endoscopique de certaines lesions tracheobronchiques. *Rev Fr Mal Respir* 7:57–60, 1979.
10. Dumon JF, Rebound E, Garbe L, et al: Treatment of tracheobronchial lesions by laser photoresection. *Chest* 81:278–289, 1982.
11. Shapshay SM, Beamis JF, Shahian DM: The use of lasers in thoracic surgery. *Chest* 87:707, 1985.
12. Unger M: Bronchoscopic utilization of the Nd:YAG laser for obstructing lesions of the trachea and bronchi. *Surg Clin North Am* 64:931–938, 1984.
13. McDougall JC, Cortese DA: Neodymium-YAG laser therapy of malignant airway obstruction: a preliminary report. *Mayo Clin Proc* 58:35–39, 1984.
14. Kvale PA, Eichenhorn MS, Radke JR, et al: YAG laser photoresection of lesions obstructing the central airways. *Chest* 87:283–288, 1985.
15. Dougherty TJ, Grindey GB, Fiel R, et al: Photoradiation therapy II, cure of animal tumors with hematoporphyrin and light. *J NCI* 55:115–121, 1975.

16. Desai SJ, Metha AC, Medendorp SV, et al: Survival experience following Nd:YAG laser photoresection for primary bronchogenic carcinoma. *Chest* 94:939–944, 1988.

17. Emslandler MP, Munteanu J, Prauer HJ, et al: Palliative endobronchial tumor resection by laser therapy. *Respiration* 51:73–79, 1987.

18. Brutinel WM, Cortese DA, McDougall JC, et al: A two-year experience with the neodymium–YAG laser in endobrachial obstruction. *Chest* 91:159–170, 1987.

19. Gelb AF, Epstein JD: Laser in treatment of lung cancer. *Chest* 86:662–666, 1984.

20. Healy GB: An experimental model for the endoscopic correction of subglottic stenosis with clinical application. *Laryngoscope* 92:1103–1115, 1982.

21. Healy GB, Fearon B, French R, et al: Treatment of subglottic hemangioma with the carbon dioxide laser. *Laryngoscope* 90:809–813, 1980.

22. Friedman EM, Healy GB, McGill TJ: Carbon dioxide laser management of subglottic and tracheal stenosis. *Otolaryngol Clin North Am* 16:871–877, 1983.

23. McElvein RB, Zorn GL: Carbon dioxide laser therapy. *Clin Chest Med* 6(2):291–295, 1985.

24. Laforet EA, Berger RL, Vaughan CW: Carcinoma obstructing the trachea: treatment by laser resection. *N Engl J Med* 294:941, 1976.

25. Andrews AH, Jr, Horowitz SL: Bronchoscopic CO_2 laser surgery. *Laser Surg Med* 1:34–35, 1980.

26. Shapshay SM, Davis RK, Vaughan CW, et al: Palliation of airway obstruction from tracheobronchial malignancy: use of the CO_2 laser bronchoscope. *Otolaryngol Head Neck Surg* 91:615–619, 1983.

27. McElvein RB, Zorn GL: Treatment of malignant disease in trachea and mainstem bronchi by carbon dioxide laser. *J Thorac Cardiovasc Surg* 86:858–863, 1983.

28. Ossoff RM, Tucker GF Jr, Duncavage JA, et al: Efficacy of bronchoscopic carbon dioxide for benign strictures of the trachea. *Am Otol Rhinol Laryngol* 96:498–501, 1985.

29. Moan J: The photochemical yield of singlet oxygen from porphyrin in difficult states of aggregation. *Photochem Photobiol* 39:445–449, 1984.

30. Kessel D, Chou TH: Tumor-localizing component of the porphyrin preparation hematoporphyrin derivative. *Cancer Res* 43:1994–1999, 1983.

31. Diamond I, Grinelli SA, McDonagh AF, et al: Photodynamic therapy of malignant tumors. *Lancet* 2:1175–1177, 1972.

32. Balchum OJ, Doiron DR, Matj AC: Photoradiation therapy of endotracheal lung cancers employing the photodynamic action of hematoporphyrin derivatives. *Laser Surg Med* 4:14–30, 1986.

33. Balchum OJ, Doiron DR: Photoradiation therapy of endobronchial lung cancer, large obstructing tumors, nonobstructing tumors and early stage bronchial cancer lesions. *Clin Chest Med* 6:255–275, 1985.

34. Cortese DA, Kinsey JH, Woolnen LB, et al: Clinical application of a new endoscopic technique for detection of in situ bronchial carcinoma. *Mayo Clin Proc* 54:635–642, 1979.

35. Profio AE, Balchum OJ: Fluorescence bronchoscopy for localization of carcinoma in situ. Presented at the Porphyrin Photoresection Workshop, Philadelphia, July 6–7, 1989.

36. Doiron DR: Photophysics of an instrumentation for porphyrin detection and activation. In Doiron DR, Gomer CJ (eds): *Porphyrin. Localization and Treatment of Tumors*. New York, Liss, 1986, pp 41–73.

37. Wilson BC, Patterson MS: The physics of photodynamic therapy. *Phys Med Biol* 31:327–360, 1986.

38. Pottier R, Trescott TG: The photochemistry and haematoporphyrin and related system. *Int T Radiat Biol* 56:421–452, 1986.

39. Benson RC Jr: Treatment of diffuse transitional cell carcinoma in situ by whole bladder hematoporphyria derivative photodynamic therapy. *J Urol* 134:675–678, 1985.

40. Dougherty TJ: An overview of the status of photoradiation therapy. In Dorion DR, Gomer CJ (eds), *Porphyrin Localization and Treatment of Tumors*. New York, Liss, 1986, pp 75–91.

41. Kato H, Konaka C, Kawaten N, et al: Five-year disease-free survival of lung cancer patients treated only by photodynamic therapy. *Chest* 90:768–770, 1986.

42. Kato H, Konaka C, Ono J, et al: Preoperative laser photodynamic therapy in combination with operation in lung cancer. *J Thorac Cardiovasc Surg* 90:420–429, 1986.

43. Hayata Y, Kato H, Amemiya R, et al: Institution of photoradiation therapy in the treatment of advanced carcinoma of trachea and bronchus. In Doiron DR, Gomer CJ (eds): *Porphyrin Localization and Treatment of Tumors*. New York, Liss, 1984, pp 759–767.

44. Kessel D, Dutton C: Photodynamic effects: porphyrin vs chlorin. *Photochem Photobiol* 40:403–405, 1984.

45. Spikes JD: Phthalocyanines as photosensitizer in biological systems and for photodynamic therapy of tumors. *Photochem Photobiol* 43:691–699, 1986.

46. Ben-Hur E, Rosenthal I: Factors affecting the photokilling of cultured Chinese hamster cells by phthalocyanines. *Radiation Res* 103:403–409, 1985.

Benign Disease

47. Kvale PA, Eichenhorn MS, Radke JR, et al: YAG laser photoresection of lesions obstructing the central airways. *Chest* 87:283–288, 1985.

48. Shapshay SM, Beamis JF Jr, Hybels RL, et al: Endoscopic treatment of subglottic and tracheal stenosis by radial laser incision and dilation. *Ann Otol Rhinol Laryngol* 96:661–664, 1987.

49. Gelb AF, Tashkin DP, Epstein JD, et al: Nd:YAG laser surgery for severe tracheal stenosis physiologically and clinically masked by severe diffuse obstructive pulmonary disease. *Chest* 91:166–169, 1987.

50. Goldberg M, Ginsberg RJ, Basiuk JP: Endobronchial carbon dioxide laser therapy. *Can J Surg* 29:180–183, 1986.

51. Benjamin B: The role of the paediatric endoscopist. *J Laryngol Otology* 100:1397–1411, 1986.

52. McGill TJ, Friedman EM, Healy GB: Laser surgery in the pediatric airway. *Otolaryngol Clin North Am* 16:865–870, 1983.

53. Friedman EM, McGill TJ, Healy GB: Carbon dioxide laser management of subglottic and tracheal stenosis. *Otolaryngol Clin North Am* 16:871–877, 1983.

54. Crockett DM, Strasnick B: Lasers in pediatric otolaryngology. *Otolaryngol Clin North Am* 22:607–619, 1989.

55. Dumon J, Reboud E, Garbe L, et al: Treatment of tracheobronchial lesions by laser photoresection. *Chest* 81:278–284, 1982.

56. Toty L, Personne C, Colchen A, et al: Bronchoscopic management of tracheal lesions using the neodymium yttrium aluminum garnet laser. *Thorax* 36:175–178, 1981.

57. Personne C, Colchen A, Leroy M, et al: Indications and technique for endoscopic laser resections in bronchoscopy. A critical analysis based upon 2,284 resections. *J Thorac Cardiovasc Surg* 91:710–715, 1986.

58. Moosdorf R, Scheld HH, Stertmann WA, et al: Laser-assisted trachea anastomoses in dogs. *Thorac Cardiovasc Surgeon* (special issue), 35:156–159, 1987.

59. Shapshay SM, Wallace KA, Kveton JF, et al: New microspot micromanipulator of CO_2 laser application in otolaryngology–head and neck surgery. *Otolaryngol Head Neck Surg* 98:179–181, 1988.

60. Ossoff RH, Duncavage JA, Gluckman JL, et al: Universal endoscopic coupler for bronchoscopic CO_2 laser surgery: a multi-institutional clinical trial. *Otolaryngol Head Neck Surg* 93:824–830, 1985.

61. Ossoff RH: Bronchoscopic laser surgery: which laser, when and why. *Otolaryngol Head Neck Surg* 94:378–381, 1986.

62. Shapshay SM, Beamis JF, MacDonald E: A new rigid bronchoscope for laser fiber application. *Otolaryngol Head Neck Surg* 96:202–204, 1987.

63. Beamis JF Jr, Shapshay SM: More about the YAG. *Chest* 87:277–278, 1985.

64. Casey KR: Preventing endotracheal fires. *Chest* 91:637, 1987.

65. Casey KR, Fairfax WR, Smith SJ, et al: Intratracheal fire ignited by the Nd:YAG laser during treatment of tracheal stenosis. *Chest* 84:295–296, 1983.

66. Dumon JF, Shapshay S, Bourcereau J, et al: Principles for safety in application of neodymium-YAG laser in bronchology. *Chest* 86:163–168, 1984.

67. Goodman RL, Hulbert WC, Ling EG: Canine tracheal injury by neodymium-YAG laser irradiation. *Chest* 91:745–748, 1987.

68. McCabe BF, Clark KF: Interferon and laryngeal papillomatosis. *Ann Otol Rhinol Laryngol* 92:2–7, 1983.

69. Breuer R, Simpson GT, Rubinow A, et al: Tracheobronchial amyloidosis: treatment by carbon dioxide laser photoresection. *Thorax* 40:870–871, 1985.

70. Williams I, Radcliffe G, Hetzel M, et al: Tracheal rhinoscleroma treated by argon laser. *Thorax* 37:638–639, 1982.

71. McLain WC III, Olsen FN, Wooldridge D, et al: Endotracheal granular cell myoblastoma. A failure of laser therapy. *Chest* 86:136–137, 1984.

72. Thaller S, Fried MP, Goodman ML: Symptomatic solitary granular cell tumor of the trachea. *Chest* 88:925–928, 1985.

SUGGESTED READINGS

Malignant Lesions

Benson RC Jr: Hematoporphyrin photosensitization and the argon dye laser. In Smith JA Jr (ed): *Lasers in Urologic Surgery*. Chicago, Year Book, 1985, pp 103–119.

Dougherty TJ, Kaufman JE, Goldfarb A, et al: Photoradiation therapy for the treatment of malignant tumors. *Cancer Res* 38:2628–2638, 1978.

Henderson BW, Dougherty TJ, Malone PB: Studies on the mechanism of tumor destruction by photoradiation therapy. In Doiron DR, Gomer CJ (eds): *Porphyrin. Localization and Treatment of Tumors*. New York, Liss, 1984, pp 601–602.

Mathews-Roth MM, Pathak MA, et al: Beta carotene therapy for erythropioetic photoporphyria and other photosensitivity disease. *Arch Dermatol* 113:1229–1232, 1977.

Ruab O: Ober die wirkung fluorezieerdev staffe auf infuroriea. *2 Biol* 19:524, 1900.

11
Palliation of Esophageal Carcinoma

Eugene Rontal
Michael Rontal
Arthur Klass

Progress in medicine and surgery has not improved the prognosis of carcinoma of the esophagus. It still remains a miserable disease. Most of the time, its course is inexorably debilitating, its prognosis dismal. Its therapeutic options are hazardous and unpleasant. In an unselected series, the 5-year cure rate was in the 5 to 6% range.[1,2] Better results in some limited series can be ascribed to preferential case selection rather than to improved cure rates in the population at risk.[3]

INCIDENCE AND PROGNOSIS

In 1983, 9000 cases of esophageal cancer were diagnosed in the United States, accounting for approximately 1% of cancers in both sexes (excluding skin and in situ tumors). The male:female ratio is 2.5:1. The disease occurs four times as often in Blacks as in Caucasians. If one excludes adenocarcinoma of the gastric cardia invading the distal esophagus—which accounts for 50% of esophageal cancers in many series—and studies only squamous cell carcinoma, then the 29% resection mortality is the highest of any routinely performed surgical procedure.[4] Factors that may be responsible for such poor results are several:

1. The esophagus is a hollow viscus and can distend without subjective awareness. Thus, dysphagia may not be sensed until at least two thirds of the circumference of the esophagus has been invaded by tumor.[5] When this happens, the disease is already stage II in the TNM classification and is generally incurable (Table 11.1).
2. The relative infrequency of the disease (3.4 per 100,000 population in the United States) renders mass screening procedures unjustified, particularly in an era of escalating health care costs and the impetus toward cost containment.

TABLE 11.1 *TNM Classification of Carcinoma of the Esophagus*

Tumor
     T1: Length less than 5 cm, nonobstructive, noncircumferential
     T2: Length greater than 5 cm, obstructive, circumferential
     T3: Extraesophageal spread
Nodal Involvement
     N0: No nodal involvement
     N1: Nodal involvement
Distant Metastases
     M0: No metastases
     M1: Distant metastases
Stage I
     T1, N0, M0
Stage II
     T2, N0, M0
Stage III
     T3 or N1 or M1

From the American Joint Committee on Cancer.

3. The delay between the onset of symptoms and diagnosis is 3 to 6 months in the United States and 7.5 months in England. Further, tumor stage and the duration of symptoms are poorly correlated—a shorter history does not confer a better prognosis.[1,6]

Surgical resection has been the time-honored treatment for cancer of the esophagus. This method provides a possible cure, accurate staging, and palliation if curative resection is not achieved. A review of surgical results based on 83,783 patients concluded that, in a population of known cancer of the esophagus, operative mortality is 29%, one-year survival is 18%, and five-year survival is 4%.[1] Such dismal results have caused some to ponder the merits of the surgical approach. Patients receiving primary radiation therapy have fared little better than those treated surgically, with a five-year survival of 6%. However, the immediate mortality, morbidity, time, and expense were less than that found with surgical treatment.[2]

ANATOMIC AND PHYSIOLOGIC CONSIDERATIONS

Normal Physiology

An understanding of the physiology, both normal and pathologic, of the esophagus explains the methods of treatment for palliation of carcinoma in this area. The act of swallowing involves the passage of food and fluid from the mouth, past the airway, into and through the esophagus, and into the stomach. To project food past the airway, the tongue and pharyngeal muscles accelerate the bolus around the epiglottis and laryngeal introitus down to the upper esophageal sphincter. The upper esophagus sphincter consists primarily of the cricopharyngeus muscle. This muscular valve of the esophagus stays closed except when food passes it. A complicated reflex neuromuscular mechanism senses the speeding bolus and times the relaxation of the cricopharyngeus muscle to permit the bolus to be deposited in the esophagus. This is a well-coordinated, active muscular action that prevents aspiration into the larynx and airway.

The 3-cm long segment of the cervical esophagus beginning with the cricopharyngeus muscle is compressed between the prevertebral muscles of the spine and the cartilaginous and laryngotracheal structures. For the swallowed bolus to pass this narrow segment, it must be forcefully propelled. Gravity is not enough to move the food bolus through this soft, unsupported segment.

Once the bolus has passed the level of the cricoid, there is little external constriction of the esophagus, which collapses. This segment of the cervical esophagus acts like the lower two thirds. In most persons, the esophageal musculature performs an active and effective stripping action. However, gravity alone will move a well-lubricated bolus down, even if the muscular wall of the esophagus does not help this passage.

Pathologic Physiology

The problems of cancerous esophageal obstruction must be viewed as a result of two factors. The obvious problem is obliteration of the lumen by tumor mass. More subtly, the loss of coordinated muscular action that overcomes anatomic and physiologic impediments to swallowing will, just as completely, prevent passage of the food bolus. Both factors must be considered in achieving resumption of oral alimentation.

In the cervical esophagus, the tumor invades the cricopharyngeus, preventing normal opening of the upper esophageal sphincter at deglutition. This is in addition to any actual obstruction of the lumen by tumor. The failure to open can be due to disruption of neurogenic reflex activity or to spastic closure of the upper esophageal sphincter by residual functioning sphincter musculature. Failure of timely opening of this segment interdicts the momentum of food bolus that is needed to overcome any resistance to passage at this level. Resistance may be due to internal closure or to external collapsing pressure as the esophagus is trapped between the laryngotracheal cartilage and the prevertebral musculature. It is also possible that the tumor infiltration of the upper esophageal sphincter stiffens the introitus to such an extent that it prevents the larynx and associated strap muscles from helping to open the introitus and the esophagus. Thus it can be seen that esophageal cancer is both an anatomic and a functional obstruction that accounts for the failure of procedures even when a well-canalized segment can be restored.

In the portion of the gullet below the upper esophageal sphincter, there is no external or internal functional mechanism to hinder the flow through the lumen. All that is needed is a rigid tube with a wide bore, which will be acted on by gravity. A tumor with its associated tissue reaction acts as the rigid wall that supports the segment. All that must be accomplished is to core a lumen.

At the upper esophageal sphincter, this simple maneuver is not enough to influence the obstruction. The lack of timely opening and the presence of external collapsing pressure defeat simple coring procedures. These factors must be considered in planning treatment. Thus lesions that are above or below the upper esophageal sphincter or extending into it can be effectively treated by the Nd:YAG or CO_2 laser. Lesions at the level of the sphincter are more difficult to treat.

Methods of Palliation

It is apparent from the foregoing that the five-year cure rate of less than 10% is the best that can be expected in an unselected population with cancer of the esophagus of all types and locations. Thus, 90% of such patients will require some type of palliation. In view of unpleasant symptoms caused by the inability to swallow saliva, food, water, and medications, no method for relief of dysphagia and obstruction has been ignored.

Ellis[7] states that palliation can be achieved surgically in nearly 85% of patients with a relatively low mortality and morbidity. Others believe that radiotherapy alone or in combination with chemotherapy provides comparable relief of dysphagia with lower morbidity and virtually no mortality. Boyce[8] recommends radiation for palliation in the majority of patients with known advanced disease. He advocates peroral dilation before and after radiation to establish and maintain luminal patency. If such methods become unacceptable to the patient, an appropriate peroral prosthesis can be inserted. With skillful insertion, one can expect a mortality as low as 2% and a perforation rate of less than 10%. Tube migration occurred in 22%, but modifications in the design of the prosthesis may lower this complication.[9] Such modifications may require that prostheses be individually fashioned rather than commercially obtained.

Others caution that prosthesis insertion is not indicated in most patients with esophageal cancer except for treatment of tracheoesophageal fistula.[10] These authors cite the higher morbidity and mortality for prosthesis insertion than for radiation therapy and emphasize the lack of data supporting superiority of the "push-through" prosthesis over radiation therapy alone or radiation therapy and bougienage. The advantage of bougienage over prosthesis insertion has not been determined, and advocates of both methods stress the need for standardized, controlled trials of this aspect of palliation.

Boyce[7] recently reviewed the role of bougienage and peroral prosthesis in palliation of advanced esophageal cancer. Pharyngostomy is mentioned only to proscribe its use. It fails to provide symptomatic relief, may cause unnecessary morbidity and mortality, and is unpleasant for the patient and family.

A more recent device for palliation of malignant strictures of the esophagus is the BICAP tumor probe.[11] A detailed review of the technique has been published by Fleischer[12] and Jensen and coworkers.[13] They conclude that both laser tumor reduction and use of the BICAP probe techniques are complementary for treatment of malignant strictures of the esophagus. Another technique that shows some promise is the use of hematoporphyrin derivative therapy, where the laser is used to destroy cancer cells that have been sensitized by a systematically administered agent (see Chapter 12). It is not clear at this time whether this will have great benefit in treatment of cancer of the esophagus.[14]

LASER PALLIATION OF ESOPHAGEAL CANCER

It is obvious that there is no single satisfactory palliative method for esophageal cancer. All of the available methods have shortcomings in terms of morbidity, mortality, and patient discomfort.

Historical Development

The use of lasers in photodestruction of bleeding and obstructing tumors of the gastrointestinal tract was a logical extension of the experience gained in controlling nontumorous bleeding lesions of the gastrointestinal tract. Numerous papers have shown lasers to be relatively safe and effective in deobstructing esophageal malignancy. Compared to the above-mentioned methods, laser palliation has a number of favorable features:

1. The procedure can generally be done with local anesthesia.
2. It does not require an operating room.
3. It may be used for recurrences after surgery or radiation.
4. It can probably be used in conjunction with other methods such as radiation and chemotherapy. The efficacy and safety of such use has not been established, but there is no theoretical contraindication.
5. Unlike radiation therapy, laser photodestruction can be used in repeated courses, conceivably on an outpatient basis, as the tumor recurs.
6. There are no systemic effects such as those associated with chemotherapy and radiation therapy.
7. Unlike radiation therapy and chemotherapy, the palliation is accomplished in a matter of days, not weeks.
8. Morbidity and mortality should be significantly lower than with any of the currently used palliative modalities.
9. Laser photodestruction can be used on tumors at all levels of the esophagus. Lesions of the cervical esophagus may be technically difficult to approach with the flexible endoscope, but modifications in technique render even such proximal lesions accessible.

The first laser device (a ruby laser) was invented in 1960 by Dr. T.H. Maiman. In 1963, McGuff and coworkers[15] reported the destruction of metastatic nodules of the liver with the ruby laser. A review of the literature published between 1963 and 1974 concerning laser applications in medicine and biology found more than 50 papers dealing with oncologic applications. In 1965, Goldman and Meyer[16] studied the transmission of laser beams to transparent rods for biomedical applications. In 1973, Nath and colleagues[17] reported the first laser endoscopy using a fiberoptic delivery system. These developments paved the way for the first transendoscopic laser coagulation in the human gastrointestinal tract. Since then, there have been worldwide investigations of the use of argon and Nd:YAG lasers in the photocoagulation of bleeding lesions of the gastrointestinal tract.

At the International Medical Laser Symposium in 1979 (Detroit, Michigan) more than 23 papers were presented pertaining to gastrointestinal laser applications. None involved gastrointestinal neoplasms, although several papers reported the use of lasers for laryngeal, tracheobronchial, and urologic tumor ablation.[18] At a similar symposium in Tokyo in 1981, the use of the Nd:YAG lasers on gastric cancers was reported. In 1982, Fleischer and Kessler[19] were the first to report use of the Nd:YAG laser for palliation of carcinoma of the esophagus. In 1985, we published our laser experience in the palliation of esophageal malignancy.[20,21]

Significance of Laser–Tissue Interactions

The theoretical basis for the application of lasers to tumor destruction can be appreciated by reviewing the principles of laser–tissue interactions (see also Chapter 2). When laser energy reaches a specific tissue, it is absorbed, reflected, scattered, and/or transmitted. When light energy is absorbed, its energy is converted to heat, which, depending on the temperatures reached, causes protein coagulation at 45 to 60°C and tissue desiccation at 90 to 100°C. Charring and vaporization are readily achieved at temperatures greater than 100°C.

The laser energy delivered to a specific tissue is a function of power, time, and surface area. The laser–tissue interaction is more complicated, since the coefficient of absorption of a specific tissue ultimately determines the amount of tissue destruction. In the control of a bleeding blood vessel, for example, one wishes to coagulate the tissue protein and produce desiccation leading to shrinkage of the perivascular tissue, producing a tourniquet effect on the bleeding vessel. This decreases linear flow and permits thermal effects to damage the vessel wall and allow thrombus to occur.

If the energy densities applied are too high, the vessel wall will be destroyed, with consequent aggravation of the bleeding. In tumor ablation, particularly when large bulky exophytic tumor is involved, volume destruction is desirable, and one can use energy densities high enough to char or vaporize. Nd:YAG laser energy, owing to its low absorption coefficient, penetrates tissues more deeply—up to 4 mm. It thus destroys a larger volume of tissue more rapidly than the continuous wave CO_2 laser. Because of the deeper penetration, however, the risk of perforation of a hollow viscus is a realistic concern. Tumor bleeding can generally be controlled with the Nd:YAG laser energy, although the large, abnormal-walled, haphazardly coursing tumor vessels may be difficult if not impossible to photocoagulate in some cases.

Because of this consideration, the experienced laser endoscopist learns to debulk no more tumor than is necessary to achieve the functional result sought. For example, in carcinomas of the cardia of the stomach obstructing the distal esophagus, the goal should be to establish a conduit through the tumor mass rather than to debulk large amounts of tumor in the cardia of the stomach. Attempts to go farther may provoke tumor bleeding as the necrosed tumor sloughs; such bleeding can be very difficult to control in that technically inaccessible area.

The standard continuous wave Nd:YAG laser generates 80 to 100 W. It must be water-cooled, usually from a high-flow wall source and drain. It is powered from a 230-V, 30-amp electrical power source. These water and electrical requirements perforce limit the transportability of the laser. However, several newer generation Nd:YAG laser generators have self-contained cooling systems that obviate the restriction of being tethered to a special water supply. As indicated above, the tissue damage caused by the Nd:YAG laser energy is more than the eye can see. Knowing when "enough is enough" is a matter of experience. It would be prudent for novices to do less at individual treatment sessions as they develop their learning curve.

The CO_2 laser energy is maximally absorbed by most tissues. Compared to the Nd:YAG and argon lasers, the CO_2 laser has an absorption coefficient in water of 778 in comparison with 0.40 for Nd:YAG and 0.001 for argon. Available power ranges up to 100 W. Power in the range of 20 to 60 W is used in both the pump (0.05 sec) and the continuous wave modes. Marked superficial tissue absorption and consequential minimal penetration permit tissues to be vaporized with visualized precision. There is minimal thermal spread into surrounding tissues. Thus, the volume of tissue removed at surgery is the final amount affected—unlike the 3- to 4-mm zone of necrotic tissue that will slough several days after an Nd:YAG laser procedure. To reemphasize, the maximum absorption of the CO_2 laser permits vaporization cell layer by cell layer. There is no worry about extended tissue penetration. Transmural burns and immediate or delayed perforation are less likely with this laser.

The continous wave CO_2 laser has little hemostatic effect for the theoretical reasons stated above. Bleeding blood vessels greater than 0.5 mm in diameter are not usually controlled by this laser. This laser thus sacrifices hemostatic control for greater precision in tissue removal.

The continuos wave CO_2 laser is used for obstructing neoplasms of the cervical esophagus via laryngoscope, an operating bronchoscope, or specially designed esophagoscopes. Because of the technical difficulty in maintaining position of a flexible fiberscope in the pharyngoesophageal introitus, when the malignant structure is within 3 to 4 cm or at the cricopharyngeus muscle, the continuous wave CO_2 energy could be delivered via operating techniques developed for ear, nose, and throat lesions.[18,21] The laser beam is reflected off gimballed mirrors controlled by a micromanipulator. A flexible fiberoptic guide to deliver CO_2 laser energy has been developed but is not yet available for clinical use.[14,22]

Surgical Procedures

Patient Selection and Preoperative Preparation

Selection of patients for use of either the CO_2 or Nd:YAG laser in treatment of carcinoma of the esophagus is important. All patients treated in our series had stage III disease in the TNM classification. Some had recurrences after resection, with or without radiation therapy or chemotherapy. Before undergoing laser surgery, all patients have a chest x-ray, esophagogram, an upper GI series, and endoscopy with histologic diagnosis of the tumor. Appropriate clinical, laboratory, and isotope scans aid in determining the extent of the disease. Computed tomography is the best noninvasive staging tool.

In patients with greater than 10% weight loss, delaying palliative therapy to allow replenishment with parenteral nutrition does not seem to improve the prognosis. Patients with evidence of esophageal retention are maintained on a clear liquid diet for at least 1 day and then are kept fasting for 12 hours before the treatment. An intravenous line is started the night before the procedure. Most procedures are performed in the standard laser facility with premedication similar to that used for routine fiberendoscopy—topical anesthetic spray and intravenous diazepam, meperidine, and antisecretory medications. Endotracheal intubation and general anesthesia are employed when patients have proximal lesions in the cervical esophagus where dilating the tissues around the larynx and cervical esophageal introitus may be difficult. It is also important if the risk of aspiration is great or if underlying medical problems mandate control by the anesthesiologist.

Equipment and Surgical Approaches

The techniques for esophageal tumor palliation employ the transendoscopic Nd:YAG laser fiber for most lesions and the CO_2 laser through the rigid endoscopes in special situations. The argon laser is not generally used because the marked absorption of argon energy by the overlying blood reduces its efficacy and has no real advantage in terms of tissue destruction over the Nd:YAG laser in this area of therapy. The Nd:YAG laser energy is delivered through a flexible quartz fiber generally in the range of 400 to 600 μm in diameter. The quartz fiber is usually passed through a 2-mm polyethylene overtube, which not only protects the fiber but allows coaxial air, water, or CO_2 gas to flow around the fiber tip, thereby reducing the buildup of debris. Debris adhering to the fiber tip enhances the meltdown of the laser fiber, which may cause endoscopic damage.

The fiber tip is usually cut so that there is an angle of divergence of approximately 8° to 12°. This angle gives a tissue spot size of about 2 mm when the fiber tip is 2 cm away, using a standard 0.6-mm diameter fiber.

The method is recent—techniques are still evolving. Since most patients seen by the laser endoscopist have obstructing cancers of the esophagus that prevent passage of even the thinnest fiberoptic endoscope, the original technique involves directing the laser energy to the proximal margin of the malignant stricture and burrowing through the tumor from above, in a prograde fashion. An alternative technique[14] is to pass a guidewire that is placed through the instrument channel of the endoscope and positioned under direct vision through the endoscope. A tapered, solid plastic bougie with a central core (Savary-Guillard dilators) is available in graded sizes and can be passed over this guidewire. There are hydrostatic balloon dilators available that can be passed over the guidewire in a similar manner.

In many malignant strictures the lumen can be dilated before laser palliation to a diameter sufficient to permit passage of a thin endoscope (9.5 to 9.8 mm in diameter). Laser tumor ablation can then take place in a retrograde fashion. By this technique, the operator has the comfort and confidence of knowing the location of the lumen so that laser energy can be directed toward tumor paralleling the long axis of the esophagus rather than perpendicularly. This technique reduces the danger of transmural penetration and perforation of the esophageal wall. The retrograde approach requires caution in locating the lumen so that the wire does not perforate the esophagus. The spring-tip wire used with the Savary-Guillard dilators minimizes this risk, but in difficult cases, the wire should be placed with fluoroscopic guidance.

This new generation of dilators and the retrograde technique have significantly enhanced the ease and safety of the laser procedure. However, it has been reported[23] that patients who had endoscopic laser therapy performed in a prograde fashion, without prior bougie dilatation, had a longer dysphagia-free interval than patients treated by the retrograde method after bougie dilatation. The investigators suggested that in the retrograde approach, less laser energy is applied when the tumor is treated tangentially, perhaps destroying the cancer less thoroughly than by coring the tumor or burrowing through it in the prograde technique. At the present stage of knowledge, prior dilation allowing retrograde tumor ablation is technically easier and may be considered safer than the prograde approach. When feasible, most laser endoscopists will use the retrograde technique.

In treating malignant strictures of the proximal third of the esophagus with the continuous wave CO_2 laser, some type of lumen finder has been used during tumor resection.[21] Most often this was a nasogastric tube. It is very important to have a feeding tube inserted as early as possible to maintain a path for laser treatment as well as feeding. These plastic tubes do not ignite because the concentration of oxygen is not high enough to support combustion.

In our series we classified lesions as being located in the upper one third and lower two thirds of the esophagus. We selected this division because the upper one third lesions have always been regarded as responding poorly to this type of palliative treatment. Lesions of the lower two thirds of the esophagus were all T2 or T3. The length of segment of the tumor was between 5 and 10 cm. It was generally circumferential. In the cervical esophagus, length of the lesion was between 3 and 5 cm.

In treating lesions in the lower two thirds of the esophagus it is desirable to have a number of fiberendoscopes with external diameters ranging from pediatric to therapeutic. One selects the endoscope with the largest biopsy/suction capability that is applicable in the individual case. Biopsy/suction channels that range from 2.5 to 5 mm in diameter are ideal because they allow the passage of larger forceps to aid in establishing a central lumen and to remove necrotic debris. In addition, their size helps in evacuating smoke.

Safety Precautions

Occasionally, a pediatric endoscope with a nasogastric tube taped to it may be used to vent the smoke. It is important to have an external smoke exhaust system available. The potential danger of the laser plume to the operator has not yet been fully defined, but there is a high probability that such hazard does exist. The potential for infection should engender concern,[24] since aerosol material is of small enough particulate size that the standard surgical mask may not filter it out. Masks with filtration size of 0.3 μm should be worn by the operator and assistants exposed to the plume. Obviously, eye shields should be worn, in addition to specific filters for the individual laser wavelength. All individuals in the room, including the patient, must have eye shields or protective filters. One individual, usually the laser technician, should be designated as the Laser Control Officer (see Chapters 3A and 3B) to ensure that all safety precautions have been instituted before the laser is turned on. An oropharyngeal suction machine readily available to the endoscopy assistant is essential to minimize aspiration.

Operative Technique

If the lumen cannot be readily found using the flexible endoscope, a guidewire may be passed transendoscopically and its location confirmed by fluoroscopy or x-ray before proceeding. Once the location of the lumen has been assured, one can proceed with bougienage dilatation. In most cases the endoscope can then be passed over the guidewire through the malignant stricture and tumor ablation can proceed via the retrograde approach. In the unlikely event that the stricture cannot be safely dilated to a lumen large enough to permit passage of the endoscope, the earlier established method of coring the lesion from the proximal side of the malignant stricture can be used. The guidewire may be left in place to mark the lumen.

The endoscope is removed and then reinserted next to the guidewire. The Nd:YAG laser fiber is then inserted through the biopsy channel of the endoscope and, under direct vision in the prograde fashion, the Nd:YAG laser energy is directed in a circumferential fashion around the guidewire, thus coring out a central lumen as one burrows deeper and deeper through the malignant stricture. Biopsy forceps can be used to remove necrotic debris, thereby unmasking further tumor. An alternative approach might be to use a contact laser with an artificial sapphire or ceramic tip. This device permits much lower laser power settings; tissue necrosis is more superficial and there is less smoke.[25] Coagulation or vaporization tips may be applied to render the desired results.

Biopsy forceps are used to scrape away necrotic tumor and remove it, thereby gradually coring out the stricture and enlarging the lumen until the endoscope can be passed through the tumor. Laser energy is then directed in a circumferential fashion at the exophytic tumor by directing the beam along the long axis of the esophagus. The laser tip should always be in view to prevent serious damage to the endoscope. As mentioned previously, debris adhering to the laser tip should be wiped or cleansed off to minimize thermal damage to the laser tip. Thermal damage necessitates replacing the fiber. This takes only about 5 minutes, but it may occur at an inappropriate moment in a prolonged procedure.

White laser tips are provided by endoscope manufacturers upon request. They prevent meltdown of the distal end of the endoscope by reflecting Nd:YAG laser energy, which is highly absorbed by the black pigment of the standard fiberendoscope but reflected by white pigment.

The laser endoscopist and the technician must be constantly alert to "flashback," indicating fiber damage, to prevent expensive damage to the endoscope. The experienced endoscopist immediately recognizes a diminution in the expected tissue effect that can indicate occlusion or damage of the laser tip.

The average power settings range from 50 to 80 W in 0.5- to 3-second impacts with a 2-mm spot size. Lower power settings are used when the prograde technique is required to establish a lumen. Higher settings are used when the operator is confident of knowing where the lumen—and thus the wall—of the esophagus is. Longer durations can be used with a moving beam, minimizing the depth of penetration at any one site.

Longer durations or the presence of blood creates charring and vaporization, obscuring the view and requiring withdrawal of the endoscope so that carbon deposits can be cleaned off the distal viewing windows. If insertion and withdrawal is required frequently, an overtube may be placed to facilitate such repetitive maneuvers and to protect the patient's airway. Extreme caution and gentleness must be employed when inserting the endoscope or bougies to minimize the risk of instrumental perforation at the site of the transmural tumor or transmural thermal damage. Probably more perforations occur from instrumentation than from laser "burnthrough."

In lesions of the proximal third of the esophagus, a laryngoscope, a rigid bronchoscope, or a recently developed rigid esophagoscope (Richard Wolf Company, Chicago, Illinois), capable of delivering both Nd:YAG and carbon dioxide laser energies, is used. Again, the laser energy is directed around the indwelling nasogastric tube, which serves as a lumen finder.

The decision that a treatment session can be safely terminated is based on experience, clinical judgment, and the individual situation. The length of lesion, the degree of obstruction, the clinical status of the patient, the ease of the particular procedure, operator fatigue, and time limits on the use of the laser facility all must be considered. About 1.5 hours per session is the average time for most operators.

Alternate-Day Treatment

For logistical and theoretical reasons, alternate-day treatments are planned, allowing time for the patient to recover and for the damaged tissue to maximally necrose and slough. This facilitates its subsequent removal. Following each treatment, dysphagia may worsen because of tissue edema. The patient is advised of this possibility and reassured of its transiency, should it occur. Slight temperature elevation and leukocytosis often occur secondary to tumor necrosis. In the absence of clinical concern for possible perforation, ice chips or a clear liquid diet can be started 6 hours after the procedure. Hemoglobin levels are monitored and banked blood is available in the event significant tumor bleeding occurs as the necrotic tissue sloughs. The usual postoperative procedures are followed. Nursing and house staff are alerted to observe for sounds of respiratory or cardiovascular distress that might signal a complication, that is, aspiration, pneumothorax, or esophagorespiratory fistula. A similar regimen is followed for subsequent therapeutic sessions.

At the time of retreatment, the results of the previous session are assessed. Debridement of necrotic tissue is achieved by gentle passage of the endoscope through the malignant stricture. Open biopsy forceps can be used to scrape necrotic tumor from the wall and push it into the distal lumen or stomach. Such gentle maneuvers will unmask further tumor, which is then photoablated with appropriate time/power settings, as described above.

The alternate-day treatment schedule is continued until a satisfactory lumen is established, usually permitting ready passage of the endoscope (12 to 15 mm in diameter).

Postoperative Care

Over the next several days, the diet is gradually increased in consistency from clear to full liquid to the maximal consistency the patient can comfortably swallow. Further necrotic tissue sloughing will occur over the next 4 to 7 days, increasing the luminal patency.

Relatively small increases in the radius of the esophageal lumen can result in a significant improvement in the case of food passage. Poiseuille's law suggests that linear flow through a tube varies directly as the fourth power of the radius. Some patients are able to eat solid foods, others can eat foods of baby food consistency, and yet others can have full liquids only. In the absence of complications, the patient is discharged several days later. If satisfactory palliation is not obtained for a reasonably long interval (more than 4 weeks) a percutaneous endoscopic feeding tube may be placed by the push-through technique via a peel-away catheter. The more standard pull-through technique for PEG placement may be technically impossible or hazardous because of the malignant stricture. The patient thus can have nutrition maintained and medications administered via the PEG while luminal patency remains adequate for swallowing saliva. All of the patients in this experience with lesions distal to the upper third could maintain adequate luminal patency to permit swallowing of saliva. Lesions involving the cricopharyngeus are a different matter; even though the technical result may have established a lumen through a high cervical esophageal lesion, disruption of the swallowing mechanism by tumor and/or therapy may preclude satisfactory swallowing.

Results

It must be remembered that in patients with carcinoma of the esophagus, the average time from diagnosis to death is about 8 months. Although there is no evidence that improving nutrition has an effect on survival, it does have a positive effect emotionally, and therefore on the quality of the remaining life. Technical or mechanical success is defined as achieving a lumen of at least 10 to 12 mm in diameter. This occurs in more than 90% of the patients. Functional success, which may be defined as the ability to maintain oral nutrition following laser therapy, occurs in 80% of cases. The diet can be liquid, pureed, and, in some cases, soft to solid.

On the average, the duration of palliation averages 4 to 8 weeks. Repeated palliation can be undertaken on an as-needed basis if the patient seeks help before near complete obstruction occurs. Generally, three alternate-day procedures on patients with carcinomas of the distal two thirds of the esophagus were necessary to achieve satisfactory luminal patency. Complications such as bleeding, sepsis, aspiration, and tracheoesophageal fistula occur about 5% of the time. Death is a rare complication from palliative laser surgery in this area.

Tracheoesophageal fistula is seen in 10% of patients with esophageal cancer and probably develops more commonly as part of the natural history of the disease rather than as a complication of therapeutic procedures. In the event of tracheoesophageal fistula, prosthesis insertion is undertaken when technically feasible. Survival averages approximately 4 weeks in patients unable to clear their pneumonia and up to $3\frac{1}{2}$ months if the aspiration pneumonia resolves. In the cervical esophagus, results seem to be somewhat more disappointing. In a recently reported study, patients have been helped very little by treatment of obstruction at the level of the cervical esophagus.[21] If the obstruction by tumor is above or below the upper cervical esophageal sphincter, then the procedures seem to be successful. In addition, complications such as pneumothorax and perforation have developed from treatment of upper esophageal sphincter lesions.

Unfortunately, a good mechanical result with adequate luminal patency may not produce a satisfactory functional result because:

1. Odynophagia is not often helped. Extension of the tumor into periesophageal tissue and nerve plexus may cause incessant pain. Analgesics and narcotics will dull the appetite and detract from the desire to eat.
2. Tumor cachexia and anorexia persist. The liver is a common site of metastasis, and involvement of that organ further aggravates anorexia.
3. The systemic effects of concurrent chemotherapy and/or radiation therapy may further blunt the patient's appetite and strength.

CONCLUSIONS

It can be seen from this discussion that deobstruction of malignancies at all levels of the esophagus may be achieved in a reasonably safe and effective manner with the Nd:YAG and continuous wave CO_2 lasers. The goal is not prolongation of life, but palliation. This relief of the dreadful sequelae of esophageal obstruction—inability to swallow saliva, to sip water, to ingest simple nutrients—is achieved in most cases. Owing to systemic effects of carcinomatosis, the functional result may not reflect an excellent technical result, but, in experienced hands, the complications of perforation, aspiration, and perioperative death are low. In the grand scheme of things, laser palliation for malignant strictures of the esophagus is a reasonable addition to the therapeutic armamentarium.

REFERENCES

1. Earlam R, Cunha-Melo JR: Oesophageal squamous carcinoma: I. A critical review of surgery. *Br J Surg* 67:381–390, 1980.
2. Earlam R, Cunha-Melo JR: Oesophageal squamous carcinoma: II. A critical review of radiotherapy. *Br J Surg* 67:457–461, 1980.
3. Pearson JG: Radiotherapy of carcinoma of the esophagus and postcricoid region in Southeast Scotland. *Clin Radiol* 17:242–257, 1966.
4. Cancer statistics, 1983. *Cancer* 33:16, 1983.
5. Edwards DAW: Carcinoma of the esophagus and fundus. *Postgrad Med* 50:223–227, 1974.
6. Younghusband JD, Aluwihare APR: Carcinoma of the esophagus: factors influencing survival. *Br J Surg* 57:422–430, 1970.
7. Ellis H Jr: Cancer of the esophagus and cardia: role of surgery in palliation. *Postgrad Med* 75:139–148, 1984.
8. Boyce HW Jr: Palliation of advanced esophageal cancer. *Semin Oncol* 11:185–195, 1984.
9. DeHartog HA, Jager FCA, Bartelsman JFWM, et al: Palliative treatment of obstructing esophageal gastric malignancy by endoscopic positioning of a plastic prosthesis. *Gastroenterology* 77:1008–1014, 1979.
10. Graham DY, Dobbs SM, Zubler M: What is the role of prosthesis insertion in esophageal carcinoma? *Gastrointest Endosc* 29:1–5, 1983.

11. Johnston JJ, Fleischer D, Betrini J, et al. Palliative bipolar electrocoagulation of obstructing esophageal cancer. *Gastrointest Endosc* 33:349–353, 1987.

12. Fleischer D: BICAP tumor probe therapy for esophageal carcinoma: a practical guide. *Endosc Rev* 5:10–29, 1988.

13. Jensen DM, Machicacdo G, Randall G, et al: Comparison of low power YAG laser and BICAP tumor probe for palliation of esophageal cancer strictures. *Gastroenterology* 94:1263–1270, 1988.

14. Rontal M, Rontal E: Laser treatment of tracheal and endobronchial lesions. In Dent TL, Strodel WE, Turcotte JG, et al. (eds): *Surgical Endoscopy*. Chicago, Yearbook Medical Publishers, 1985, pp 391–406.

15. McGuff T, Bushnell D, Soroff H, et al: Studies of the surgical applications of laser. *Surg Forum* 13:143–145, 1963.

16. Goldman JA, Meyer R: Transmission of laser beams through various transparent rods for biomedical applications. *Nature* 205:892–894, 1965.

17. Nath G, Gorisch W, Kreitmair A, et al: Transmission of a powerful argon laser beam through a fiberoptic flexible gastroscope for operative gastroscopy. *Endoscopy* 5:213–215, 1973.

18. *Lasers in surgery and medicine:* Abstracts of papers presented at the 5th International Congress of Lasers in Medicine and Surgery. Detroit, MI, October 7–9, 1983. Abstracts 119, 120, 121, 122, 161, 249, 250, 253.

19. Fleischer D, Kessler F: Endoscopic Nd:YAG laser therapy for carcinoma of the esophagus: a new form of palliative treatment. *Gastroenterology* 85:600–606, 1983.

20. Klass A: Laser palliation of carcinoma of the esophagus. In Dent TL, Strodel WE, Turcotte JG, et al. (eds): *Surgical Endoscopy*. Chicago, Yearbook Medical Publishers, 1985, pp 85–97.

21. Rontal E, Rontal M, Jacob HJ, et al: Laser palliation for esophageal carcinoma. *Laryngoscope* 96:846–850, 1986.

22. Rontal M, Rontal E, Fuller T, et al: Flexible nontoxic fiberoptic delivery system for the carbon dioxide laser. *Ann Otol Rhinol Laryngol* 94:357–360, 1985.

23. Rutgeerts P, Vantrappen G, Broeckaert L, et al: Palliative Nd:YAG laser therapy for cancer of the esophagus and gastroesophageal junction: impact on the quality of remaining life. *Gastrointest Endosc* 34:87–90, 1988.

24. *Official Newsletter*. American Society for Laser Medicine and Surgery, 3:6, 1989.

25. Joffe SN: Artifical sapphire probe for contact photocoagulation and tissue vaporization with the neodymium:YAG laser. *Med Instrum* 19:173, 1985.

SUGGESTED READING

Beatty JD, DeBoeer G, Rider WD: Carcinoma of the esophagus: pretreatment assessment and correlation of radiation treatment parameters with survival and identification and management of radiation treatment failure. *Cancer* 43:2254–2267, 1979.

Halvorsen RA, Thompson WM: Computed tomographic evaluation of esophageal carcinoma. *Semin Oncol* 11:113–126, 1984.

Kelsen D: Chemotherapy of esophageal cancer. *Semin Oncol* 11:159–168, 1984.

Kranser N, Beard J: Laser radiation of tumors of the oesophagus and gastric cardia. *Br Med J* 288:829, 1984.

Lightdale CU, Winawer SJ: Screening, diagnosis and staging of esophageal cancer. *Semin Oncol* 11:101–112, 1984.

Moss AA, Schnyder P, Thoeni RF, et al: Esophageal carcinoma: pretherapy staging by computed tomography. *AJR* 136:1051–1056, 1981.

Picus D, Balfe DM, Koehler RE: Computed tomography in the staging of esophageal carcinoma. *Radiology* 146:436–438, 1983.

Thompson WM, Halvorsen RA, Foster WL, et al: Computed tomography for staging of esophageal and gastroesophageal cancer: a reevaluation. *AJR* 141:951–958, 1983.

Ying-K'Ai W, Kuochun H: Chinese experience in the surgical treatment of carcinoma of the esophagus. *Ann Surg* 190:361–365, 1979.

12
Photodynamic Therapy in Head and Neck Cancer

Jack L. Gluckman
Robert P. Zitsch, III

Photodynamic therapy (PDT) is a relatively new therapeutic method. It employs a photosensitizing drug that selectively localizes in tumors and, on activation by exposure to light, causes necrosis of the tumor. Like all new cancer therapies this technique has generated great enthusiasm and initially was heralded as the long-sought panacea for this most dreaded of all diseases. Time and experience have tempered this sentiment. However, it does appear to be effective in many situations, although much basic research is required before its exact role in contemporary cancer therapy can be defined. Two ingredients are necessary for this technology to be effective—the photosensitizer and the activating light.

A *photosensitizer,* by definition, is a chemical capable of absorbing light and thereby causing an intracellular molecular reaction. It has long been known that many substances have this property, including tetracycline,[1] berberine sulfate,[2] acridine orange,[3] fluorescein,[3] rhodamine,[4] and several porphyrins.[5-7] Use of such a photosensitizer in a biologic system was first described at the turn of the century by Raab,[8] who reported the effect of acridine dye on paramecium incubated and exposed to light. In 1903, Tappenier and Jesionek[9] were the first to use this process in the treatment of malignant disease. They treated skin cancers using topical eosin as a photosensitizer, together with white light as the activating light.

Of the photosensitizers, porphyrins have attracted the greatest interest because in addition to behaving as a photosensitizer, they are retained preferentially by malignant tissue and are detectable by fluorescence. In 1924, Policard[10] first reported a reddish-orange fluorescence in certain malignant tumors and attributed the phenomenon to the accumulation of endogenous porphyrins as a result of secondary infection by hemolytic bacteria. In 1942, Auler and Banzer[6] injected hematoporphyrin into experimental rats in which tumors had been implanted. He observed tumor fluorescence upon exposure to ultraviolet light. In 1948, Figge and coworkers[7] studied the uptake of porphyrins in a wide range of tumors and tissue. They demonstrated that porphyrins accumulate not only in tumors but in traumatized tissue, lymph nodes, and embryonic tissue. This was confirmed by Rasmussen-Taxdall and coworkers[11] who, however, demonstrated a selective uptake of hematoporphyrin by tumor cells.

In 1960, a new preparation called hematoporphyrin derivative (HPD) was first used by Lipson.[12] This contained a mixture of several porphyrins and caused red fluorescence in tissues exposed to violet light. Fluorescence was noted in bronchial and esophageal tumors after systemic injection of this substance.[13] Using ultraviolet light, Lipson subsequently demonstrated an 80% correlation between tumor fluorescence and biopsy-proven malignancy.[14] Tumors that failed to fluoresce were found to be submucosal or inaccessible to light exposure.

In 1966, hematoporphyrin used as a photosensitizer, together with light from a xenon lamp, was noted to have a therapeutic effect when Lipson and colleagues[15] reported that partial tumor destruction followed use of the light to illuminate an ulcerating breast cancer. Since that time numerous animal experiments have confirmed the tumoricidal effect of this treatment.[16-18] Because of dissatisfaction with hematoporphyrin, some work has commenced using other photosensitizers, although this remains mostly at a basic research level.

DRUGS

Hematoporphyrin Derivative (HPD), Dihematoporphyrin Ether (DHE)

Hematoporphyrin derivative (HPD) is a mixture of several porphyrins derived from hemoglobin. Some known components of HPD, that is, hematoporphyrin (HP), hydroxyethylvinyldeuteroporphyrin (HVD), and protoporphyrin (PROTO), have been shown not to be effective tumor photosensitizers, and much activity was devoted to isolating the active ingredient.[19-22] In 1981, Dougherty and colleagues[23] discovered the active photosensitizing component to be bis-1-[8-(1-hydroxyethyl) deuteroporphyrin-3-yl] ethyl ether (Fig. 12.1) by using high-performance liquid chromatography, gel exclusion chromatography, and nuclear magnetic resonance spectroscopy. This substance, which is now known as dihematoporphyrin ether (DHE), is composed 45% of hematoporphyrin. It reached equivalent tissue levels at half the dosage of HPD and caused significantly less skin photosensitivity. DHE, therefore, has become the preferred hematoporphyrin derivitive for both diagnostic and therapeutic purposes.

Although not ideal, DHE appears to fulfill many of the criteria for a satisfactory photosensitizer for use in the diagnosis and treatment of malignant disease in humans, for example: (1) absence of any systemic toxicity, (2) activation by light at wavelengths that are transmitted by human tissue, and (3) concentration in malignant tissue generally at a higher level than in surrounding tissue.

Absence of Systemic Toxicity

In both animals and humans HPD was found to be nontoxic, apart from generalized temporary skin photosensitivity on exposure to light.[15,24] The purified form, DHE, causes even less skin photosensitivity.

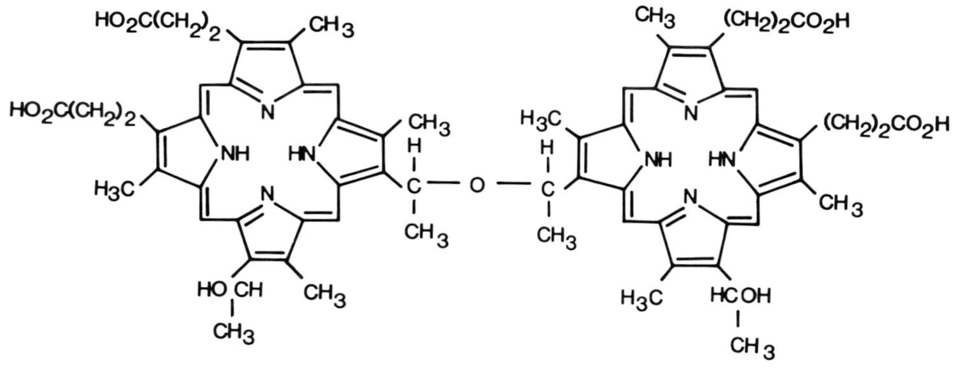

Bis −1− [8−(1−hydroxyethyl) deuteroporphyrin−3−yl] ethyl ether

Figure 12.1. Structure of dihematoporphyrin ether (DHE).

Light Activation

When tissue containing DHE is exposed to light, the resultant photochemical reaction causes cell necrosis. The degree of necrosis depends on the light penetration through tissue. In general, the longer the light wavelength, the greater the tissue penetration.

Although DHE can be excited by absorption of light over several wavelengths, the greatest absorption unfortunately occurs at around 400 nm, with smaller peaks at 500, 540, 580, and 630 nm (Fig. 12.2). Light at 400 nm would thus appear ideal, but it will only penetrate up to 1 mm and therefore it is not practical for use as an activator for photodynamic therapy. Light at 630 nm represents the best available wavelength because it allows tissue penetration of 5 to 20 mm.[25,26]

Tissue Uptake

Initially, DHE was thought to be selectively taken up by neoplastic tissue[6,7,15,24,27,28]; however, it is now recognized to be taken up by all tissues, particularly liver, spleen, kidney, lung, skin, and muscle.[29] The serum half-life following injection is 3 hours, and during this period the hematoporphyrin is evenly distributed throughout the stroma and parenchyma of the normal tissue. Once the serum level begins to fall, normal parenchymal cells and stroma begin to clear hematoporphyrin, though it is retained in the macrophage cell system and the cells of the reticuloendothelial system for longer periods.

The retention in tumor, however, remains relatively high for several days. The reason for preferential retention in tumors is not clear. Bugelski and associates[30] theorized that tumors have a high vascular permeability with an inefficient lymphatic clearance. Therefore, protein-bound substances such as DHE are trapped by these tumors. The concentration in tumor is always higher than in muscle and skin. Concentration in liver, kidney, and spleen, however, is at all times higher than in tumor. This is because of uptake by reticuloendothelial cells, which include macrophages, mast cells, and liver Kupfer cells.

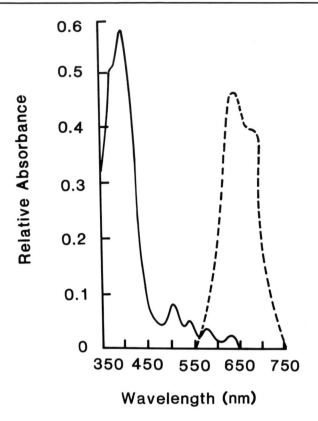

Figure 12.2. Absorption spectrum (*solid line*) and red fluorescence spectrum (*dotted line*) of HPD.

Tumors appear to concentrate HPD predominantly in the vascular stroma with the ratio of stroma to tumor cells being approximately 5:1[30] (Fig. 12.3). After 5 to 7 days, tumor cells demonstrate reduced amounts of hematoporphyrin, whereas the stroma continues to demonstrate high levels.

Rhodamine-123

Another photosensitizing agent undergoing comprehensive evaluation is rhodamine-123, more specifically designated methyl-O-(6-amino-3'-imino-3H-xanthen-9-yl) benzoate monohydrochloride. It is a cationic, lipophilic mitochrondrial dye with a maximal light absorption at a wavelength of 511 nm. Rhodamine-123 is a single member of a group of rhodamine compounds that have been used in the past as histologic stains. Certain members of this group, including rhodamine-123, are selectively concentrated in the mitochondria of cells. The selective uptake and fluorescent characteristics of rhodamine-123 form a combination of physical properties that have been employed to localize mitochondria in living cells.[31]

Figure 12.3. Fluorescence microscopy of spontaneous murine mammary tumor demonstrating DHE in tumor capsule.

In 1982, Summerhayes and colleagues[32] first demonstrated that rhodamine-123 is taken up and retained differently by normal cells and tumor cells. Certain carcinomas were observed to accumulate more rhodamine-123 and to retain it for longer periods than do most normal cells. A clear reason for this differential in uptake and retention, however, has not yet been elucidated.

The first in vivo investigations of the potential use of rhodamine-123 for cancer chemotherapy were published in 1983,[33] with the selective uptake by tumor cells providing the basis for these investigations. It was shown that, in nonlethal doses, rhodamine-123 exhibited significant and measurable antitumor activity in mice. Further toxicity studies demonstrated that the concentrations necessary to produce antitumor effects were also cytotoxic for normal fibroblasts.[34] Therefore, the role of rhodamine-123 strictly as a cancer chemotherapeutic agent appears to be limited.

More promising, however, is the potential of rhodamine-123 as a photosensitizer of tumor cells. The first such use, in combination with the argon laser, was reported in 1986.[35] The argon laser's energy wavelength of 514.5 nm permits it to be used to destroy rhodamine-sensitized tumor cells.[34]

These successful in vitro studies have led to further in vivo investigations of the tumoricidal effects of rhodamine-123 photodynamic therapy. Castro and coworkers[4] demonstrated complete eradication without regrowth of human squamous cell carcinoma transplanted to nude mice by using rhodamine-123 photodynamic therapy. The effect occurred with a nontoxic dosage (1 mg/ml) of the photosensitizer at temperatures as low as 36°C.

Several features of this form of photodynamic therapy make it appealing for future use in humans. The effectiveness of permanent tumor eradication in the animal model is remarkable. The results seem to be dependent purely on a photochemical reaction, since they are achieved at nontoxic doses of rhodamine-123 at normal temperatures. Furthermore, no known phototoxicity reactions are commonly observed as with hematoporphyrins. Further studies will be necessary, however, before its use for the treatment of human malignancy can be evaluated.

Other Photosensitizers

The early clinical successes achieved with the hematoporphyrins have stimulated a search for additional photosensitizers. Other promising photochemosensitizers with a potential for clinical use are sulfonated metallophthalocyanines, diaziquone, berberine, *N,N'-bis*-(2-ethyl-1,3-dioxolane)kryptocyanine (EDKC), Nile blue A (NBA), tetra-(4-sulfonatophenyl)porphine (TPPS), silicon naphthalocyanine, hypocrellin A, and prophycenes.

Metals that have been complexed to form sulfonated metallophthalocyanines possessing photochemosensitizing characteristics are zinc, gallium, cerium, and aluminum.[36,37] Each of these seems to exhibit preferential uptake by certain malignancies in rodent studies, leading to selective necrosis of the tumors when exposed to energy from an argon dye laser.

Another compound that has been intensively investigated recently is TPPS. This agent has been used topically to sensitize neoplastic skin lesions in patients, followed by treatment with an argon-pumped dye laser. Patients treated in this fashion had an overall cure rate of 76%.[38] However, other animal studies with the agent suggest a lack of specificity for tumor tissue, prompting the authors to recommend caution.[39]

Nile blue A is a cationic dye that exhibits selective localization in experimetnal tumors in mice.[40] Systemically administered, NBA facilitates tumor necrosis when melanoma or squamous cell carcinoma tumors in mice are irradiated with an argon-pumped dye laser.

In vitro studies with leukemia cells confirm diaziquone as another photosensitizing agent.[41] Berberine has similarly shown an inhibition of gastric cancer cell growth in vitro when irradiated with light of wavelength 320 to 450 nm.[42] Another agent with photosensitizing characteristics selective for carcinoma cells is EDKC, a cyanine dye.[43]

Finally, other compounds exist that possess physical and chemical properties suggesting a potential for clinical use. These are hypocrellin A,[44] silicon naphthalocyanine,[45] and prophycenes.[46] Scant data on the use of these agent are currently available.

None of these newer photosensitizers has so far been extensively evaluated either in animals or patients. Therefore the systemic, local, and phototoxic reactions that may occur with their use are not known. It is hoped that some of these agents will exhibit better tumor specificity, and consequently more complete and selective tumor eradication with fewer side effects, than is currently available with hematoporphyrins.

INSTRUMENTATION

Light Source

The other essential component for photodynamic therapy is the light source. In general, two types of light sources are available—lamps and lasers. Historically, lamps were the light source of choice. Raab[8] and Tappenier and Jesionek,[9] at the turn of the century, used white light for their work. Many subsequent workers used blue-violet light to fluoresce and treat tumors,[14,24] while others used red light.[15,16]

The major disadvantage of the lamp is that it emits a broad spectrum of light, which must be filtered to obtain monochromatic light. The light is noncoherent and therefore of limited brightness, so it must be focused by a system of mirrors and lenses to be effective. The only obvious advantage of a lamp as opposed to a laser is the low cost.

Lasers are the preferred source of light. Since they emit monochromatic coherent light, the power is greater and can be channeled down a single optical fiber. The fiber may then be used for surface illumination or, if necessary, can be implanted into the substance of the tumor via a needle. The laser most commonly used for therapy is the argon ion pumped dye laser.

TYPES OF LASERS USED IN PHOTODYNAMIC THERAPY

Argon Ion Pumped Dye Laser

The argon ion pumped dye laser consists of a 5- to 20-W argon ion laser that pumps a dye laser to produce light at 630 nm. The dye laser may use rhodamine B or kiton red. It converts the wavelength of the blue-green beam (454 to 514.5 nm) from the argon laser to the red-orange range (630 nm). This may produce 1 to 4 W when tuned to 630 nm, depending on the power emitted by the argon tube. The light is then coupled to single or multiple optical fibers for delivery.

Gold Vapor Laser

The gold vapor laser produces a pulsed beam at 627.8 nm, so no dye laser is required. At this time it is not clear whether this pulsed effect is advantageous, by enhancing the tumor necrosis, or deleterious, by causing damage to surrounding normal tissue. The use of pulsed lasers is being actively investigated with a view to improving the effectiveness of tumor ablation.

Since the gold vapor laser is a relatively new development, and as such is only available in a few centers, its effect on a tumor and its surrounding tissue in photodynamic therapy has not yet been established. It may be potentially more effective than the argon ion dye laser, but current research is inconclusive.[47]

Argon Laser

The argon laser, in its own right, has been used in animal experiments together with rhodamine-123 as a photosensitizer. This delivers light at 514 nm, but at higher power output of up to 10 W.[4]

DELIVERY SYSTEMS

A fiberoptic system is used to deliver the laser energy during photodynamic therapy. The best fibers are long, flexible rods made of silicone-quartz covered with a protective coating. The distal end of the optical quartz fiber may be modified in several ways to obtain optimal light delivery. These applicators direct the light to the lesion in a pattern depending on the configuration of the tip. The flat-cut applicator delivers a spot field of light and is used for surface application (Fig. 12.4A).

Lenses may be used to improve the light distribution within the spot, and diffusers may be fashioned to produce a desired distribution pattern. For example,

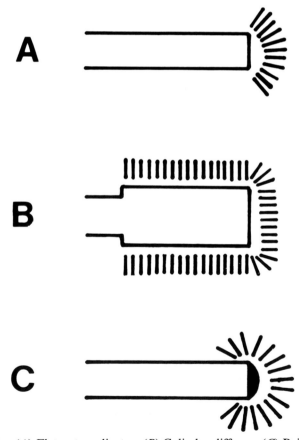

Figure 12.4. (*A*) Flat cut applicator. (*B*) Cylinder diffuser. (*C*) Point diffuser.

the cylinder diffuser is used to treat a hollow viscus such as the trachea and the esophagus (Fig. 12.4B). The point diffuser is used to illuminate spherical cavities such as the oral cavity (Fig. 12.4C).

LIGHT DOSIMETRY

Calculating the optimal amount of light to be delivered to an affected area is referred to as dosimetry. The exposure time required for tumor ablation depends on laser *power output* in watts, *dose rate* measured in W/cm^2, and *light dose* in joules/cm^2. This relationship is expressed in the following equation:

$$\text{Exposure time (seconds)} = \frac{\text{light dose (J/cm}^2)}{\text{dose rate (W/cm}^2)}.$$

At this stage in the development of this technology, the calculation of optimal light dosage is inexact and depends on many variables. As experience is gained, it is hoped that this process will become easier.

PHOTODYNAMIC THERAPY (PDT)

Although intensive research has been devoted to the technology of photodynamic therapy, some extremely fundamental problems remain unresolved. For example, neither the exact mode of action, the optimal instrumentation and drug to be used, nor the dosimetry of light required in any given patient treatment is currently understood. Because most of the animal and human experience reported so far has been gained using DHE and the argon dye-pumped laser, this form of photodynamic therapy is described here. Different drugs and different wavelengths will certainly become available as this technology evolves.

Mode of Action

Although the mode of action of photodynamic therapy is not clear, some understanding of the mechanism at a cellular and subcellular level has been acquired through numerous in vitro and in vivo animal experiments. In experimental tumors exposed to photodynamic therapy two possible macroscopic reactions may occur: The tumor may become hemorrhagic, or it may become blanched.

It is generally accepted that the mechanism that causes cells to necrose after exposure to light is a process of energy transfer. The singlet oxygen produced by the excited triplet state of the hematoporphyrin causes irreversible oxidation of some essential cellular components.[48] This reaction requires oxygen, although there may be a nonoxygen-dependent process that may also result in cell necrosis.[49]

Another possible mechanism of tumor necrosis is ischemia secondary to an effect on tumor vasculature. It has been demonstrated in animal tumors that blood flow becomes sluggish after photodynamic therapy; the red cells coagulate, and ultimately the vessels may rupture.[30] Exactly why the tumor vasculature is damaged is unknown, but, as had already been demonstrated, the highest uptake of HPD and DHE is in the vascular stroma. The tumor cell necrosis may therefore result from ischemia or from a direct cytotoxic effect.

There is a striking similarity between the effects produced by photodynamic therapy and those produced by hyperthermia. However, at the lower power produced by the laser, thermal damage does not appear to be a factor. In animal work, both the cure rate and depth of necrosis can be enhanced by combining heat with photodynamic therapy.[50]

TECHNIQUE

There are two basic approaches to the administration of photodynamic therapy: surface illumination and interstitial implantation. At this stage in the development of PDT technology, not even the most rudimentary aspects of the ideal therapy have been clearly determined. We use the following regimen.

The drug of choice, DHE (2.0 mg/kg body wt), is given intravenously 72 hours before therapy. It is administered by intravenous piggyback with 5% dextrose water. The infusion is maintained for 1 hour after injection of the drug while the patient is observed for any adverse reaction. Although 72 hours remains the traditional delay before therapy to allow for clearance of the drug by normal tissue, some physicians have successfully treated patients 3 hours after administration of DHE.[51] The patient should take precautions to guard against skin photosensitivity: avoiding sunlight and bright artificial light, wearing protective clothing, and using sunscreen preparations. These measures should be continued for 4 to 6 weeks after therapy.

If the lesion to be treated is accessible, the procedure is performed without anesthesia, usually with the fiber being held in place by a mechanical holder (Fig. 12.5). If the lesion is inaccessible, surface illumination is administered through an endoscope, under general anesthesia if necessary. In treating a bulky lesion, the fiber may be implanted directly into the tumor with a 15-gauge needle. A circumferential tumor necrosis of approximately 2-cm diameter will be achieved. The size of the tumor and depth of infiltration dictate which approach to use.

THE CLINICAL APPLICATION OF PHOTODYNAMIC THERAPY

Background

The efficacy of photodynamic therapy in the treatment of cancer has long been demonstrated in both animal experiments and the clinical setting. Although little work has been done in cancer of the head and neck, the modality has been used in other areas with varied success.

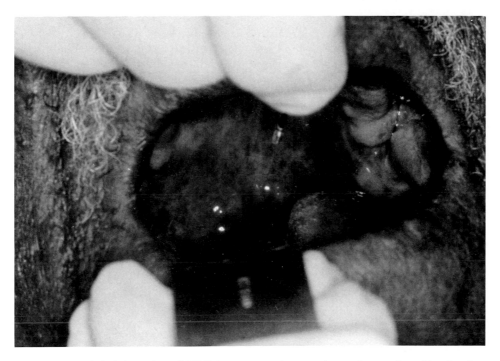

Figure 12.5. Administration of PDT in an outpatient setting, using surface illumination.

Dermatology

Basal cell cancer, squamous cell cancer, malignant melanoma, metastatic cancer, Kaposi's sarcoma, Bowen's disease, and mycosis fungoides have all been treated with PDT with encouraging results.[52-56] Careful appraisal of the reported results, however, is confusing, as there appears to be little consistency in the type or size of the tumor treated and the technique of application. The following facts are apparent.

Small superficial tumors respond extremely well even in areas previously exposed to ionizing radiation. The optimal therapeutic dosage for these superficial tumors appears to be 20 to 35 J/cm^2 administered 72 hours after injection of HPD. Higher doses appear to affect normal tissue, although the effect may be thermal effect rather than pharmacologic. Larger tumors benefited only if the tumor was localized and even then, if deeply infiltrating, were best treated with a combination of superficial and interstitial implantation of the laser. In tumors that are very large, multiple simultaneous and/or sequential implantations of fibers are necessary for debulking tumor, but this achieves very little in influencing the course of the disease. Complications other than generalized photosensitivity are rare, but pain and edema may develop in the surrounding tissues, particularly at higher doses of light. Previous ionizing radiation did not appear to be a contraindication to therapy.

Bronchology

Photodynamic therapy was first used for cancer of the bronchus in 1980, with an excellent result.[57] Since then a number of series have reported predictably varied responses. A review of 73 cases by Hayata and coworkers[58] revealed that PDT was effective in superficial lesions, but if deep invasion had occurred, it is contraindicated. Reasons for failure included an inability to assess depth of invasion accurately and an inadequate light delivery system. PDT has also been successfully used in the palliative ablation of advanced tumors obstructing a mainstream bronchus.[59] This was performed using surface illumination or, in the case of large tumors, interstitial implantation. Accumulation of secretions frequently necessitated prophylactic repeat bronchoscopy a few days after therapy to clear the necrotic debris. Severe delayed hemorrhage has also been reported.

Esophagus and Stomach

Early cancers of the esophagus and stomach are potentially curable with the application of photodynamic therapy; however, this would be a most rare scenario. Palliative ablation of larger lesions has been successfully accomplished.[60-62]

Urology

It is in the field of urology that photodynamic therapy has made its most spectacular advances. The lesions that have benefited most are diffuse carcinoma in situ or very superficial bladder cancers, particularly if they are multicentric.[51] Bladder cancer appears to concentrate dihematoporphyrin ether well, and the normal urothelium shows marked resistance to PDT damage. Larger tumors can undergo palliative ablation with some success.[63]

Gynecology

Promising results have been reported following the treatment of vaginal cancers with surface and interstitial application of PDT.[64,65] Its use in recurrent cervical, vaginal, and endometrial cancers has also been reported.[66]

Neurology

The major thrust in neurology appears to be adjuvant intraoperational therapy for residual tumor following resection.[67] A major problem has been the development of postoperative cerebral edema.

Ophthalmology

The use of PDT technology in the management of choroidal malignant melanoma has been described.[68] The preliminary nature of the reports is stressed, but the results have been encouraging. No side effects on the retina have been observed.

Head and Neck

Review of the literature devoted to the use of photodynamic therapy in cancer of the head and neck reveals that initially this modality was used predominantly in advanced cancer for palliation, particularly in those lesions that are not treatable by, or are refractory to, more conventional therapy.[69-72] Although these lesions have frequently demonstrated spectacular response, it is unrealistic to expect local therapy to influence the course of this extensive disease.

The PDT technique has, however, proved reasonably valuable as a palliative procedure. Many treatment failures with local recurrence result in swelling, pain, and discomfort, thus severely compromising the patient's quality of life. In most reported instances in which the clear intent was to produce palliation, this was successfully accomplished in a high percentage of cases. For example, in Keller and Doiron's series,[72] clearly defined palliative goals were accomplished in two thirds of the cases, particularly with regard to debulking the tumors, thereby improving swallowing, respiration, and so on. Schuller and coworkers[70] noted marked relief of pain. Although many of these responses were transient, a major potential advantage of this therapy is that it can be administered repeatedly. Occasionally, complete responses and even isolated cures were achieved. Because of the poor tissue penetration accomplished by surface illumination (maximum of 1 to 2 cm), the preferred method of administration for palliation of these large tumors is interstitial implantation with multiple fibers.

Another potential use of PDT could be the intraoperative treatment of residual disease after resection. Schuller and coworkers[70] attempted this approach; however, in two of three reported cases, the treatment was unsuccessful.

Our experience in using PDT to treat advanced recurrent head and neck cancer has been somewhat unrewarding, and for this reason a change in philosophy evolved. Our current sentiment is that the true role of PDT in head and neck cancer is in the management of superficial mucosal and cutaneous cancers.[73,74]

Rationale for the Use of PDT for Treatment of Early Cancers

For the following reasons, photodynamic therapy may represent the ideal method of treating superficial cancer of the mucosa of the upper aerodigestive tract.

1. The anatomy of the upper aerodigestive tract frequently allows adequate visualization of the lesion but renders adequate endoscopic excision or ablation cumbersome and difficult. A technique that requires only visualization and "no-touch" ablation would be potentially a vast improvement over more conventional means.

2. Theoretically, because of the selective uptake of the drug and therefore selective necrosis of the tumor, the anxiety regarding frozen section control would be rendered unnecessary, provided complete exposure to the lesion can be achieved.

3. In most circumstances, this procedure requires no anesthesia and can be performed in an office setting. In certain situations, general anesthesia may be necessary to achieve access to the tumor.

4. Certain lesions may preferentially be treated in this manner, that is, field cancerization with large areas of superficial premalignant and malignant change, and multicentric

malignancies. This phenomenon is well documented in the mucosa of the upper aerodigestive tract and is extremely difficult to treat.[75-77] The PDT technique allows relatively large areas to be treated with preservation of normal tissue.

5. If recurrent or persistent cancer should develop, the lesions may easily be retreated as frequently as necessary to attain ablation. This is in sharp contradistinction to other modalities, for example, radiation therapy.

Many of the above criteria are equally applicable to cutaneous malignancies, and PDT may represent the best therapy for multiple superficial lesions of the skin.

LIMITATIONS OF PHOTODYNAMIC THERAPY

There appears to be little doubt that photodynamic therapy causes tumor necrosis; however, the exact role of this therapy in contemporary head and neck cancer management remains ill-defined. The reasons for this include lack of experience with this technique as well as rather obvious limitations of the technology itself. As experience widens, it appears that large lesions do not respond satisfactorily to PDT and that the ideal lesion is the relatively superficial cancer. Unfortunately, it is impossible at this stage to predict exactly how large a tumor can be treated effectively by this method, because the tumor necrosis is dependent on numerous factors, many of which are ill-understood. These factors have to do with tumor ablation, problems of technology, and complication, each of which is in turn affected by additional considerations.

Unpredictable Tumor Ablation

The uptake of HPD (DHE) by the tumor remains unpredictable. As has already been said, the intratumoral distribution of hematoporphyrin in induced animal tumors has only recently been determined. Uptake has been demonstrated in the perivascular stroma, but it is still unclear whether the tumor cells themselves take up the hematoporphyrin. Whether or not these findings can be extrapolated to spontaneous tumors occurring in humans has not been established. In addition, it appears that anoxic necrotic tumor may not take up DHE, in which case the effectiveness of this therapy would be severely compromised. Whether or not all types of tumor take up the drug equally also remains to be determined. A further problem is that following injection of the drug the optimal time to administer the laser therapy is still not apparent, that is, we do not know when the tumor:background tissue ratio is optimal for therapy. Ongoing research may lead to the development of a more specific and effective photosensitizer.

Light penetration also affects tumor ablation. The depth of light penetration depends on a number of factors, including the wavelength of light and the instrumentation used to deliver the light. The type of laser used affects this parameter.

Effective tumor ablation also requires the ability to expose the whole field of growth to light. In the upper aerodigestive tract, the complex nature of the anatomy may render adequate exposure of the tumor to the light extremely difficult. In addition, it is often hard to differentiate on gross examination what represents benign, premalignant, and malignant change. Therefore, in dealing with extensive areas of "condemned mucosa," it is necessary to design a technique that will allow the whole area to be treated without compromising normal tissue.

Problems Related to Technology

The overall inconvenience of the technique, that is, expense, specialized instrumentation, and special training, must be weighed against the potential advantages, particularly when dealing with superficial lesions that could be treated by simpler alternative therapies. Other technical difficulties are related to the drug being used for photosensitization and to the laser itself.

Hematoporphyrin, even in its purified form, is a less than ideal photosensitizing drug in humans, with the most significant drawback being that photosensitivity may last up to 30 days. In addition, the unsatisfactory absorption spectrum and the nonspecific tissue uptake obviously impair the effectiveness of this technology.

Finally, the argon ion pumped dye laser, which is the type most commonly used in PDT, is cumbersome, temperamental, and capable only of low power output. The gold vapor laser ultimately may become the laser of choice to deliver light at this wavelength.

Complications

Complications include edema, local pain, and skin photosensitivity. *Edema* has not been a major problem in our own experience. However, if an extensive area is treated, or if too high a power is used, edema may develop. The use of high power may create a thermal effect that would predispose to edema. Great care should be taken to avoid contact between the applicator tip and the tissue, as this may also induce a thermal effect.

Local pain has not been highlighted in the literature, but it has been a constant finding in our experience. The reasons for this are obscure, but it may be due to local fat necrosis, or even tumor necrosis; in certain situations, these could cause severe complications such as marked laryngeal edema and even permanent laryngeal stenosis.

By far the most common problem, however, is *skin photosensitivity,* which may last from 4 to 6 weeks following the administration of hematoporphyrin. This reaction is usually mild and easily managed by taking appropriate precautions. Occasionally, however, it may be severe and may cause considerable discomfort (Fig. 12.6).

CONCLUSION

Photodynamic therapy has the potential to be an exciting new advance in the fight against cancer. Unfortunately, at this time little is known about even the most basic aspects of this technology. We are confident, however, that with time, PDT will find a defined role in cancer management. What exactly this role will be will depend

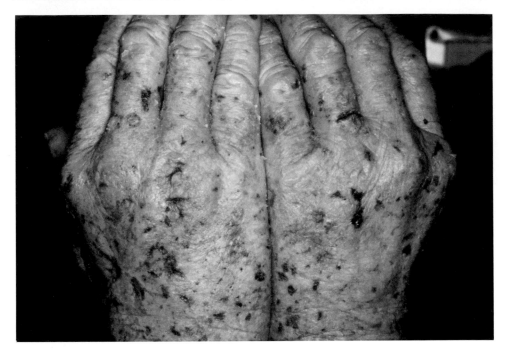

Figure 12.6. An extreme example of skin photosensitivity after exposure to 3 hours of intense sunlight.

not only on determining which tumors will ideally respond to the PDT modality but also on rendering this rather complex and expensive therapy "user friendly." This will probably require different photosensitizers, lasers, and methods of administration. We hope that multicenter trials will be instituted to aid in the evaluation of this technology.

REFERENCES

1. Rall DD, Loo TL, Lane M, et al: Appearance and persistence of fluorescent material in tumor tissue after tetracycline adminstration. *J Natl Cancer Inst* 19:79–86, 1957.
2. Mellors RC, Glassman A, Papanicolaou GN: A microfluorimetric scanning method for the detection of cancer cells in smears of exofoliated cells. *Cancer* 5:458–468, 1952.
3. Tomson SH, Emmett EA, Fox SH: Photodestruction of mouse epithelial tumors after acridine orange and argon laser. *Cancer Res* 34:3124–3127, 1974.
4. Castro DJ, Saxton ER, Fetterman H, et al: Phototherapy with argon lasers and rhodamine-123 for tumor eradication. *Otol Head Neck Surg* 98:581–588, 1988.
5. Moore GE: *Diagnosis and Localization of Brain Tumors: A Clinical and Experimental Study Employing Fluorescent and Radioactive Tracer Methods.* Springfield, IL, Charles C Thomas, 1953.
6. Auler H, Banzer G: Untersuchungen über die Rolle der Porphyrin bei geschwulstkranken Menschen und Tieren. *Z Krebsforsch* 53:65–68, 1942.

7. Figge FHJ, Weiland GS, Manganiello LOJ: Cancer detection and therapy. Affinity of neoplastic embryonic and traumatized regenerating tissues for porphyrins and metalloporphyrins. *Proc Soc Exp Biol Med* 68:640–641, 1948.

8. Raab O: Über die Wirkung fluoreszierenden Stoffe auf Infusoria. *A Biol* 39:524, 1900.

9. Tappenier H, Jesionek A: Therapeutische reosuche mit fluoreszierenden Stoffe. *Muench Med Wochenschr* 1:2042, 1903.

10. Policard A: Etudes sur les aspects offerts par des tumeurs expérimentals examinée à la lumière de Woods. *CR Soc Biol* 91:1423, 1924.

11. Rasmussen-Taxdall DS, Ward GE, Figge FH: Fluorescence of human lymphatic and cancer tissue following high doses of intravenous hematoporphyrin. *Cancer* 8:78–81, 1955.

12. Lipson RL: The photodynamic and fluorescent properties of a particular hematoporphyrin derivative and its use in tumor detection. Master's thesis, Minneapolis, University of Minnesota, 1960.

13. Lipson RL, Baldes EJ, Olsen AM: Hematoporphyrin derivative: a new aid of endoscopic detection of malignant disease. *J Thorac Cardiovasc Surg* 42:623, 1961.

14. Lipson RL, Baldes EJ, Olsen AM: A further evaluation of the use of hematoporphyrin derivative as a new aid for the endoscopic detection of malignant disease. *Dis Chest* 46:676, 1964.

15. Lipson RL, Gray MJ, Baldes EJ: Hematoporphyrin derivative for detection and management of cancer. *Proc 9th Int Cancer Cong* p 398, 1966.

16. Dougherty TJ, Grindey GB, Fiel R, et al: Photoradiation therapy. II. Cure of animal tumors with hematoporphyrin and light. *J Natl Cancer Inst* 55:115, 1975.

17. Dougherty TJ: Activated dyes as anti-tumor agents. *J Natl Cancer Inst* 52:1333–1336, 1974.

18. Diamond I, Granelli S, McDonaugh AF, et al: Photodynamic therapy of malignant tumors. *Lancet* 2:1175–1177, 1972.

19. Moan J, Evensen JF, Christensen T, et al: Chemical composition of hematoporphyrin derivatives: tumor localizing and photosensitizing properties of its main components. *Abstracts of the 10th Annual Meeting of the American Society of Photobiology, Vancouver, BC,* 1982, pp 173–174.

20. Moan J, Christensen R, Sommer S: The main photosensitizing components of hematoporphyrin derivative. *Cancer Lett* 15:161–166, 1982.

21. Kessel D: Components of hematoporphyrin derivatives and their tumor-localizing capacity. *Cancer Res* 42:1703–1706, 1982.

22. Berenbaum M, Bonnet R, Scoundes PA: In vivo biological activity of the components of hematoporphyrin derivative. *Br J Cancer* 45:571–581, 1982.

23. Dougherty TJ, Potter WR, Weishaupt KR: The structure of the active component of hematoporphyrin derivative. In Doiron D, Gomer CD (eds): *Porphyrins in Tumor Phototherapy.* New York, Plenum, 1984, pp 301–314.

24. Lipson RL, Pratt JH, Blades EJ, et al: Hematoporphyrin derivative for the detection of cervical cancer. *Obstet Gynecol* 24:78, 1964.

25. McCaughan JS, Guy JT, Hawley P, et al: Hematoporphyrin derivative and photoradiation therapy of malignant tumors. *Lasers Surg Med* 3:199–209, 1983.

26. Doiron DR, Svassand LO, Profio AE: Light dosimetry in tissue: application to photoradiation therapy. In Kessel D, Dougherty TJ (eds): *Porphyrin Photosensitization.* New York, Plenum, 1983, pp 63–76.

27. Gregorie HB, Horger EO, Ward JL, et al: Hematoporphyrin derivative fluorescence in malignant neoplasma. *Ann Surg* 167:820–827, 1968.

28. Winkelman J, Rasmussen-Taxdal DS: Quantitative determination of porphyrin uptake by tumor tissue following parenteral administration. *Bull Johns Hopkins Hosp* 107: 228–233, 1960.

29. Gomer CJ, Dougherty TJ: Determination of (3H) and (14C) hematoporphyrin derivative distribution in malignant and normal tissue. *Cancer Res* 39:146–151, 1979.

30. Bugelski PJ, Porter CW, Dougherty TJ: Autoradiographic distribution of hematoporphyrin derivative in normal and tumor tissue of the mouse. *Cancer Res* 41:4606–4612, 1981.

31. Johnson LV, Walsh ML, Chen LB: Localization of mitochondria in living cells with rhodamine-123. *Proc Natl Acad Sci USA* 77:990–994, 1980.

32. Summerhayes IC, Lampidis TJ, Bernal SD, et al: Unusual retention of rhodamine-123 by mitochondria in muscle and carcinoma cells. *Proc Natl Acad Sci USA* 79:5292–5296, 1982.

33. Bernal SC, Lampidis TJ, McIsaac RM: Anticarcinoma activity in vitro of rhodamine-123, a mitochondrial-specific dye. *Science* 222:169–172, 1983.

34. Castro DJ, Saxton RE, Fetterman HR, et al: Rhodamine-123 as a new photochemosensitizing agent with the argon laser: "non-thermal" and thermal effects on human squamous carcinoma cells in vitro. *Laryngoscope* 97:554–561, 1987.

35. Marchesini R, Melloni E, Dasdia T, et al: Photosensitizing properties of rhodamine-123 on different human tumor cell lines. *Laser Surg Med* 6(2):163, 1986.

36. VanLier JE, Brasseur M, Ali H, et al: Sulfonated metallophthalocyanines: new agents for photodynamic therapy. *Lasers Surg Med* 6:230–231, 1986 (abstract).

37. Straight RC, Spikes JD, et al: Phthalocyanine dyes as photodynamic sensitizers in vivo: localization, retention and phototoxicity in a mouse tumor model. *Photochem Photobiol* 43(suppl):63S, 1986 (abstract).

38. Sacchini V, Melloni E, Marchesini R, et al: Topical administration of tetrasodium-meso-tetraphenyl-porphinesulfonate (TPPS) and red light irradiation for the treatment of superficial neoplastic lesions. *Tumori* 73:19–23, 1987.

39. Jori G, Reddi E, Romandini P, et al: Studies of the possible utilization of tetra-(4-sulfonatophenyl)porphine in the photodynamic therapy of tumors. *Lasers Surg Med* 6:231, 1986 (abstract).

40. Oseroff AR, Ohuoha D, Ara G, et al: Selective photochemotherapy of melanoma and human squamous cell carcinoma using cationic photosensitizers. *J Invest Dermatol* 88:510, 1987 (abstract).

41. Kessel D, Thompson P: Photosensitization of leukemia L1210 cells with diaziquone. *Cancer Res* 46:5587–5588, 1986.

42. Wang MX, Huo LM, Yang HC, et al: An experimental study of the photodynamic activity of berberine in vitro of cancer cells. *J Tradit Chin Med* 6:125–127, 1986.

43. Oseroff AR, Ohuoha D, Ara G, et al: Intramitochondrial dyes allow selective in vitro photolysis of carcinoma cells. *Proc Natl Acad Sci USA* 83:9729–9733, 1986.

44. Cheng LS, Wang JZ: Photodamage in human erythrocyte membranes, induced by new photosensitizer hypocrellin A. *Shin Yen Sheng Wu Hsueh Pao* 18:89–97, 1985.

45. Firey PA, Rodgers MAJ: Photo-properties of a silicon naphthalocyanine: a potential photosensitizer for photodynamic therapy. *Photochem Photobiol* 45:535–538, 1987.

46. Aramendia PF, Redmond RW, Nonell S, et al: The photophysical properties of porphycenes: potential photodynamic therapy agents. *Photochem Photobiol* 44:555–559, 1986.

47. Bellnier DA, Lin LW, Parrish JA: Hematoporphyrin derivative and pulse laser photoradiation. In Doiron D, Gomer C (eds): *Porphyrin Localization and Treatment of Tumors.* New York, Alan R. Liss, 1984, pp 533–540.

48. Weishaupt KR, Gomer CJ, Dougherty TJ: Identification of singlet oxygen as a cytotoxic agent in photoactivation of a murine tumor. *Cancer Res* 36:2326–2329, 1976.

49. Grossweiner LI, Goyal GG, Richard P: Effects of aggregation and sensitizer binding on liposome membrane photosensitization by hematoporphyrin and hematoporphyrin derivative. *Am Soc Photobiol* p 91, 1982 (abstract).

50. Waldow SM, Henderson BW, Dougherty TJ: Potentiation of phototherapy by heat. *Lasers Surg Med* 5:83–99, 1985.

51. Benson RC: The use of hematoporphyrin derivative (HPD) in the localization and treatment of transitional cell carcinoma of the bladder. In Doiron DR, Gomer C (eds): *Porphyrin Localization and Treatment of Tumors.* New York, Alan R. Liss, 1984, pp 795–804.

52. Forbes I, Cowled A, Leong AS-Y, et al: Phototherapy of human tumors using hematoporphyrin derivative. *Med J Aust* 2:489, 1980.

53. Kennedy J: HPD photoradiation therapy for cancer at Kingston and Hamilton. In Kessel D, Dougherty TJ (eds): *Porphyrin Photosensization.* New York, Plenum, 1983, pp 53–62.

54. Tokuda Y: Primary skin cancer. In Hayata Y, Dougherty TJ (eds): *Lasers and Hematoporphyrin Derivative in Cancer.* New York, Igaku-Shoin Medical Publishers, 1983, p 88.

55. Wile AG, Dahlman A, Burns RG: Laser photoradiation therapy of cancer following hematoporphyrin sensitization. *Lasers Surg Med* 2:163, 1982.

56. Tomio L, Calzavara F, Zorat PL, et al: Photoradiation therapy for cutaneous and subcutaneous malignant tumors using hematoporphyrin. In Doiron DR, Gomer C (eds): *Porphyrin Localization and Treatment of Tumors.* New York, Alan R. Liss, 1984, pp 829–840.

57. Hayata Y, Kato H, Konaka C, et al: Fiberoptic bronchoscopic laser photoradiation for tumor localization in lung cancer. *Chest* 52:10, 1982.

58. Hayata Y, Kato H, Hememiya R, et al: Indications for photoradiation therapy in early stage lung cancer on the basis of post-PRT histological findings. In Doiron DR, Gomer C (eds): *Porphyrin Localization and Treatment of Tumors.* New York, Alan R. Liss, 1984, pp 747–758.

59. Balchum O, Doiron DR, Huth G: HPD photodynamic therapy for obstructing lung cancer. In Doiron DR, Gomer C (eds): *Porphyrin Localization and Treatment of Tumors.* New York, Alan R. Liss, 1984, pp 727–745.

60. Aida M, Hirashima T: Cancer of the esophagus. In Hayata Y, Dougherty TJ (eds): *Lasers and Hematoporphyrin Derivative in Cancer.* New York, Igaku-Shoin Medical Publishers, 1983, pp 57.

61. Aida M, Kawaguchi M: Gastric cancer. In Hayata Y, Dougherty TJ (eds): *Lasers and Hematoporphyrin Derivative in Cancer.* New York, Igaku-Shoin Medical Publishers, 1983, pp 65.

62. McCaughan JS: Photoradiation of malignant tumors presensitized with hematoporphyrin derivative. In Doiron DR, Gomer C (eds): *Porphyrin Localization and Treatment of Tumors.* New York, Alan R. Liss, 1984, pp 805–827.

63. Hiazumi H, Misaki T, Miyoshi N: Photodynamic therapy of bladder tumors. In Hayata Y, Dougherty TJ (eds): *Lasers and Hematoporphyrin Derivative in Cancer.* New York, Igaku-Shoin Medical Publishers, 1983, pp 85.

64. Ward BG, Forbes IJ, Wowled PA, et al: The treatment of vaginal recurrences of gynecologic malignancy with phototherapy following hematoporphyrin derivative treatment. *Am J Obstet Gynecol* 142(3):3562, 1982.

65. Soma H, Akiya K, Nutahara S, et al: Treatment of vaginal carcinoma with laser photoradiation following administration of hematoporphyrin derivative. Report of a case. *Ann Chir Gynaecol* 71:133, 1982.

66. Rettenmaier M, Berman M, DiSaia P, et al: Photoradiation therapy in gynecology. In Doiron DR, Gomer C (eds): *Porphyrin Localization and Treatment of Tumors*. New York, Alan R. Liss, 1984, pp 767–775.

67. McCulloch GA, Forbes IJ, Lee See K, et al: Phototherapy in malignant brain tumors. In Doiron DR, Gomer C (eds): *Porphyrin Localization and Treatment of Tumors*. New York, Alan R. Liss, 1984, pp 709–717.

68. Bruce RA: Photoradiation of choroidal malignant melanoma. In Doiron D, Gomer C (eds): *Porphyrin Localization and Treatment of Tumors*. New York, Alan R. Liss, 1984, pp 777–784.

69. Dahlman A, Wile AG, Burns RG, et al: Laser photoradiation therapy of cancer. *Cancer Res* 43:430–434, 1983.

70. Schuller DE, McCaughan JS, Rock RP: Photoradiation in head and neck cancer. *Arch Otolaryngol* 3:351–355, 1985.

71. Wile AG, Novotny J, Mason GR: Photoradiation therapy of head and neck cancer. *Am J Clin Oncol* 6:39–63, 1984.

72. Keller GS, Doiron DJ: Photodynamic therapy in otolaryngology/head and neck surgery. Presented at the course on PDT at Western Institute for Laser Treatment, October, 1984.

73. Gluckman JL, Waner M, Shumrick K, et al: Photodynamic therapy. A viable alternative to conventional therapy for early lesions of the upper aerodigestive tract. *Arch Otol Head Neck Surg* 112:949–952, 1986.

74. Gluckman JL, Weissler MC: Role of photodynamic therapy in the management of early cancers of the upper aerodigestive tract. *Laser Med Sci* 1:217–219, 1986.

75. Gluckman JL, Crissman JD, Donegan JO: Multicentric squamous cell carcinoma of the upper aerodigestive tract. *Head Neck Surg* 3:90–96, 1980.

76. Gluckman JL, Crissman JD: Survival rates in 548 patients with multiple primary neoplasms of the upper aerodigestive tract. *Laryngoscope* 93(1):71–74, 1983.

77. Gluckman JL: Synchronous multiple primaries of the upper aerodigestive system. *Arch Otolaryngol* 105:597–598, 1979.

13
Microvascular Laser Welding

Scott Shapiro
Michael C. Dalsing

The areas of interest to the head and neck surgeon in the field of microvascular laser welding revolve around the repair of nerves and vascular structures. This chapter reviews the possible benefits and shortcomings of these techniques. Comparison with the standard suturing methods provides a basis for determining whether the laser can benefit individual surgeons in their practice. Some clinical applications have been attempted, but this area should generally be considered experimental at present.

LASER-ASSISTED MICROVASCULAR ANASTOMOSIS

Artery: End-to-End

The technique of a laser-assisted microvascular anastomosis (LAMA) for arterial repair has been performed with each of the three readily available medical lasers: CO_2 (carbon dioxide), argon, and Nd:YAG (neodymium:yttrium-aluminum-garnet). In end-to-end anastomosis two to four stay sutures are placed equidistantly around the artery ends to approximate the two edges. Before laser welding, the two ends are generally approximated more closely by exerting gentle traction on sequential stay sutures. The laser energy is then used to seal the two vessel edges together to form a stable anastomosis (Fig. 13.1).

Each medical laser achieves an effective seal under different parameters. The CO_2 laser is often used in continuous mode or in 0.1-second pulses at a power level of 60 to 120 mW with a spot size of 150 to 300 μm.[1-11] The argon laser requires a power level of 300 to 800 mW with a 150- to 400-μm spot.[12-14] The Nd:YAG is used with a power output of 10 to 20 W and a spot of 0.2 to 0.3 mm.[15,16] Effective welding is indicated by a flattening of the everted edges and a slight tannish discoloration of the vessel wall when using the CO_2 and Nd:YAG

273

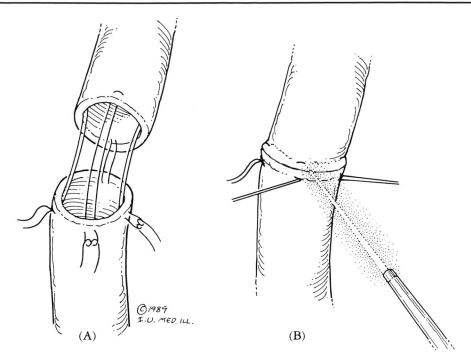

Figure 13.1. (*A*) Placement of stay sutures (2–4 in number). (*B*) Gentle traction on adjacent tied stay sutures sets edges for laser welding.

lasers. The stay sutures are usually left in place indefinitely after laser welding has been accomplished.

Several investigators have found laser welding to be more time-effective than the corresponding suture method of repair. Frazier and coworkers[1] performed end-to-end laser anastomoses in approximately 20 minutes, whereas it took them 30 minutes to complete a suture anastomosis. Two other investigators[2,3] could complete the laser-assisted repair in 5 to 6 minutes with the suture repair taking 10 to 15 minutes.

Guo and Chao[4] reported a doubling of the laser repair time when the suture method was substituted. Technical speed alone is not a prerequisite for a successful anastomosis, but a short duration may sometimes be important in reducing critical ischemia.

Maintaining a patent anastomosis is critical to tissue viability. The patency rate of 1- to 2-mm arteries repaired with a laser is statistically similar to that for the suture method of arterial anastomosis. Serure, et al. found the patency rate to be 100% for both types of repair.[2] The patency rate was 93% for both methods in the experience of Guo and Chao,[4] and was 78% and 84%, respectively, for laser and conventional methods when studied by Fried and Moll.[5] However, Frazier and coworkers[1] observed a 100% patency rate in the laser-repaired arteries, but 80% of suture repairs were stenotic or occluded after 13 weeks when studied in growing swine. Flemming and associates[3] demonstrated 90 and 97.1% patency rates for laser repair versus suture repair, which statistically favors the suture method. Although the laser method of repair has not always been found to be superior to the

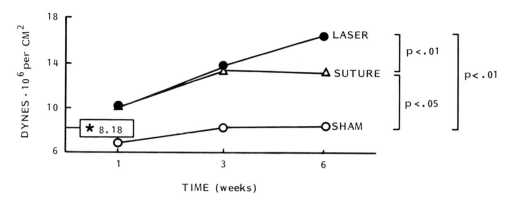

Figure 13.2. Comparison of the tensile strength of laser versus suture arterial anastomoses. (Printed with permission: Hartz RS, et al: Mechanical properties of end-to-end laser-assisted and sutured arterial anastomoses under axial loading. *Surg Forum* 36:457–459, 1985.)

suture method, it is generally quite acceptable and may be superior when continued growth of the vessel is a factor.

One of the concerns involved in using the laser as a repair tool was the question of anastomotic strength. White and Dalsing and colleagues[6] have found the laser-assisted microvascular arterial repair to be quite stable at physiologic blood pressures of 82-100 mm Hg while withstanding wall tensions of 2.47×10^5 to 2.91×10^5 dynes/cm². Extending this observation to 6 weeks, Hartz and coworkers[17] have found this repair to have tensile strength comparable and possibly superior to the conventional suture anastomosis (Fig. 13.2). Using the argon laser instead of the milliwatt CO_2, Gomes and coworkers[12] determined that the initial laser repair had a lower bursting pressure than the suture repair. Eventually, however, the laser repair was just as strong as the conventional type. Even on initial study the laser anastomosis had a bursting pressure well over 500 mm Hg, significantly higher than any normal physiologic stress. The use of a blood bond or fibrin glue sealant might improve the initial bursting strength even further.[7,8] It appears that the laser forms a secure seal that should be adequately resistant to disruption, even with severe fluctuations in blood pressure.

Histologic study of the two types of arterial anastomoses gives some insight into the effect of these methods on living tissues. Careful observation of the area of laser anastomosis suggests that the mechanism of repair involves the coagulation of adventitial and medial tissues into an amorphous glue (Fig. 13.3).[4-6,9,10,12-14,16] Whether the bond is mainly a rearrangement of collagen bonds, fibrin bonds, or fibrinogen polymerization is not yet clear. Interestingly, over time the amorphous coagulum is reabsorbed, leaving a rather normal-appearing arterial wall.[1,4,13,16] Others have found the vessel wall to be replaced with scar or to have a continued defect in the normal wall layers.[2,4-6,8,9,14,18-20] In contrast, the suture-repaired arteries initially demonstrate pressure necrosis throughout the wall where sutures have been placed. In long-term follow-up, the sutures are found to cause a foreign body

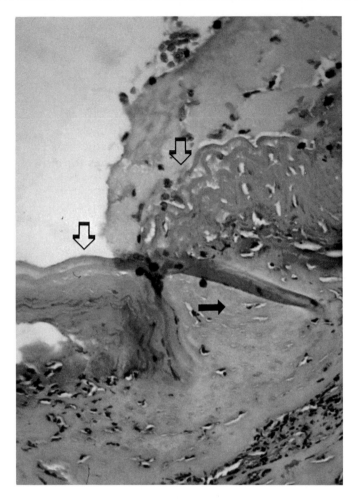

Figure 13.3. High-power photomicrograph of microvascular anastomosis using the Nd:YAG laser, which clearly demonstrates the amorphous coagulum (dark arrows) that seals the edges. Open arrows point to the luminal surface.

giant cell reaction that does not regress with time.[2,4,5,11] These tissue reactions demonstrate damage to the vessel wall, which might lead to aneurysms or detrimental hyperplasia.

The formation of an aneurysm would eventually jeopardize the vascular repair and therefore is undesirable. Aneurysm formation has been reported with microsuture arterial anastomoses with an incidence of up to 48%.[21] However, this seems an extremely high rate in view of more recent studies that compare the laser and suture methods of arterial repair.

Frazier and coworkers[1] found no aneurysms in either type of repair in the miniature swine model, nor did Fried and Moll[5] in the rat femoral artery model.

Guo and Chao,[4] studying the autotransplantation of rabbit saphenous arteries, could demonstrate no abnormal dilatation of laser-assisted anastomoses but found a 4.2% rate in the suture repairs.

Three investigative groups, also using the CO_2 laser, could find no problems with the suture repairs but did see a 6.3 to 18.6% rate of aneurysmal formation in the laser repairs.[2,11,20] Flemming and coworkers[3] discovered aneurysms in 38.3% of laser repairs and in 14.3% of conventional suture anastomoses.

Aneurysms have also been reported to occur in 8 to 20% of cases with the use of the argon or Nd:YAG lasers.[13-15,19] The precise reason for this discrepancy is not known but probably involves the precision of repair, the laser power used, and the method of handling these delicate tissues. It is imperative that before clinical use, each microvascular surgeon learn the proper techniques for a successful repair to minimize the risk of aneurysmal degeneration.

Subintimal or intimal hyperplasia seems to occur following vascular injury as one step in the process of healing. Approximately 20 years ago, Baxter and associates[22] observed that sutures damage the vessel wall, especially the internal elastic lamina, and that effective healing involves a hyperplastic response (subintimal hyperplasia). Quigley and coworkers[23] demonstrated a prohibitive effect of the laser on early intimal proliferation but could see a stimulatory effect at 6 weeks of follow-up. Studying both the suture and the laser-assisted anastomoses, McCarthy and colleagues[11] could see a six- to eight-cell hyperplastic response at 8 weeks in both types of repair. Up to 1 year later, this same group could still observe hyperplasia in both methods of anastomosis without detrimental compromise of the vessel lumen.[24] Other investigators have found the hyperplasia to be slightly worse in the conventional suture repair, with total resolution in 6 weeks.[5] Another researcher[4] found this tissue response in laser-treated vessels only in areas of severe damage. Frazier and coworkers,[1] studying the growing miniature swine, did not observe hyperplasia as a problem in the laser specimens. In summary, some degree of intimal hyperplasia may result from vascular injury, but this response is not excessive, nor is it confined to the laser-assisted arterial vascular anastomosis.

The endothelium, although initially destroyed at the site of arterial anastomosis, is quickly reestablished to cover the area of repair in both the suture and laser repairs. Reepithelialization is usually complete in 10 days to 3 weeks.[2,5,6,9-11,13,14] The thermal injury was neither beneficial nor detrimental to the process of intimal repair in the models studied.

Artery: End-to-Side

The technique of laser-assisted end-to-side microvascular anastomosis is quite similar to the end-to-end technique. Four stay sutures of small-diameter vascular suture are placed at each apex and in the center of the posterior and anterior walls. By exerting a slight amount of tension on adjacent stay sutures before laser energy application, the edges are positioned for precise welding. The medical laser is then fired to weld the intervening tissue edges together (Fig. 13.4).

The power used by us for the CO_2 laser was 70 to 100 mW, with a spot size of 300 μm. One investigator used the Nd:YAG laser in a pulse mode at 5 W with a spot size of 600 μm and a power duration of 0.3 sec.[25] Jain[26] used the Nd:YAG laser at 17 W with a duration of 0.1 sec and a spot size of 0.3 mm. Jain did not use stay sutures but simply approximated the vessel edges with microforceps and then

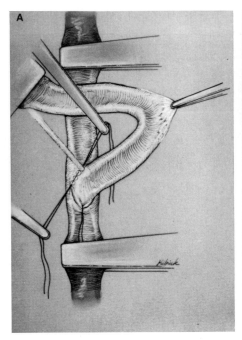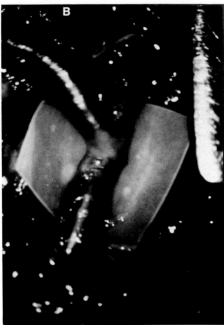

Figure 13.4. (*A*) Artist's representation of techniques employed during laser application. (Printed with permission: Shapiro SA, et al: The laser in vascular and neural welding. *Neurosurgery* 22:475–493, 1987.) (*B*) Intraoperative photograph of a completed Nd:YAG anastomosis.

applied the laser power for welding. As is usual for these microvascular repairs, the lasers were often connected to a microscope with a micromanipulator for precise laser application.

The laser anastomosis can take less than 5 minutes.[27] The resulting early patency rate was 85 to 100%, with the lower rate in Nd:YAG laser anastomoses.[25,27] Angiography (Fig. 13.5) and operative visualization were used to determine patency rates. These repairs can undoubtedly withstand physiologic arterial pressure, as demonstrated by the continued patency observed over at least a 2-month period.[25,27] Jain[25] reported that the anastomoses achieved can withstand blood pressures up to 200 mmHg but did not mention the method used to support this statement.

The histology of the laser repair paralleled that seen in the end-to-end laser anastomosis. Both light microscopy and scanning electron microscopy were employed in the histologic evaluation of these repairs. Intimal thickening was noted rarely.[25] The most consistent feature at the area of anastomosis was a coagulation necrosis of the media and adventitia with only minimal endothelial involvement. In contrast, the anastomoses performed with the Nd:YAG laser showed a more extensive transmural coagulation with some extension along the wall, indicating conduction of the laser energy laterally.[27] The phenomenon may be due to the deeper penetration achieved with the Nd:YAG laser. Endothelial healing seemed to progress in a standard fashion.

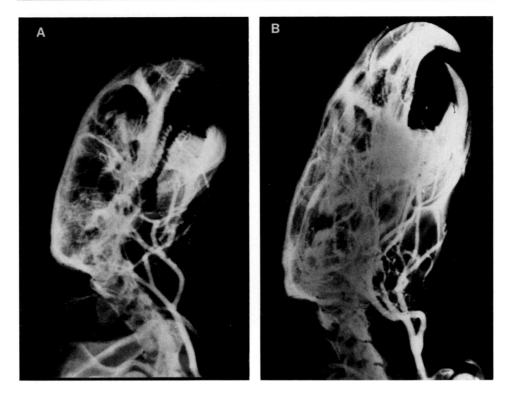

Figure 13.5. (A) Lateral angiogram of normal Nd:YAG anastomosis at 2 months. (B) Lateral angiogram of Nd:YAG anastomosis at 2 months, demonstrating anastomotic dilatation.

Jain[26] found no problems with arterial aneurysms in animals over a follow-up of up to 2 months. In contrast, our group noted aneurysmal degeneration in 10% of CO_2-repaired arteries and 25% of those welded with Nd:YAG laser.[26,27] In those vessels not demonstrating an aneurysmal change, the internal elastic membrane could be well visualized by light microscopy.[26] Aneurysms seemed to occur in vessels that required reexposure to the laser for adequate hemostasis or in those in which tension was greater than usual because the donor artery was short. Figure 13.6A depicts a small anastomotic aneurysm occurring between the stay sutures. Histologically, the area of dilatation shows a loss of smooth muscle cells and elastic fibers (Fig. 13.6B). The neck and dome of the aneurysm are composed of fibrotic tissues and myointimal cells. The higher rate of aneurysmal formation noted in the Nd:YAG specimens may reflect the more early extensive coagulation necrosis noted at the site of repair.

Jain[28] has reported on the use of the Nd:YAG laser to perform extracranial–intracranial bypass operations in five patients. Follow-up to 9 months on these patients was extensive. No aneurysmal degeneration was found on angiography, and anastomoses were patent.[28] Most other investigators have not ventured into the clinical arena, but have instead confined their investigation to determining the best type of laser, laser parameters, and technique to ensure a long-term predictable result.

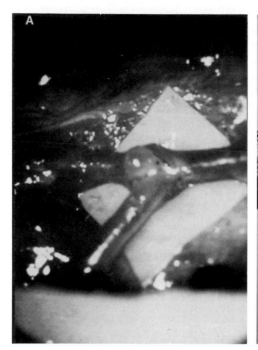
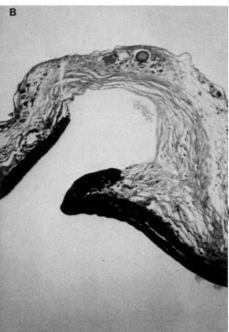

Figure 13.6. (*A*) Intraoperative photograph of Nd:YAG anastomotic site, demonstrating an aneurysm at 6 months. (*B*) Photomicrograph of Nd:YAG aneurysm seen in Figure 6A (elastic stain, × 125).

Vein: End-to-End

The technique of venous anastomosis is very similar to that of the end-to-end arterial repair. The vein is divided and gently reapproximated with four small-diameter stay sutures placed equidistant from each other. The CO_2 laser power setting is usually lower than in the artery repair, typically stated to be 70 to 80 mW. One author, however, used a setting of 200 mW.[3,5,11] Gomes and coworkers[12] set the power level of the argon laser at 0.8 to 1.4 W, but they were working with the dog saphenous vein, which is over 2 mm in diameter in larger canines. Spot sizes of 150 to 300 μm have been employed.[3,5,11] Adjacent stay sutures are held under mild tension to evert and approximate the vein edges, after which the laser energy is applied to complete the anastomosis.

The laser venous repair can be performed more quickly than the conventional suture method.[3,5] Furthermore, the overall patency rate of the two techniques is quite similar, having been reported to be 82.2 to 86% for the laser and 81 to 97.9% for the suture repairs.[3,5] In a rabbit model with a vena cava diameter of 4 to 6 mm, the patency rate was 96% for the laser-assisted anastomoses and 95% for the suture.[11]

Baxter and associates[22] explored the histology of microvascular anastomoses of 0.8- to 1.0-mm diameter veins in the rabbit model. Histologically, they found venous repairs to be similar to arterial repairs in terms of damage to the wall by sutures and the eventual sequence of healing. The rate of luminal surface repair was appreciably slower, however, with no endothelialization being noted for 4 to 6 weeks. Subintimal hyperplasia was much less prominent than in comparable arterial healing, which is consistent with the small medial component in vein walls. Baxter's group also noted that even though the entire venous wall may appear completely necrotic early in the healing process, this situation did not affect the patency of the venous repair.[22]

McCarthy and associates[11] noted full-thickness necrosis of the vein wall following the laser-assisted venous anastomosis, but, again, patency did not appear to be affected. An endothelial-like covering was evident at 2 weeks in both the laser and suture repairs, and the intimal thickening was less than in the arterial repair, no matter which method of anastomosis was used.[11] Fried and Moll[5] merely state that the laser and suture methods of venous repair are quite similar histologically for all observation periods. Venous repairs were unlike their arterial counterparts in that no intimal hyperplasia was noted in the repair of rat femoral veins by either sutures or laser.[5] Endothelial healing was evident in 2 to 3 weeks. A significant foreign body giant cell reaction was seen in the area of anastomosis; it was more conspicuous in the conventional technique.[5,11] In distinction, the amphorous coagulum present with the laser method of repair slowly resolves over time.[11]

There appears to be little difference between the suture and laser methods of venous repair except for the amount of foreign body reaction around the joined areas. No recent study confirmed the delay in endothelial repair suggested by Baxter and coworkers[22] in either the suture or the laser-assisted venous anastomoses.

Although aneurysms are a problem for the arterial microvascular anastomosis, venous aneurysmal formation either is not observed or is less frequently a problem.[3,5,11] In the rabbit vena cava model, slight fusiform dilatation was noted in only 7% of laser-assisted repairs, whereas it was seen in 15% of suture repairs.[11] In summary, the major difference between arterial and venous repairs is the amount of subintimal hyperplasia resulting from the healing process.

LASER-ASSISTED NEURAL ANASTOMOSIS

In laser-assisted neural anastomosis, cut nerve ends are approximated, with 9-0 or 10-0 nylon sutures and the laser is used to weld the remaining free epineural surface. Fischer and colleagues[29,30] studied the repair of rat sciatic nerves exposed through a posterior thigh approach. The nerve on both sides was transected with a scalpel. On one side, the nerve ends were repaired with four 10-0 nylon microepineural sutures. On the other side, the nerve was gently pulled together with one 10-0 suture, and the ends were welded with a CO_2 laser. The power setting was 5 W in a pulsed mode of 0.5 sec duration with a spot size of 0.6 mm. The laser was directed tangentially because the spot size was considered too large. Shapiro and associates[27] compared the laser and conventional suture repair of nerves after transection with both the scalpel and the laser in a dog ulnar nerve model. The laser-assisted repair was accomplished using a power setting of 100 mW with a spot

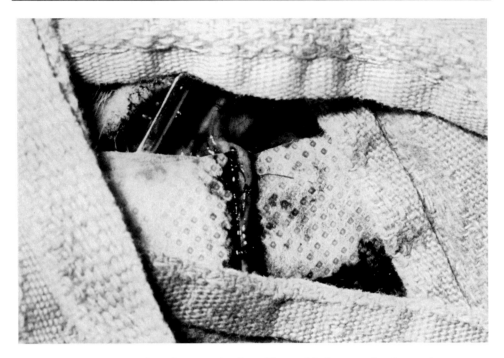

Figure 13.7. Intraoperative photograph of a milliwatt CO_2 laser-assisted neural anastomosis acutely completed on a dog ulnar nerve.

of 300 μm and multiple bursts of 0.1 to 0.3 milliseconds. Three to four 9-0 epineural stay sutures were positioned equidistantly around the nerve edges for precise approximation. Gentle traction on adjacent sutures prior to laser welding provided even more precise edge alignment. No brownish discoloration or desiccation occurred (Fig. 13.7). The conventional method of repair required eight 9-0 interrupted sutures.

The anastomotic integrity rate was 80 to 85%.[27,29,30] Interestingly, the four neural anastomotic disruptions noted by Shapiro and colleagues[27] were in those nerves transected with the laser and then repaired with the laser. Therefore, the integrity rate was 100% for all other groups, including those transected with a knife and then repaired with a laser-assisted technique. This may not be unexpected in view of the fact that the nerves already had undergone a coagulation event prior to attempted welding, and we know that such tissue does not weld like fresh collagenous tissue. The neurosurgical group at the Indiana University Medical Center is conducting an ongoing sciatic nerve study on the rat model. After a 6-month follow-up they noted 100% integrity when using similar laser parameters without the use of stay sutures (Fig. 13.8). The suture repairs were intact in all cases as well.

Clinical functional evaluation of dogs with repaired ulnar nerves evaluated fanning of the claws, withdrawal to pinprick along the ulnar aspect of the paw, and gait pattern.[27] An independent examiner rated the response on a scale of 0 to 4, with 0 representing no response and 4 representing a normal sensory and motor function. All animals had a normal gait at the 12-week examination. The results

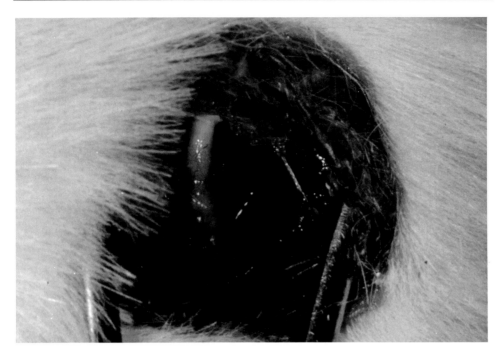

Figure 13.8. Intraoperative photograph of a sutureless milliwatt CO_2 laser-assisted neural anastomosis of a rat sciatic nerve at 6 months.

regarding withdrawal to pinprick and claw fanning were variable and bore no consistent relationship to recorded nerve action potentials in these animals.

Well-defined nerve action potentials were recorded in 85% of the laser-repaired nerves and 78% of the sutured group in the studies of Fischer and associates.[29,30] Nerve action potentials were recorded across both the laser and suture anastomoses in 11 rats. The stimulus intensities required to elicit a threshold and a maximal response were then compared. The voltage needed to generate a threshold averaged 14.2 V in the laser repairs and 14.8 V in the suture group. An action potential of maximal amplitude was produced by average stimulus intensities of 71.8 and 84.5 V in the laser-treated and suture-repaired animals, respectively.

The ongoing study of the sutureless laser anastomoses of the rat sciatic nerve at Indiana demonstrates nearly normal latency across the laser repairs—an improvement over conventional microepineural anastomosis. In the dog ulnar nerve study, the ulnar nerve was exposed 3 cm above and below the anastomotic site without disturbing the anastomosis.[25] Bipolar stimulating and recording electrodes were then placed proximal and distal to the repair, and nerve action potentials were obtained. The nerve was stimulated, usually at the site where the nerve passed through the cubital tunnel, and recorded proximally at a distance 2 to 3 cm from the point of stimulation. There was an obvious difference between laser-*transected* nerves and scalpel-transected nerves. The laser-transected nerves produced action potentials with lower amplitudes than the knife-transected nerves, regardless of the method of anastomosis. However, the method of nerve *repair* could not be distinguished on the basis of the postrepair nerve action potential.

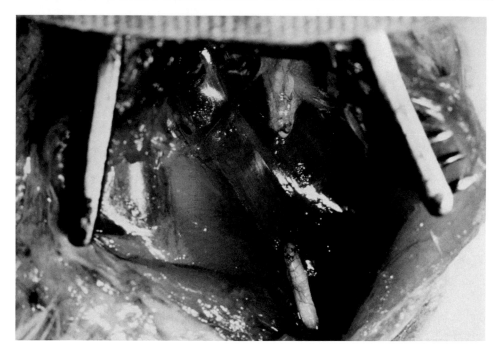

Figure 13.9. Intraoperative photograph of a rat sciatic CO_2 laser neurectomy with subsequent milliwatt CO_2 laser "sealing."

The thrust of this discussion concerns the use of the laser for the anastomosis of nerves. Nevertheless, one final comment must be made on the theory that laser "sealing" of sectioned nerve endings may reduce neuroma formation.[31,32] Both Shapiro and coworkers[27] and Fischer and coworkers[33] have shown that neuroma formation in the rat model is aggravated by laser neurectomy (Fig. 13.9). The ensuing carbonaceous debris and attendant giant cell inflammation may contribute to this increased neuroma formation (Fig. 13.10). Using the milliwatt CO_2 at lower energy fluence, the Indiana group found none of the carbonaceous debris nor giant cell inflammatory reaction seen with higher power settings. The rate of neuroma formation was the same, however.

When using a 5-W power setting on the CO_2 laser, Fischer and associates[29,30] found dense carbonaceous deposits of varying size in the anastomotic zone of the laser-repaired nerves. These deposits were typically walled off by macrophages and multinucleated giant cells. The histology of suture-repaired nerves, however, demonstrated an even more elaborate and complex reaction around sutures with a more abundant resulting scar formation. Furthermore, the density of myelinated nerve fibers in regions very close to the carbonaceous deposits seemed similar to that in other endoneurial areas devoid of this foreign material, whereas the density of the regenerated myelinated nerve fibers around sutures was generally reduced and exhibited a disorganized pattern. Proximal to the anastomosis, the histologic morphology of the two methods of repair was quite similar. Distal to the repair, the vasculature of the laser-treated nerves appeared more prominent than in the conventional suture method but was otherwise similar. Morphometric analysis of

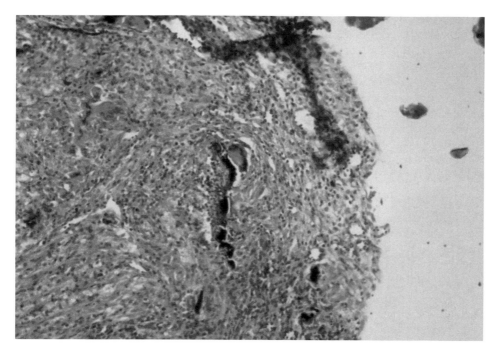

Figure 13.10. Photomicrograph of a longitudinal section of the nerve in Figure 9, harvested at 9 weeks, demonstrating the multinucleate giant cell inflammatory response with ingested carbonaceous debris in the distal neuroma (H&E, × 100).

myelinated nerve fibers both proximal and distal to the anastomosis revealed that the laser had no deleterious effect on the degree of retrograde axonal degeneration or regenerative potential as compared with the suture technique.

Histologic study of the ulnar nerves by Shapiro and coworkers[27] demonstrated good preservation of basic nerve architecture in the scalpel-transected, suture-repaired nerves. There was a minimal cellular reaction confined to the areas around the sutures. Following knife transection, laser-repaired specimens also showed good preservation of nerve histology with no carbonaceous debris or cellular reaction. In some instances, mild disruption of the normal axonal architecture was seen with resultant whorling neuromatous changes.

The laser-cut, sutured group was distinctive in the more pronounced disruption of the axons with frequent whorling neuroma formation and fibrotic collagenous response.

Those specimens both transected and repaired with the laser demonstrated the greatest architectural disruption, with prominent neuroma development. There was even some carbonaceous debris with resultant fibrotic reaction seen in these specimens (Fig. 13.10).

It would appear that transection of the nerves with the laser is detrimental to the nerves' ability to heal. When performed with controlled laser energy, however, the anastomosis is histologically similar to the suture method but is without the foreign body inflammatory reaction seen at the areas of suture placement.

Work by Maragh and associates[34] compared the tensile strength of laser-assisted nerve repairs with the conventional suture technique. The rat sciatic nerve was the experimental model. The laser-assisted method of repair was found to be less strong for the first 4 days after repair, but thereafter nerves repaired with both techniques were comparable in terms of tensile strength.

The Neurosurgery Unit at Indiana University has recently performed an intracranial facial nerve laser anastomosis with the milliwatt CO_2. Technically, the repair was quite effective in this difficult area of surgical reconstruction. The long-term clinical outcome remains to be determined.

CONCLUSION

The laser-assisted microvascular anastomosis is more time-effective than suturing, with a patency rate similar to the conventional suture method. Although tensile strength may initially be inferior to that obtained with the suture method, it is sufficient to withstand any pressures observed in vivo. Furthermore, the strength of the laser weld increases with time, to compare very favorably with the conventional methods of repair. Histologically, the laser-repaired vessels show less inflammatory reaction at the site of repair than the suture specimens. Hyperplasia is not a problem unique to the laser anastomosis and, in fact, may be less of a problem in the maturing animal when the laser is used. Luminal surface healing is similar with both methods of repair. The major problem with laser repairs may be the presence of aneurysmal degeneration, which in some series was more frequent than in the suture-repaired vessels. This problem may be overcome when a more detailed study of laser types and laser parameters reveals the optimal penetration of laser energy for a precise, nondamaging weld. Certainly, laser-assisted microvascular welding has a role in vascular repair when speed of anastomosis or growth is an important consideration.

The laser anastomosis of nerves is feasible. Its patency is similar to the suture method of repair. The laser should not be used to trim or clean the nerve end, however, since this leads to more heat damage and an insecure anastomosis. With currently available milliwatt laser units, however, fewer problems associated with coagulated debris and the resultant scarring occur than are created by the foreign body giant cell reaction generated by suture placement. The functional results in animals have been at least as good in the laser repairs as in those performed in the conventional manner. These facts have encouraged further clinical use of the laser for microanastomoses.

REFERENCES

1. Frazier OH, Painvin GA, Morris J, et al: Laser-assisted microvascular anastomoses: angiographic and anatomopathologic studies on growing microvascular anastomoses: preliminary report. *Surgery* 97:585–590, 1985.
2. Serure A, Withers EH, Thomsen S, et al: Comparison of carbon dioxide laser-assisted microvascular anastomosis and conventional microvascular sutures anastomosis. *Surg Forum* 34:634–636, 1983.

3. Flemming AFS, Colles MJ, Guillianotti R, et al: Laser-assisted microvascular anastomosis of arteries and veins: laser tissue welding. *Br J Plast Surg* 441:378–388, 1988.

4. Guo J, Chao YD: Low power CO_2 laser-assisted microvascular anastomosis: an experimental study. *Neurosurgery* 22:540–543, 1988.

5. Fried MP, Moll ERS: Microvascular anastomoses. *Arch Otolaryngol Head Neck Surg* 113:968–973, 1987.

6. White JV, Dalsing MC, Yao JST, et al: Tissue fusion effects of the CO_2 laser. *Surg Forum* 36:455–457, 1985.

7. Wang SU, Grubbs PE, Base S, et al: Effect of blood bonding on bursting strength of laser-assisted microvascular anastomoses. *Microsurgery* 9:10–13, 1988.

8. Grubbs PE, Wang SU, Marini C, et al: Enhancement of CO_2 laser microvascular anastomoses by fibrin glue. *J Surg Res* 45:112–119, 1988.

9. Thomsen S, Morris JR, Neblett CR, et al: Tissue welding using a low energy microsurgical CO_2 laser. *Med Instrum* 21:231–237, 1987.

10. Quigley MR, Bailes JE, Swaan HC, et al: Microvascular anastomosis using the milliwatt CO_2 laser. *Lasers Surg Med* 5:357–365, 1985.

11. McCarthy WJ, Hartz RS, Yao JST, et al: Vascular anastomoses with laser energy. *J Vasc Surg* 3:32–41, 1986.

12. Gomes OM, Macruz R, Armelin E, et al: Vascular anastomosis by argon laser beam. *Texas Heart Inst J* 10:145–149, 1982.

13. Godlewski G, Pradal P, Rouy S, et al: Microvasular carotid end-to-end anastomosis with the argon laser. *World J Surg* 10:829–833, 1986.

14. Godlewski G, Ruoy S, Dauzat M: Ultrastructural study of arterial wall repair after argon laser micro-anastomosis. *Lasers Surg Med* 7:258–262, 1987.

15. Ulrich F, Durselen R, Schober R: Long-term investigations of laser-assisted microvascular anastomoses with the 1.318-μm Nd:YAG laser. *Lasers Surg Med* 8:104–107, 1988.

16. Niijima KH, Yonekawa Y, Handa H, et al: Nonsuture microvascular anastomosis using an Nd:YAG laser and a water-soluble polyvinyl alcohol splint. *J Neurosurg* 67:579–583, 1987.

17. Hartz RS, LoCicero J, Shih SR, et al: Mechanical properties of end-to-end laser-assisted and sutured arterial anastomoses under axial loading. *Surg Forum* 36:457–459, 1985.

18. Bailes JE, Quigley MR, Cerullo LJ, et al: Review of tissue welding applications in neurosurgery. *Microsurgery* 8:242–244, 1987.

19. Pribil S, Powers SK: Microvascular laser anastomosis of rat carotid vessel. Association for the Advancement of Medical Instrumentation (AAMI) 20th Annual Meeting, Boston, MA, May, 1985.

20. Quigley MR, Bailes JE, Kwaan HC, et al: Aneurysm formation after low power carbon dioxide laser-assisted vascular anastomosis. *Neurosurgery* 18:292–299, 1986.

21. Maxwell GP, Szabo Z, Buncke JH: Aneurysms after microvascular anastomoses. *Plast Reconstr Surg* 63:824–849, 1979.

22. Baxter TJ, O'Brien BM, Henderson PN, et al: The histopathology of small vessels following microvascular repair. *Br J Surg* 59:617–622, 1972.

23. Quigley MR, Bailes JE, Kwaan HC, et al: Comparison of myointimal hyperplasia in laser-assisted and suture-anastomosed arteries. *J Vasc Surg* 4:217–219, 1986.

24. McCarthy WJ, LoCicero J, Hartz RS, et al: Patency of laser-assisted anastomoses in small vessels: one-year follow-up. *Surgery* 102:319–326, 1987.

25. Sartorius CJ, Shapiro SA, Campbell RL, et al: Experimental laser-assisted end-to-side microvascular anastomosis. *Microsurgery* 7:79–83, 1986.

26. Jain KK: Sutureless end-to-side microvascular anastomosis using neodymium:YAG laser. *J Vasc Surg* July/Aug:240–243, 1983.

27. Shapiro SA, Sartorius CJ, Campbell RL: The laser in vascular and neural welding. *Neurosurgery* 22:475–493, 1987.

28. Jain KK: Sutureless extra-intracranial anastomosis by laser. *Lancet* 2:816–817, 1984.

29. Beggs JL, Fischer DW, Shetter AG: Comparative study of rat sciatic nerve microepineurial anastomoses made with carbon dioxide laser and suture techniques: Part 2. *Nu Sci* 18:266–269, 1986.

30. Fischer DW, Beggs JL, Kenshalo DL, et al: Comparative study of microepineurial anastomoses with the use of CO_2 laser and suture techniques in rat sciatic nerves: Part 1. *Nu Sci* 17:300–308, 1985.

31. Ascher PW: Der CO_2 Laser in der Neurochirugie. *Fortschr Med* 98:253–254, 1980.

32. Holzer P, Ascher PW: Laser Surgery of Peripheral Nerves. In Kalpin T (ed): *Laser Surgery III: Proceedings of the Third International Congress for Laser Surgery.* Tel Aviv, OT-Paz, 1980, pp 149–153.

33. Fischer DW, Beggs JL, Shetter AG, et al: Comparative study of neuroma formation in the rat sciatic nerve after CO_2 laser and scalpel neurectomy. *Nu Sci* 13:287–294, 1983.

34. Maragh H, Hawn R, Gould J, et al: Is laser repair comparable to microsuture coaptation? *J Reconstr Microsurgery* 4:189–195, 1988.

Index

Page numbers followed by *t* refer to tables.
Page numbers followed by *f* refer to figures.